Textbook of Zoonoses

Textbook of Zoonoses

Jasbir Singh Bedi
Guru Angad Dev Veterinary and Animal Sciences University
Punjab, India

Deepthi Vijay
Kerala Veterinary and Animal Sciences University
Kerala, India

Pankaj Dhaka
Guru Angad Dev Veterinary and Animal Sciences University
Punjab, India

WILEY Blackwell

This first edition first published 2022

Registered Offices
John Wiley & Sons, Inc., 111 River Street, Hoboken, NJ 07030, USA
John Wiley & Sons Ltd, The Atrium, Southern Gate, Chichester, West Sussex, PO19 8SQ, UK

Editorial Office
9600 Garsington Road, Oxford, OX4 2DQ, UK

For details of our global editorial offices, customer services, and more information about Wiley products visit us at www.wiley.com.

Wiley also publishes its books in a variety of electronic formats and by print-on-demand. Some content that appears in standard print versions of this book may not be available in other formats.

Library of Congress Cataloging-in-Publication Data

Names: Bedi, Jasbir Singh, 1978- author. | Vijay, Deepthi, 1988- author. |
Dhaka, Pankaj, 1988- author.
Title: Textbook of zoonoses / Jasbir Singh Bedi, Deepthi Vijay, Pankaj
Dhaka.
Description: Hoboken, NJ : Wiley-Blackwell, 2022. | Includes
bibliographical references and index.
Identifiers: LCCN 2022009992 (print) | LCCN 2022009993 (ebook) |
ISBN 9781119809517 (paperback) | ISBN 9781119809524 (adobe pdf) |
ISBN 9781119809531 (epub)
Subjects: MESH: Zoonoses
Classification: LCC RC113.5 (print) | LCC RC113.5 (ebook) | NLM WC 950 |
DDC 616.95/9--dc23/eng/20220323
LC record available at https://lccn.loc.gov/2022009992
LC ebook record available at https://lccn.loc.gov/2022009993

Cover Design: Wiley
Cover Images: © KristinaVelickovic/Getty Images, carduus/Getty Images, CSA Images/Getty Images, Sunny_nsk/Shutterstock.com, Serkan OZBAY/Shutterstock.com

Set in 9.5/12.5pt STIXTwoText by Straive, Pondicherry, India
Printed and bound by CPI Group (UK) Ltd, Croydon, CR0 4YY

C9781119809517_230622

We dedicate this book to our colleagues and families who remain a constant source of inspiration and support throughout our life journey. We express our gratitude to GOD ALMIGHTY for blessing us with such wonderful companies.

Contents

Preface

Zoonoses are infections that are naturally transmissible between animals and humans. Zoonotic diseases need special attention, as most of the emerging infectious diseases of epidemic and pandemic potential belong to this category. Zoonoses have a substantial socioeconomic impact not only on the rural population of the world where the human–animal interface is quite porous, but also many of these infections are emerging due to the unsustainable expansion of our cities and other anthropogenic activities disturbing the biodiversity (e.g. deforestation, climate change, wars and conflicts, etc.).

How Did the Idea for Writing the Book Come Up?

There are few textbooks on zoonoses along with the information available on the websites of public health agencies. Our students and professional colleagues used to ask us 'Where can we get the required information on all the relevant zoonoses in one place?'. Our attempts to address this query inspired us to collect and present this *Textbook on Zoonoses* in a logical format, covering the required information for each zoonosis. The COVID-19 pandemic has made this the best possible time to write this book to further spread knowledge and awareness of zoonoses.

Who Should Use this Book?

Most zoonoses are multifaceted in origin, involving the interaction(s) of host(s) (both human and animal), agent and environment-related factors. Therefore, the effective tackling of zoonoses needs a 'One Health' approach, where collaborations between various professionals can produce synergistic effects for efficient prevention and control.

We hope this textbook will be of help to all public health professionals, mainly veterinary and medical professionals, to inspire learning and development of expertise in the field of zoonoses.

Book Content and Our Expectations

The book has six sections on bacterial, viral, parasitic, fungal, rickettsial and prion zoonoses. Each chapter describes the aetiology, epidemiology, clinical symptoms in humans and animals, diagnosis, treatment options, and prevention and control strategies of the mentioned disease. By using this book as reference material, we hope that public health students and professionals across relevant disciplines will develop a deep appreciation of the epidemiological and clinical characteristics of various zoonoses, which will enable them to play a valuable part in the 'One Health' taskforce of regional, national and global importance.

Jasbir Singh Bedi
Deepthi Vijay
Pankaj Dhaka

Acknowledgements

We express our gratitude to our mentors at the Guru Angad Dev Veterinary and Animal Sciences University, Ludhiana; Kerala Veterinary and Animal Sciences University, Pookode; Indian Veterinary Research Institute, Bareilly; Rajiv Gandhi College of Veterinary and Animal Sciences, Pondicherry; and Royal Veterinary College, London, for giving us the solid professional ground on which we stand today.

This book stands on the shoulders of the knowledge imparted by the zoonoses and public health experts across the world, which we relied upon throughout the drafting of this textbook. We would also like to thank our families for patiently allowing us the time and wholeheartedly supporting us to finalise this text.

Jasbir Singh Bedi
Deepthi Vijay
Pankaj Dhaka

About the Authors

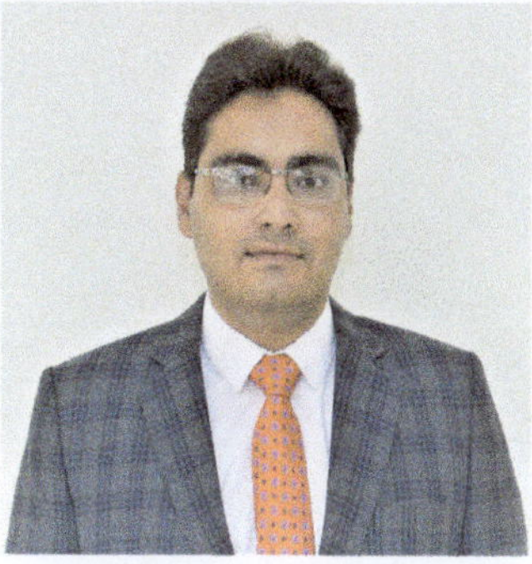

Dr Jasbir Singh Bedi is currently Director, Centre for One Health, Guru Angad Dev Veterinary and Animal Sciences University, Ludhiana, India. Dr Bedi has served as an academician and researcher for the last 20 years in the areas of zoonoses and veterinary public health, and has been associated with research projects on zoonoses, food safety and antimicrobial resistance.

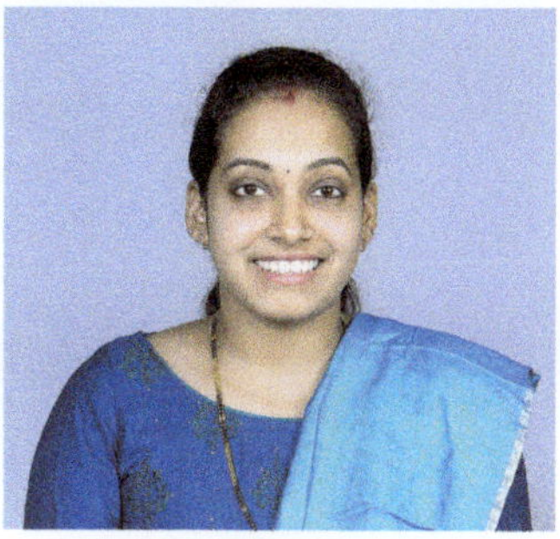

Dr Deepthi Vijay is an Assistant Professor at the Department of Veterinary Public Health, College of Veterinary and Animal Sciences, Kerala Veterinary and Animal Sciences University, Mannuthy, Kerala. Dr Deepthi has 7 years' in the academic areas of veterinary public health and epidemiology, with research expertise in various zoonoses and antimicrobial resistance in the animal health sector.

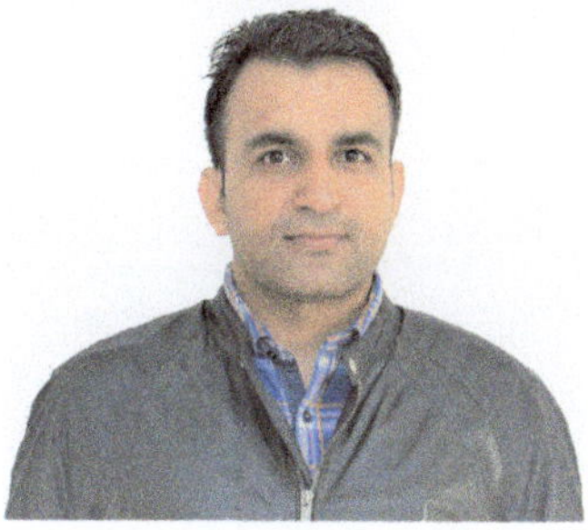

Dr Pankaj Dhaka is an Assistant Professor at the Centre for One Health, Guru Angad Dev Veterinary and Animal Sciences University, Ludhiana, India. Dr Dhaka is involved in the academic and research activities of undergraduate and postgraduate students in the areas of epidemiology of zoonoses, farm biosecurity and antimicrobial resistance.

Introduction to Zoonoses

What are Zoonoses?

The word 'zoonoses' is derived from the Greek words *zōon* meaning 'animal' and *nosos* means 'disease' (the singular is 'zoonosis' and plural is 'zoonoses').

The term 'zoonoses' was coined by Rudolf Virchow during his study on *Trichinella* in 1855, to indicate the infectious disease link between animal and human health [1]. As described by the World Health Organization (WHO), 'A zoonosis is any disease or infection that is naturally transmissible from vertebrate animals to humans' [2].

Overview on Zoonoses

Since the Agricultural Revolution, humans have been afflicted by zoonoses. The classic zoonoses, such as rabies, plague, leptospirosis, brucellosis, bovine tuberculosis, cysticercosis, echinococcosis, toxoplasmosis and yellow fever, have been well known for centuries and are still causing major socio-economic effects in many parts of the globe. In recent years, new zoonotic entities (e.g. Lyme borreliosis, enterohaemorrhagic *Escherichia coli,* cryptosporidiosis, Ebola, Nipah, severe acute respiratory syndrome coronavirus (SARS-CoV), Middle East respiratory syndrome (MERS), influenza viruses of animal origin (swine flu – H1N1), hantavirus, etc. are posing a serious threat to the globalised world. Among other issues, there is also concern regarding the potential 'bio-weaponisation' of many of the zoonotic pathogens, some of which have been used this way historically (e.g. anthrax and glanders).

A wide variety of animal species, domesticated, peridomesticated, and wild, can act as reservoirs for these pathogens. Therefore, considering the wide variety of animal species involved and the often complex natural history of the pathogens concerned, effective surveillance, prevention and control of zoonotic diseases pose challenges to public health.

The awareness of zoonoses is very important, more especially among occupationally at-risk groups like farmers, pet owners, veterinarians, etc. In this regard, 'World Zoonoses Day' is held every year on July 6. The day commemorates 6 July 1885, when the renowned microbiologist Louis Pasteur successfully administered the first vaccine against the rabies virus.

Classification of Zoonoses

As per the joint WHO/Food and Agricultural Organization (FAO) Expert Group on zoonoses, the zoonoses can be grouped into three categories.

Textbook of Zoonoses, First Edition. Jasbir Singh Bedi, Deepthi Vijay, and Pankaj Dhaka.

A) **Classification of zoonoses based on aetiological agents:** Zoonoses can be caused by a range of pathogens such as viruses, bacteria, fungi and parasites. In a study, out of the listed 1415 pathogens known to infect humans, 61% were found to be zoonotic [3]. The classification of zoonoses based on the category of aetiological agents is given in Table I.1.

B) **Classification of zoonoses based on the reservoir host(s):** Zoonoses can be classified based on the reservoir host(s) and the life cycle of the infecting pathogen. The reservoir of an infectious agent is the habitat in which the agent normally lives, grows and multiplies. The reservoirs for zoonotic pathogens include humans, animals and the environment. Our incomplete understanding of the reservoirs can hamper the control of zoonoses (e.g. it is important to know the possible wildlife reservoirs of rabies in a given area). Based on reservoir hosts, zoonoses can be classified as follows.

- *Anthropozoonoses*: The zoonotic diseases which can be transmitted to humans from lower vertebrates. Therefore, these infections primarily affect animals but can be naturally transmitted to humans (e.g. rabies, brucellosis, Q fever, leptospirosis, ringworm, etc.).
- *Zooanthroponoses (also known as 'reverse zoonotic disease transmission')*: Those zoonotic diseases which can be transmitted to lower vertebrate animals from infected humans. Therefore, these infections are primarily of human origin (e.g. methicillin-resistant *Staphylococcus aureus*, *Cryptosporidium parvum*, *Ascaris lumbricoides*, etc.).
- *Amphixenoses*: The zoonoses which are maintained in both humans and lower vertebrate animals, which may be transmitted in either direction (e.g. *Staphylococcus* infection, *E. coli* infection, salmonellosis, etc.).

C) **Classification based on the transmission cycle:** The transmission of zoonotic pathogens can occur through reservoir hosts (e.g. bats shedding Nipah virus into date palm collection vessels), and in other instances, can be facilitated by intermediate hosts (e.g. Nipah virus infection from bats to pigs in Malaysia resulting in pig-to-pig and pig-to-human transmission by aerosol route) or via insect vectors (e.g. West Nile virus as a mosquito-borne disease). Therefore, it is important to understand the transmission cycle of the pathogen for proper implementation of surveillance systems and control measures. Based on the requirement of intermediate host and inanimate objects, zoonoses can be categorised as follows.

Table I.1 Classification of zoonoses based on aetiological agents.

Sl. No.	Type	Examples
1	Bacterial zoonoses	Anthrax, brucellosis, coxiellosis, plague, leptospirosis, tuberculosis, Lyme disease, zoonotic tuberculosis, etc.
2	Viral zoonoses	Rabies, yellow fever, Ebola, Japanese encephalitis, zoonotic coronaviruses, Nipah, Rift valley fever, etc.
3	Parasitic zoonoses	Toxoplasmosis, taeniasis, cryptosporidiosis, echinococcosis, trichinellosis, leishmaniasis, etc.
4	Fungal zoonoses	Aspergillosis, blastomycosis, coccidioidomycosis, cryptococcosis, histoplasmosis, etc.
5	Rickettsial zoonoses	Epidemic typhus, endemic typhus, scrub typhus, tick typhus, Rocky Mountain spotted fever, etc.
6	Prions	New variant Creutzfeldt–Jakob disease (nvCJD)

- *Direct zoonoses:* Those zoonotic diseases which are perpetuated in nature by a single vertebrate species (e.g. anthrax, rabies, Q fever, etc.).
- *Cyclozoonoses:* Zoonotic diseases which require two or more vertebrate hosts to complete the transmission cycle. These can be further classified as follows.
  - Obligatory cyclozoonoses: The zoonotic diseases in which the involvement of humans as a host is compulsory to continue the transmission cycle (e.g. taeniasis).
  - Non-obligatory cyclozoonoses: The zoonotic diseases in which humans are accidentally involved in the transmission cycle of the pathogen (e.g. hydatidosis).
- *Metazoonoses:* The zoonotic diseases which require both vertebrate and invertebrate hosts to continue their transmission cycle. This can be further classified as shown in Table I.2.
- *Saprozoonoses:* The zoonotic diseases which require an inanimate object(s) for the completion of the transmission cycle are known as saprozoonoses. These can be further classified as follows.
  - Saproanthropozoonoses: The zoonoses which can transfer from animals to humans through inanimate substances (e.g. erysipeloid).
  - Saproamphixenoses: The zoonoses which can be shared between humans and animals through inanimate objects (e.g. histoplasmosis).
  - Saprometanthropozoonoses: These zoonoses require vertebrate hosts and invertebrate hosts as well as inanimate objects for the completion of their life cycle (e.g. fascioliasis).

Other Classifications

Classification According to the Ecosystem in which Pathogens Circulate [4]

- **Synanthropic zoonoses:** The zoonotic diseases which transmit through the urban (domestic) cycle where the sources of infection(s) are domestic and synanthropic animals (e.g. urban rabies, cat-scratch disease and zoonotic ringworm through pets).
- **Exoanthropic zoonoses:** The zoonotic diseases which transmit through the sylvatic cycle in natural foci through feral or wild animals (e.g. arboviruses, wildlife rabies, Lyme disease and tularaemia). **Note:** Some zoonoses can circulate in both urban and sylvatic cycles (e.g. yellow fever and Chagas disease).

Major Transmission Routes of Zoonoses

Generally, disease results from the interaction(s) of the host (person or animal), agent (e.g. bacteria, virus, parasite or fungi) and the environment (e.g. contaminated feed and/or water supply, dirty

Table I.2 Classification and examples of metazoonoses.

Type	Number of invertebrate hosts	Number of vertebrate hosts	Examples
I	1	1	Yellow fever, plague
II	2	1	Paragonimiasis
III	1	2	Clonorchiasis
IV	Transovarian transmission		Tick-borne encephalitis

farm conditions). The diseases can be transmitted directly or indirectly. A disease can be transmitted directly from animal to human (i.e. direct transmission) (e.g. rabies through dog bite). Indirect transmission can occur through common vehicles such as contaminated air or water supply, or by vectors such as mosquitoes, or inanimate objects. Some of the important modes of transmission for zoonotic diseases are listed below.

- Direct contact of a susceptible host with infected animals (e.g. scabies, brucellosis, leptospirosis, etc.).
- Direct transmission through animal bites (e.g. rabies) and scratches (e.g. cat-scratch fever).
- Transmission through contaminated animal food products, mainly due to improper food handling and inadequate cooking practices (e.g. *Salmonella* spp., *Clostridium perfringens*, *E. coli*, etc.).
- Faeco–oral transmission from animals to humans (e.g. salmonellosis, *E. coli*, *Toxoplasma gondii*, etc.).
- **Vector-borne transmission:** Vectors such as mosquitoes, ticks, fleas and lice can transmit zoonotic diseases to humans (e.g. yellow fever, Kyasanur forest disease, plague, etc.).
- **Air-borne transmission:** Air-borne transmission results from the inhalation of small particles (droplet nuclei) which are considered to have diameters $\leq 5\,\mu m$ (e.g. influenza viruses).
- Indirect transmission through contaminated soil (e.g. roundworm eggs can survive for years in contaminated soil). Allowing the faeces to dry out and disintegrate contaminates the soil which increases the risk of exposure to pathogens [5].
- Indirect transmission through contaminated water sources (e.g. *Cryptosporidium* spp., cholera, rotavirus infection, leptospirosis, etc.).

Note: Some occupational groups (e.g. farmers, butchers, veterinarians) are at high risk of exposure to zoonotic pathogens due to their frequent exposure to livestock which may result in increased occurrence of transmission. Further, these high-risk groups can also become carriers of zoonotic pathogens that may spread in the community.

References

1 Brown, C. (2003). Virchow revisited: Emerging zoonoses. *ASM News-American Society for Microbiology* 69 (10): 493–497.

2 World Health Organization (2020). Zoonoses. www.who.int/topics/zoonoses/en/

3 Taylor, L.H., Latham, S.M., and Woolhouse, M.E. (2001). Risk factors for human disease emergence. *Philosophical Transactions of the Royal Society of London. Series B: Biological Sciences 356* (1411): 983–989.

4 Hubálek, Z. (2003). Emerging human infectious diseases: anthroponoses, zoonoses, and sapronoses. *Emerging Infectious Diseases 9* (3): 403.

5 Beeler, E., and May, M. (2011). The link between animal feces and zoonotic disease. LA County Department of Public Health. June–July 2011, pp. 4–5. http://publichealth.lacounty.gov/vet/docs/Educ/AnimalFecesandDisease.pdf)

Understanding Concepts and Terms Related to Zoonoses

Globally, zoonoses are responsible for severe socio-economic losses, affecting global food security networks and thereby posing an increasing public health threat to our interconnected world. The endemic zoonoses are responsible for the majority of human cases of illness as well as for the reduction in livestock production in many parts of the world. In a study, 56 zoonoses were found to be responsible for around 2.5 billion cases of human illness and 2.7 million human deaths a year [1].

The emergence of novel zoonotic pathogens is one of the greatest challenges to global health security in the twenty-first century. The importance of zoonotic diseases can be observed from the fact that out of 1415 species known to be pathogenic to humans, 61% (868/1415) are considered to be zoonotic. And, out of 175 pathogenic species which are considered to be 'emerging' pathogens, 75% (132/175) are considered zoonotic [2]. In general, viruses account for a significant proportion of emerging infectious diseases (EIDs), and the majority have zoonotic origin, including ebolaviruses, human immunodeficiency virus (HIV), hantaviruses, Hendra and Nipah viruses, severe acute respiratory syndrome (SARS) coronavirus, influenza A viruses and severe acute respiratory syndrome coronavirus 2 (SARS-CoV-2). These listed viruses are RNA viruses, which are considered as the primary aetiological agents of emerging infectious diseases (44% of total EIDs) due to their higher ability to infect new host species with exceptionally short generation times. The RNA viruses are also characterised by their rapid evolutionary rates due to the frequent error-prone replication cycles [3].

Important Terms

Emerging Infectious Diseases

These are the diseases that have not occurred before (e.g. SARS in 2003, COVID-19) or have occurred previously but affected only small numbers of people in isolated places but now are rapidly increasing in incidence or geographical range (e.g. Zika was discovered in 1947 but the major epidemic was in 2015–2016) or have occurred throughout the human history but only recently been recognised as a distinct disease due to infectious agent (e.g. the causative agent of Lyme disease was discovered in 1982) [4].

Re-emerging Infectious Diseases

These are the diseases that once were major health problems globally or in a particular country, and then declined dramatically, but are again becoming health problems for a significant proportion of the population (e.g. malaria, rabies, cholera, tuberculosis) [4].

Textbook of Zoonoses, First Edition. Jasbir Singh Bedi, Deepthi Vijay, and Pankaj Dhaka.

Neglected Zoonotic Diseases

Neglected zoonotic diseases are a subset of neglected tropical diseases. The term 'neglected' highlights that 'these diseases affect mainly poor and marginalised populations in low-resource settings'. Examples include rabies, echinococcosis, taeniasis/cysticercosis, schistosomiasis, etc. Addressing this group of diseases requires collaborative, cross-sectoral efforts of human and animal health systems and a multidisciplinary approach that considers the complexities of the ecosystems where humans and animals coexist [5]. Ongoing efforts to establish the 'One Health' framework will be helpful in addressing these neglected zoonoses.

Transboundary Animal Diseases (TADs)

These may be defined as those epidemic diseases which are highly contagious or transmissible and have the potential for very rapid spread, irrespective of national borders, causing serious socio-economic and possibly public health consequences [6]. Globalisation, land encroachment and climate change contribute to outbreaks of such animal diseases, some of which are transmissible to humans, such as brucellosis, bovine tuberculosis, parasitic illnesses, anthrax, bovine spongiform encephalopathy and influenza viruses [6].

Endemic, Epidemic and Pandemic Diseases

- An *endemic* is defined as the habitual presence of a disease within a given geographic area. It may also refer to the usual occurrence of a given disease within an area (e.g. rabies and brucellosis in India).
- An *epidemic* is defined as the occurrence of disease above the normal expectancy in a region/country (e.g. Ebola outbreak in West African countries during 2014).
- A *pandemic* refers to a worldwide epidemic covering larger geographical regions (e.g. H1N1 outbreak in 2009; COVID-19 outbreak of 2019–2021).

Public Health Emergencies of International Concern (PHEIC)

A PHEIC is defined in the International Health Regulations (2005) as 'an extraordinary event which is determined to constitute a public health risk to other States through the international spread of disease and to potentially require a coordinated international response' [7]. This definition implies a situation that:

- is serious, sudden, unusual or unexpected
- carries implications for public health beyond the affected state's national border
- may require immediate international action.

Factors Responsible for the Emergence of Infectious Diseases [8]

Different determinants can contribute to the emergence of novel zoonotic agents. Among the factors that shape the emergence of zoonoses are human demographics and behaviour; technological developments, industrialisation and agricultural activities; unsustainable economic development and land use; international trade and travel; commerce-related activities; military expeditions and wars; microbial adaptation and change; and breakdown of public health measures due to natural or man-made calamities. Some examples of zoonoses emergence and responsible factors are described in Table 1 and Figure 1.

Table 1 Brief description of various factors associated with emerging infectious diseases.

Factors	Examples of specific factors	Examples of diseases
Ecological changes	Agricultural land use, depletion of human–wildlife interface, deforestation, changes in the ecosystem and associated biodiversity loss, and global climate change	Vector-borne diseases (e.g. Zika, dengue, etc.), schistosomiasis, Rift Valley fever, scrub typhus, leptospirosis, Lyme disease, hantavirus pulmonary syndrome, etc.
Human demographics and behaviour	Rapid population growth and migration (movement from rural regions to cities); war or civil conflicts	Leptospirosis, HIV, dengue, malaria, cholera, etc.
International travel and trade	Globalisation leading to the worldwide movement of goods and people	Dissemination of mosquito vectors (e.g. dengue, malaria), rodent-borne diseases, dissemination of O139 *Vibrio cholerae* in many parts of the globe
Technological advancement and industrial influences	Globalisation of food supplies; changes in food processing pattern and packaging; drugs causing immunosuppression; widespread misuse of antibiotics and dissemination of resistant bugs	Food-borne outbreaks of *E. coli* O157:H7 through contaminated beef, Creutzfeldt–Jakob disease from contaminated batches of human growth hormone
Microbial adaptation and changes	Microbial evolution, selection pressure on microbes and response to selection in the environment	The antibiotic-resistant phenomenon in bacteria, 'antigenic drift' and 'antigenic shift' in segmented RNA viruses
Breakdown in public health measures	Curtailment or reduction in prevention programmes including vaccinations; inadequate sanitation and vector control measures	Extensively drug-resistant tuberculosis; cholera in refugee camps during a natural disaster or war-related breakdown in public health infrastructure

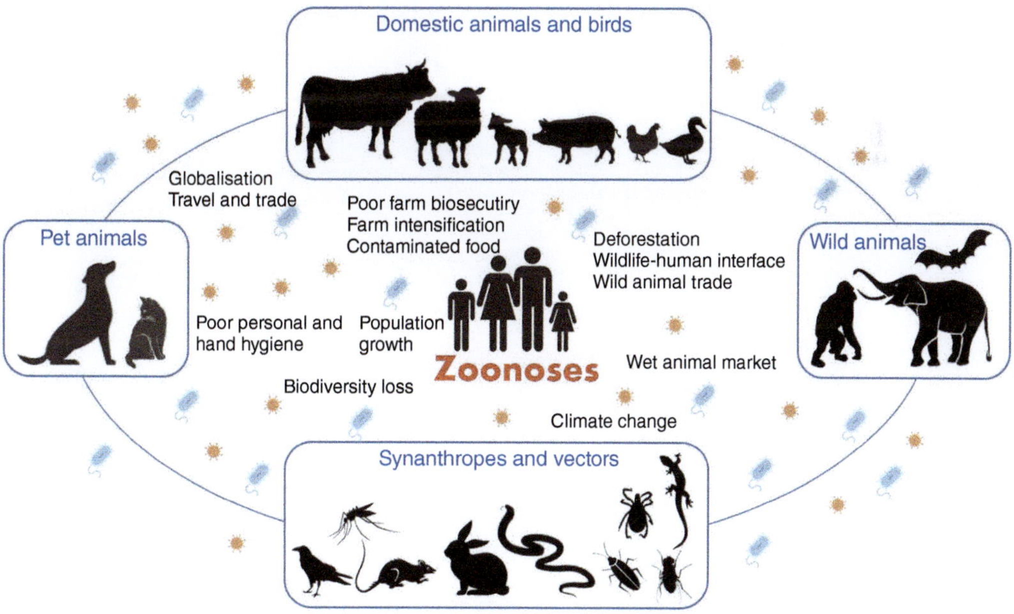

Figure 1 The important factors for emergence of zoonoses in humans.

References

1 Grace, D., Mutua, F., Ochungo, P., et al. (2012). Mapping of poverty and likely zoonoses hotspots. Zoonoses Project 4. Report to the UK Department for International Development. Nairobi, Kenya: ILRI2012. https://hdl.handle.net/10568/21161

2 Taylor, L.H., Latham, S.M., and Woolhouse, M.E. (2001). Risk factors for human disease emergence. *Philosophical Transactions of the Royal Society of London. Series B: Biological Sciences 356* (1411): 983–989.

3 Woolhouse, M.E. and Gowtage-Sequeria, S. (2005). Host range and emerging and re-emerging pathogens. *Emerging Infectious Diseases 11* (12): 1842.

4 National Institutes of Health (2007). Understanding emerging and re-emerging infectious diseases. National Institutes of Health, Bethesda, MD. www.ncbi.nlm.nih.gov/books/NBK20370/

5 World Health Organization (2021). Neglected zoonotic diseases. www.who.int/neglected_diseases/zoonoses/infections_more/en/

6 Food and Agricultural Organization (FAO) (2021). Transboundary animal diseases. www.fao.org/ag/againfo/programmes/en/empres/diseases.asp

7 World Health Organization (2021). IHR Procedures concerning public health emergencies of international concern (PHEIC). www.who.int/ihr/procedures/pheic/en/

8 Morse, S.S. (2001). Factors in the emergence of infectious diseases. In: *Plagues and Politics* (ed. F. Mullan), 8–26. London: Palgrave Macmillan.

Section 1

Bacterial Zoonoses

1

Anthrax

Etymology

The word 'anthrax' is derived from the Greek word *anthrakis* which means 'coal'. This is linked with the characteristic dark necrotic skin-eschar in the cutaneous form of anthrax in humans.

Synonyms

Siberian plague, black bane, charbon, splenic fever, ragpicker's disease, hide porter's disease, wool sorters' disease, Cumberland disease, malignant pustule, malignant carbuncle and Milzbrand.

Aetiology and Pathogen Characteristics

Anthrax is an anthropozoonotic infection caused by *Bacillus anthracis*. The organism is a Gram-positive, aerobic or facultative anaerobic, non-motile, non-haemolytic, spore-forming, rod-shaped bacteria. The organism develops a capsule in the body of the host.

Sporulation

Spores are the dormant form of bacteria that are highly resilient, with resistance to temperature extremes, drought and UV light, possibly due to the protection of DNA in a crystalline core. In the case of *B. anthracis*, sporulation may initiate due to poor nutrient availability and in the presence of oxygen. Some of the characteristics of *B. anthracis* include the following.

- Spores can survive in dry soil for 60 years [1]; the longest reported survival of spores, i.e. 200 ± 50 years, is from bones retrieved during archaeological excavations at Kruger National Park in South Africa [2].
- The pathogen is categorised as a Centers for Disease Control and Prevention (CDC) 'category A' biological agent. The spores can be used as bioweapons due to their size of 2–6 microns diameter, which is an ideal size for impinging on the human lower respiratory tract. Moreover, anthrax spores lend themselves well to aerosolization.

Textbook of Zoonoses, First Edition. Jasbir Singh Bedi, Deepthi Vijay, and Pankaj Dhaka.

Historical Overview on Anthrax

- **1834:** The first case of human anthrax was detected in 1834 in the USA, and in 1938, Delafond demonstrated the causal organism microscopically in the blood of animals.
- **1877:** Robert Koch discovered the anthrax bacillus and also hypothesised Koch postulates.
- **1881:** Louis Pasteur developed the first whole-cell anthrax vaccine.
- **1930s:** Discovery of Sterne-type vaccines. The vaccine is based on an avirulent non-encapsulated strain 34F2 (pXO1^{+ve} and pXO2^{-ve}), which can stimulate a protective immune response. The Sterne strain is currently the predominant strain used for immunisation of domesticated animals against anthrax. It is administered to livestock in a dose containing up to 10 million viable spores.
- **1979:** Anthrax outbreak in Sverdlovsk (USSR) caused 61 deaths and 11 non-fatal cases in 6 weeks. Some researchers concluded the outbreak could have resulted from the accidental spread of anthrax spores by the wind from a microbiology facility at the local military compound [3].
- **2001:** Use of anthrax spores in a bioweapon attack in the USA by mailing of spores to seven locations, which resulted in 22 cases of anthrax (including five deaths) [4].
- **2009:** The first outbreak of injectional anthrax was reported in heroin users in Scotland. The source of contamination was proposed to be goat skins that were used to transport the heroin [5].

Pathogenesis and Virulence Factors

The bacterium *B. anthracis* is likely to be evolved from *Bacillus cereus* that acquired two extrachromosomal plasmids, pXO1 and pXO2, from the environment through lateral genetic transfer.

The plasmid **pXO1** encodes tripartite toxin complex as follows.

1) **Protective antigen** (PA, 83 kDa): This permits the entry of toxins into the host cell.
2) **Oedema factor** (EF, 90 kDa): This is responsible for oedema toxin (PA + EF). Due to this toxin, the calmodulin-dependent adenylate cyclase increases intracytoplasmic levels of cAMP that lead to alteration of water homeostasis which results in oedema. The oedema toxin can induce lethality in the host mainly by targeting hepatocytes.
3) **Lethal factor** (LF, 89 kDa): This is responsible for lethal toxin (PA + LF). It is a zinc metalloprotease toxin that can cause the hyperinflammatory condition in macrophages by activating the oxidative burst pathway and release of reactive O_2 intermediates. It cleaves and inactivates mitogen-activated protein kinase kinases (MAPKKs) 1–4, 6 and 7, which play a crucial role in responses to diverse stimuli, such as mitogens, heat shock, proinflammatory cytokines and cellular stresses. It is responsible for the production of proinflammatory cytokines (TNF-α and IL-1β). The lethal toxin causes lethality by targeting the cardiovascular system, in particular cardiomyocytes and vascular smooth muscle cells.

The plasmid **pXO2** encodes proteins that synthesise a poly-γ-D-glutamic acid capsule which confers resistance to phagocytosis.

Transmission Cycle

Most mammals are susceptible to anthrax. The disease is most commonly seen in herbivores (e.g. cattle, sheep, goats) whereas pigs, equines, dogs and camels are reported to be moderately susceptible. The disease has also been commonly reported in wild animals (e.g. lion, hyena, elephant, jackal, giraffe, zebra, etc.).

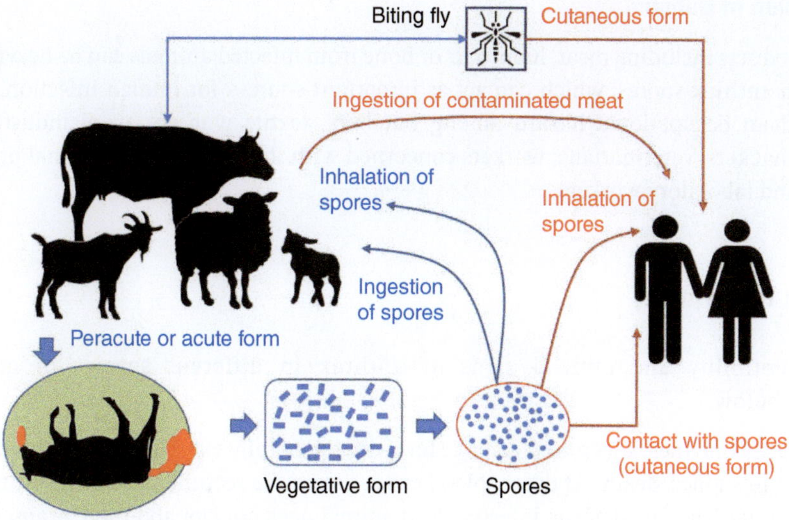

Figure 1.1 The transmission cycle of anthrax between animals and humans.

Herbivores are considered the primary host for anthrax. Upon the death of the host, bacteria in the carcass are exposed to air through haemorrhages, opening of the carcass by scavengers, etc. On exposure, the bacteria sporulate and persist in the soil for prolonged periods which can be the source of infection to other animals or humans. The soil can act as a long-term reservoir for spores of anthrax bacilli. In addition, regions with high humidity, alkaline soils and a high amount of organic matter are categorised as 'incubator areas' for the survival or persistence of anthrax spores. An overview of the transmission cycle of anthrax in animals and humans is provided in Figure 1.1.

Factors Affecting the Transmission of Anthrax

Transmission in Animals

- Ingestion of contaminated fodder, water and processed feed (meat/bone meal, meat scraps).
- Inhalation of spores during wallowing in contaminated water sources.
- Climatic conditions may influence the animal's contact with spores.
  - Grazing closer to contaminated soil in dry periods when grass is sparse increases the chances of animal contact with spores.
  - Enforced grazing at restricted sites (contaminated areas/burial sites) when water sources become scarce is also considered an important risk factor.
- Spiky grass and grits can cause orogastrointestinal lesions in animals which can be infected by germination of spores.
- Calcium-rich soils with neutral-to-alkaline pH can act as favourable sites for spore development. Such regions are also known as 'anthrax belts'.

  Note: *Role of calcium in spore formation*: calcium is integral to the dehydration of vegetative cell genome precursors, which is necessary for its effective long-term storage in spore form.
- Mechanical transmission of the pathogen can occur by biting flies (e.g. *Hippobosca* spp., *Tabanus* spp.).
- The use of contaminated surgical instruments for dehorning and docking may cause disease transmission.

Transmission in Humans

Animal products including meat, hide, hair or bone from infected animals can be heavily contaminated with anthrax spores, which can act as important sources for human infection. Anthrax is considered an occupational hazard among butchers, textile workers, wool industry workers, farmers, knackers, veterinarians, workers concerned with the processing of animal products (e.g. tannery) and laboratory workers.

Anthrax in Animals

The susceptibility and clinical signs of anthrax in different species of animals are described below.

- **Herbivores** (bovines, sheep, and goats): Herbivores generally exhibit per-acute infection which may lead to sudden death. At death, blood exudes from the rectum and other natural openings of the animal. The blood of the infected dead animal does not clot and there is absence of rigor mortis in the carcass. It has been found that the blood of the infected animal may contain $>10^8$ bacilli/mL [6].
- **Horses**: Equines mainly exhibit acute symptoms and die within 2–3 days of infection. In some animals, biting flies may transmit the pathogen and cause large oedematous lesions on breast, abdomen, neck and shoulders.
- **Pigs**: Pigs are more resistant to anthrax than bovines and mainly exhibit localised signs which include oedema of the throat, pharyngeal and cervical lymph nodes.
- **Dogs and cats:** Dogs and cats are considered to be resistant to anthrax. Dogs that have scavenged anthrax carcasses may suffer from severe inflammation and oedematous swelling of the throat, stomach, intestine, lips, jowl, tongue and gums.
- **Birds**: In birds, apoplectic type of death is observed due to anthrax whereas less acute cases may exhibit carbuncular lesions on comb or extremities.

Anthrax in Humans

The clinical forms of anthrax in humans are described below.

1) **Cutaneous anthrax:** The cutaneous form of anthrax is responsible for 95% of global human cases and is mainly reported in developing countries following contact with infected animals and their products. Cutaneous anthrax usually develops 1–7 days after exposure, but incubation periods as long as 17 days have been reported [7]. The characteristic clinical signs are anthrax eschars on exposed regions of the body, i.e. face, neck, hands and wrists. Malignant oedema is a rare complication of the cutaneous form which is characterised by severe oedema, induration, multiple bullae and symptoms of shock (Note: The common description of this form as 'malignant pustule' is a misnomer because the lesion is not purulent and painless.)
2) **Inhalation anthrax:** This occurs mainly due to inhalation of spores (size $<5\,\mu m$) which reach the lower respiratory tract. The incubation period ranges from 1 to 60 days.

The alveolar macrophages then phagocytise these spores and transport them to hilar and mediastinal lymph nodes, where they germinate, proliferate and spread systemically. There is also the possibility that spores gain entry to subepithelial and lymphatic tissues in the upper airways where germination occurs and vegetative forms can spread. The initial symptoms are fever, cough, myalgia, malaise, chest pain and acute respiratory distress. However, in the septicemic form, severe cases involve high fever, dyspnoea, cyanosis, haemorrhagic mediastinitis and effusion followed by rapid progression of shock. In untreated cases, the mortality rate is nearly 100%.

3) **Gastrointestinal anthrax:** Gastrointestinal anthrax mainly occurs after consumption of contaminated meat from infected animals. The two forms of gastrointestinal anthrax are:
   - **oropharyngeal form:** characterized by the development of oral or oesophageal ulcers followed by regional lymphadenopathy, oedema and sepsis
   - **lower gastrointestinal form**: exhibits intestinal lesions mainly in the terminal ileum or caecum.
4) **Injectional anthrax:** The heroin (drug)-associated anthrax resulting from direct injection or injection under the skin, or 'skin popping', among persons who inject drugs (PWIDs) is a distinct form of anthrax which was reported during the 2009–2010 outbreak in Scotland and England and again during 2012–2013 in northern Europe and Germany [5].

Laboratory Diagnosis

Growth Media and Biochemical Characteristics of *B. anthracis*

- **Selective media:** Polymyxin-lysozyme-EDTA-thallous acetate (PLET) agar.
- **On blood agar:** Non-haemolytic colonies with irregular borders.
- **In liquid medium:** Inverted fir tree appearance.
- **On nutrient agar:** Medusa head or comet tail appearance.
- **McFadyean reaction:** Polychrome methylene blue stain (blue bacilli with purple capsule).

Table 1.1 Differences between *B. anthracis* and other bacilli (anthracoid).

Characteristics	Anthrax	Other bacilli
Capsule	Present	Absent
Motility	Non-motile	Motile
On blood agar	Non-haemolytic	Haemolytic
Gelatin liquefaction	Slow	Rapid
Susceptibility to penicillin	Susceptible	Not susceptible
Susceptible to γ phage	Susceptible	Not susceptible
Animal pathogenicity	Pathogenic	Non-pathogenic

Diagnostic Tests

- **Ascoli test:** This is a thermostable antigen precipitin test developed in 1911. It is an old method but is still used in several countries to detect residual antigens in animal tissue(s). It is not a highly specific test as the antigens being detected are shared by other *Bacillus* spp.
- **McFadyean reaction:** The McFadyean stain remains important for the rapid diagnosis of anthrax. It is a staining procedure for blood or tissue smears from dead animals. The capsular material of the organism can be detected by the McFadyean reaction which involves staining with polychrome methylene blue. The positive observation includes blue rods in a background of purple/pink-stained capsular material.
- **Molecular diagnosis:** Polymerase chain reaction (PCR) is commonly used to target the specific genes of the organism. In addition, molecular typing of the isolates can be carried out by appropriate tools including DNA microarrays, pulsed-field gel electrophoresis (PFGE), multilocus variable number tandem repeat analysis (MLVA), etc.
- **Serology:** The commonly used serological procedure is enzyme-linked immunosorbent assay (ELISA) in microwell plates coated with protective antigen (PA) and lethal factor (LF). Other tests including direct fluorescent assay (DFA) and fluorescence resonance energy transfer (FRET) assay can be used as per availability.

Vaccination

Animals

Globally, the Sterne strain 34F2 anthrax vaccine (non-capsulating [$pXO1^+/pXO2^-$]) is used in animals. This vaccine affords immunological protection primarily due to antibodies specific for the protective antigen (PA). In vaccinated animals, observation of the withholding period for meat (i.e. 3–6 weeks before slaughter) is highly important for human consumption. There is no withholding period for milk in vaccinated animals.

Humans

In humans, immunisation with live spores has been limited to the former USSR and China. Other cell-free human vaccines like Biothrax™ are available in the UK and USA.

Treatment in Humans

The drugs commonly used for anthrax treatment are ciprofloxacin and doxycycline (usually administered together) [8]. It is important to start oral antibiotics within 24 hours of exposure. Advocated antibiotics course durations are:

- 60 days – without vaccine
- 30 days – with three doses of vaccine.

Prevention and Control Measures

The epidemiology of anthrax involves livestock, wildlife, human and environmental components. This complex cycling of the pathogen makes anthrax an ideal example for discussion in the One

Health context. Therefore, prevention and control measures should target the relevant chain of transmission. Some of the measures are listed below.

In Animals

- Vaccination of livestock to generate herd immunity in endemic areas.
- Restrict grazing on contaminated pastures.
- Proper quarantine of imported animals.
- Respect import bans from endemic areas.
- Implementation of laws on prohibition of slaughter and consumption of meat and animal products from infected animals.
- Adequate tracing and destruction of contaminated meat and animal products.
- During an outbreak:
  - avoid opening or postmortem of 'suspected' dead animals
  - plug orifices of dead animals with cotton soaked in carbolic acid/lysol
  - safe disposal of the carcass as per the guidelines
  - disinfect the site of the dead animal with lysol or 3–5% formaldehyde
  - disinfect slaughter sites, processing factories and retail outlets as per the guidelines.

In Humans

- Rapid detection and confirmation of cases by laboratory diagnostics is essential.
- Robust surveillance and tracing of cases should be the priority in endemic areas.
- Appropriate medical interventions during outbreaks.
- Community education and awareness programmes for occupational risk groups.

Environment

Environmental contamination from stray or wild animal carcasses or even from soil disturbance over historic animal graves is possible. Therefore, extra care is required in endemic regions, especially in context with an extensive livestock production system.

References

1 Inglesby, T.V., O'Toole, T., Henderson, D.A. et al. (2002). Anthrax as a biological weapon, 2002: updated recommendations for management. *JAMA 287* (17): 2236–2252.

2 De Vos, V. and Turnbull, P.C. (2004). Anthrax. In: *Infectious Diseases of Livestock, with Special Reference to Southern Africa*, 2e, vol. 3 (eds. J.A. Coetzer, G.R. Thomson and R.C. Tustin), 1788–1818. Cape Town: Oxford University Press Southern Africa.

3 Meselson, M., Guillemin, J., Hugh-Jones, M. et al. (1994). The Sverdlovsk anthrax outbreak of 1979. *Science 266* (5188): 1202–1208.

4 Jernigan, D.B., Raghunathan, P.L., Bell, B.P. et al. (2002). Investigation of bioterrorism-related anthrax, United States, 2001: epidemiologic findings. *Emerging Infectious Diseases* 8 (10): 1019.

5 Abbara, A., Brooks, T., Taylor, G.P. et al. (2014). Lessons for control of heroin-associated anthrax in Europe from 2009–2010 outbreak case studies, London, UK. *Emerging Infectious Diseases* 20 (7): –1115.

6 Baillie, L. and Read, T.D. (2001). *Bacillus anthracis*, a bug with attitude! *Current Opinion in Microbiology 4* (1): 78–81.

7 Centers for Disease Control and Prevention (2020). Travel-Related Infectious Diseases. Chapter 4-Anthrax. https://wwwnc.cdc.gov/travel/yellowbook/2020/travel-related-infectious-diseases/anthrax

8 Turnbull, P.C.B. (ed.) (2008). *Anthrax in Humans and Animals*, 4e. World Health Organization https://apps.who.int/iris/handle/10665/97503.

2
Brucellosis

Brucellosis, one of the most prevalent but neglected zoonoses worldwide, is caused by infection with Gram-negative bacteria of the genus *Brucella*. The most common species causing brucellosis in humans are *Brucella melitensis* (main reservoirs: goats and sheep), *Brucella abortus* (main reservoirs: cattle/other Bovidae) and *Brucella suis* (main reservoir: pigs). Human exposure mainly occurs through direct contact with infected animals, consumption of contaminated food (especially unpasteurised milk and milk products) or inhalation of contagious aerosols.

Synonyms

In humans: Mediterranean fever, undulant fever, Malta fever, melitococcosis, rock fever of Gibraltar, and gastric fever.

In animals: Contagious abortion, infectious abortion, epizootic abortion, Bang disease (in cattle), slinking of calves and ram epididymitis.

Historical Context

- **1884:** Dr David Bruce differentiated between brucellosis (Malta fever) and typhoid outbreaks in Malta. Later, in 1887, Dr Bruce isolated *B. melitensis* (*Micrococcus melitensis* at that time) from the spleen of a British soldier who died from a febrile illness (Malta fever).
- **1897:** Danish veterinarian L.F. Benhard Bang discovered Bang's bacillus or bacillus of cattle abortion, later named *B. abortus*, which was considered as the principal causative agent of brucellosis in cattle and undulant fever in humans.
- **1905:** Themistocles Zammit demonstrated the zoonotic nature of brucellosis by isolating *B. melitensis* from goat's milk. The discovery that healthy goats could be carriers of the disease has been considered as one of the greatest advances in the study of epidemiology.
- **1941:** The first live attenuated 'strain 19 vaccine' was licensed for brucellosis.

Textbook of Zoonoses, First Edition. Jasbir Singh Bedi, Deepthi Vijay, and Pankaj Dhaka.

Characteristics of the Organism

Brucellosis is considered as one of the most prevalent zoonoses affecting farm animals and humans, with considerable socio-economic and trade losses. The genus *Brucella* is composed of Gram-negative, aerobic, facultative intracellular, non-motile, non-spore-forming, partially acid-fast microorganisms. These organisms lack flagellae, capsules, endospores or native plasmids.

There are currently 12 species of *Brucella*, four of which (*melitensis*, *abortus*, *suis* and *canis*) have zoonotic potential of public health significance [1]. As per the Centers for Disease Control and Prevention (CDC) classification, the *Brucella* species causing brucellosis are categorised as 'group B' pathogens due to their low infective dose (i.e. 10 bacteria) and potential of the aerosol route of transmission. A list of *Brucella* species and their natural hosts is provided in Table 2.1 [1].

Survivability Factors

Brucella spp. are quite sensitive to commonly used disinfectants and easily killed by the milk pasteurisation process. The organism cannot survive acidity below pH 4. However, *Brucella* can survive in various environmental conditions for long periods when there is an adequate combination of humidity and temperature.

Some of the common vehicles of the pathogen and associated survivability periods are listed below [2].

Table 2.1 List of *Brucella* species and their natural hosts.

Sl	*Brucella* species	Colony	Natural host	Zoonoses	Year of isolation
1	*B. melitensis* (*bv.* 1–3)	Smooth	Goat and sheep	+++	Bruce (1893)
2	*B. abortus* (*bv.* 1–6, 7, 9)	Smooth	Cattle	++	Schmidt (1901)
3	*B. suis* biovar:				Huddleson (1929)
	1–3	Smooth	Pig	++	
	2	Smooth	Wild boar, hare	+	
	4	Smooth	Reindeer, caribou	++	
	5	Smooth	Rodent	–	
4	*B. ovis*	Rough	Sheep	–	Buddle (1956)
5	*B. neotomae*	Smooth	Desert rat	+	Stoenner and Lackman (1957)
6	*B. canis*	Rough	Dog	+	Carmichael and Bruner (1968)
7	*B. ceti* (*B. delphini*)	Smooth	Dolphins	+	Foster et al. (2007)
8	*B. pinnipedialis*	Smooth	Seals	+	Foster et al. (2007)
9	*B. microti*	Smooth	Wild voles	(?)	Scholz et al. (2008)
10	*B. inopinata*	Smooth	Human	++	Scholz et al. (2009)
11	*B. papionis*	(?)	Baboons (*Papio* spp.)	(?)	Whatmore et al. (2014)
12	*B. vulpis*	(?)	Red foxes (*Vulpes vulpes*)	(?)	Scholz et al. (2016)

Source: From El-Sayed and Awad (2018) [1].

- Dust: 15–40 days
- Tap water: up to 60 days
- Wet soil: up to 70 days
- Goat's cheese: up to 180 days
- Liquid manure: up to 2 years

Pathogenesis

Brucella spp. have a type IV secretion system named *VirB* and periplasmic cyclic β-1,2-glucans. This enables *Brucella* to redirect their intracellular trafficking to avoid fusion and intracellular killing in lysosomes, and thus reach their final replicating niche in the endoplasmic reticulum. After entry into the endoplasmic reticulum, *Brucella* extensively replicates without restricting basic cellular functions or generating programmed cell death. It has been suggested that the smooth, non-endotoxic lipopolysaccharides help in blocking the development of innate and specific immunity during the early stage of infection, and protect the pathogen from the microbicidal activities of the immune system [3].

In cattle, sheep, goats and swine, susceptibility to brucellosis is high in sexually mature animals. Young animals are often resistant but latent infections can occur and such animals when matured may present a hazard as a carrier. The protection in brucellosis is usually short-term and incomplete, and lifelong immunity does not occur, so reinfections can be possible.

Note: Erythritol sugar is considered important for determining tissue tropism of *B. abortus*. It is a well-known fact that bovine placental tissue is rich with erythritol, and during gestation, *B. abortus* replicates intensively in placental trophoblasts, which may induce disruption of placental integrity and abortion.

Brucella spp. infect humans as an incidental host, where the pathogen can multiply within phagocytic cells. In humans, *Brucella* may gain entry via ingestion or inhalation, or through conjunctiva or skin abrasions. The intracellular lifestyle of *Brucella* limits exposure to the host innate and adaptive immune responses and sequesters the organism from the effects of some antibiotics. The unique features of pathology in infected hosts are typically divided into three distinct phases: (i) the incubation phase before clinical symptoms, (ii) the acute phase during which the pathogen invades and disseminates in host tissue, and (iii) the chronic phase that can eventually result in severe organ damage and death of the host.

Brucellosis in humans typically presents with high-grade undulating fever. However, chronic brucellosis may affect many organs, leading to arthritis, orchitis, hepatitis, encephalomyelitis and endocarditis. The low number of virulent organisms required for infection (infectious dose of 10–100 organisms) combined with the capacity for aerosolisation renders *Brucella* spp. as a category B pathogen and potential agent for bioterrorism [4].

Transmission of Brucellosis in Animals

The pathogen is generally associated with but not obligated to specific hosts. For example, in cattle, *B. suis* and *B. melitensis* infections can occur if cattle are in contact with infected pigs and goats. The disease is highly contagious and the infected animals act as the main source of the disease in the herd. *Brucella* can also pass through abraded/injured skin and all mucous membranes. Factors such as wide host range and resistance of *Brucella* spp. to environmental factors and the host immune system facilitate its survival in the population for prolonged periods.

The natural infection in animals occurs mainly through the following mechanisms.

- Ingestion of food or water contaminated by uterine discharges, aborted foetus or foetal membranes, and even through licking the genitalia of infected animals.
- Skin or mucous membrane contamination and udder inoculation from infected milking cups.
- Infected males can spread the infection among females through natural mating (common in sheep and pigs, rarely in cattle) and artificial insemination (if the semen is not screened for the pathogen).
- Intensive mixed livestock farms in endemic regions may facilitate cross-species infection.

Notes:

- Aborted foetus, placental membranes or fluids and other vaginal discharge after abortion (or calving) of infected animals are highly contaminated (10^{13} micro-organisms have been estimated in 1 g of placenta) [5].
- It is important to bear in mind that dogs can acquire infection with *B. abortus*, *B. melitensis* or *B. suis* from aborted ruminants or swine, usually by ingesting foetal or placental material and they can then excrete these pathogens which may pose a serious hazard to humans and livestock. Hence, proper biosecurity of farms must be a priority in *Brucella* control programmes.

Transmission in Humans

Brucellosis is considered an important occupational zoonosis. Farmers, veterinarians, abattoir workers, meat industry workers and personnel involved in laboratory brucellosis research are at-risk groups. An overview of transmission of brucellosis in animals and humans is shown in Figure 2.1. The important transmission routes for brucellosis in humans are as follows.

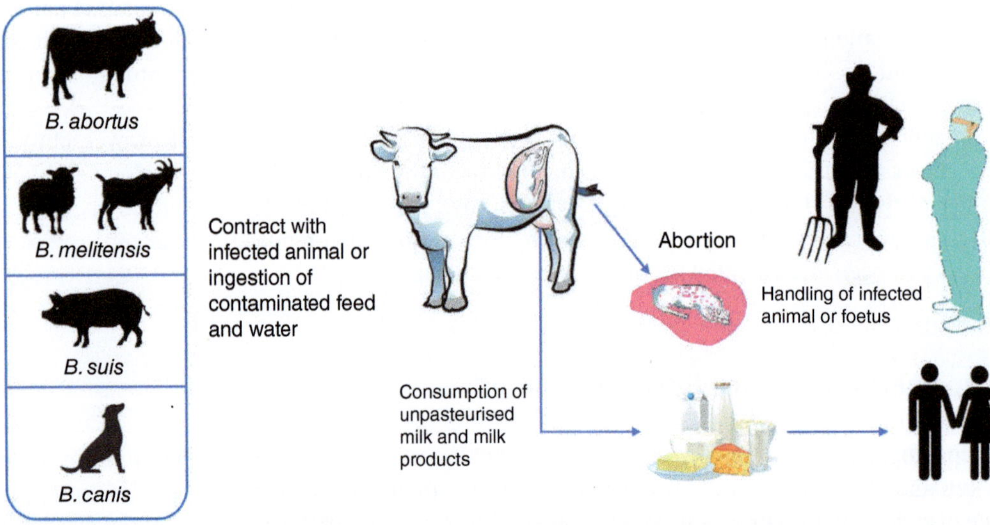

Figure 2.1 An overview of the transmission cycle of brucellosis in animals and humans.

- Contact with an infected animal(s) or their secretions. The risk activities involve close contact with infected animals such as handling aborted animals, clinical examination of the uterus, shearing, vaccination and treatment of infected animals.
- Transmission via inhalation of aerosols generated through contaminated secretions during abortions of infected animals.
- Accidental inoculation with live vaccine strains, especially among veterinarians during vaccination.
- Other risky practices in some regions of the world include skinning of stillborn lambs, kids and aborted foetuses, or crushing the umbilical cord of newborn lambs and kids with the teeth.
- Laboratory-acquired infections (LAIs) of brucellosis by aerosol transmission are widely accepted as a potential biohazard. This mainly occurs due to low awareness or availability of biohazard precaution measures which include improper handling of the pathogen without biosafety level-3 cabinets (BSL-3).
- The alimentary route of transmission of brucellosis includes consumption of unpasteurised dairy products or improperly cooked contaminated meat and meat products.
- Rare transmission of brucellosis between humans may occur through the breach in placental barrier, lactation, sexual intercourse or blood and bone marrow transfusion.

Clinical Signs of Brucellosis in Animals

Characteristic but not specific signs of brucellosis in most animal hosts include late-term abortion (third trimester) or premature birth, infertility, retention of placenta, stillbirth or weak offspring. Infected cows usually abort once, but some animals may abort during subsequent pregnancies. Other important clinical signs include the following.

- In many cases, *Brucella* localises in the supramammary lymph nodes and mammary glands of infected animals and results in secretion of the pathogen in milk throughout their lives. The disease has been associated with decrease in average milk yield of infected animals.
- In males, the infection can cause swelling of the testicles (orchitis), epididymitis and arthritis. Hygroma of knee joints is a common clinical outcome.
- In horses, *Brucella* causes bursitis (also known as fistulous withers and poll evil [swelling of neck or back due to inflammation of the supraspinous bursa]).
- In pigs, late-term abortion, prolonged bacteraemia, lameness, paralysis, spondylitis and metritis are the prominent signs.
- In dogs, abortion occurs in the last trimester of pregnancy with prolonged vaginal discharge. Male dogs suffer from epididymitis, periorchitis and prostatitis.
- Wildlife animals may also exhibit abortion, infertility, debilitation and even death. Predators such as crows, vultures and bears may act as vectors in disease transmission.

Disease in Humans

Brucella spp. are stealth microbes which exhibit induction of chronic infections in humans. The clinical spectrum of the disease ranges from asymptomatic to severe, life-threatening forms. The incubation period usually lasts 1–4 weeks, but depending on the virulence of the organism, route of entry, infective dose and host resistance, the incubation period may be as long as several months. The pathogenic and invasive species of *Brucella* for humans in descending order are: *B. melitensis* > *B. suis* > *B. abortus* > *B. canis*.

Clinical Symptoms

- Fever, headache, night sweats, extreme fatigue, malaise, chills, weight loss, joint pain, back pain and orchitis. Besides the general manifestations of illness, brucellosis can involve any organ or tissue of the body (e.g. osteoarticular brucellosis, genitourinary localisation, neurological complications, etc.). In chronic illness, splenomegaly and hepatomegaly are possible.
- The most characteristic among these symptoms is the triad comprising:
  - *fever* (may be continuous, intermittent, remittent or irregular)
  - *sweating* (intensive sweating with the characteristic smell of wet hay, mainly at night, and diaphoresis may be present)
  - *arthralgia* (arthralgias are of differing intensity and may have migratory patterns).
- Although cardiac involvement is rare (0–2% of symptomatic patients), endocarditis remains the most common cause of death from brucellosis.
- Brucellosis during pregnancy is associated with poor foetal prognosis and may result in abortion, miscarriage, prematurity and foetal death.

Diagnosis of Brucellosis

Isolation of the Pathogen

The isolation of *Brucella* from blood, bone marrow, lymph nodes or cerebrospinal fluids is considered the gold standard test for the diagnosis of brucellosis. However, isolation by cultural technique remains a challenging task as detection requires prolonged incubation due to the organism's slow doubling time and requires specialised laboratory facilities. *Brucella* is a class III pathogen, so proper handling in BSL-3 cabinets is advisable.

Brucella can grow on many of the available standard media (e.g. blood agar, chocolate agar, trypticase soy agar, serum-dextrose agar). Bovine or equine serum may be needed for growth by various strains. The organism grows slowly in culture, so subcultures should be made every 5 days onto the solid medium. Good growth is observed at 37 °C with raised and convex, smooth and circular colonies of 0.5–1 mm in diameter.

Notes:

- The classic biphasic Castañeda method, which is based on a solid and liquid phase in the same blood culture bottle, avoids the need for repeated subcultures. However, the recovery time of *Brucella* from blood culture can still take up to 30 days.
- Incubation under 5–10% CO_2 is a distinguishing feature for *B. abortus* isolates.

Serological Diagnosis

Serological antibody tests measure the ability of serum to agglutinate a standardised amount of killed *B. abortus* cells and reflect the presence of antibodies against the O-side chain (derived from lipopolysaccharide). During infection, *Brucella*-specific IgM appears by the end of the first week of the disease followed by IgG antibodies. The serum agglutination test, also referred to as standard tube agglutination test (STAT), is commonly used for the diagnosis of acute brucellosis.

Note: The 2-mercaptoethanol (2-ME) *Brucella* agglutination test is identical to the STAT test except for the addition of 2-ME that disrupts disulfide bonds. This makes IgM antibodies inactive and permits *Brucella* agglutination only by IgG (resistant to 2-ME disruption). This inactivation characteristic of 2-ME is useful in predicting recovery from brucellosis and determining the adequacy of antibiotic therapy.

Other useful serological tests include:

- Rose Bengal plate agglutination test (RBPT)
- counter immunoelectrophoresis (CIE)
- Coombs' test
- immuno-capture agglutination test
- latex agglutination
- enzyme-linked immunosorbent assay (ELISA).

Limitations

- The currently used serological tests were originally developed and validated for use in cattle. Therefore, when applied to other species, they are inaccurate and unpredictable and need revalidation as per local strains.
- These serological tests are not useful for the diagnosis of *B. canis* (a naturally O-side chain deficient strain).
- Human brucellosis is generally confirmed by the following parameters:

  agglutination titre > 1:160, CF titre > 1:4 and/or ELISA titre > 1:20.

Molecular Diagnosis

The DNA-based assays targeting genus- and species-specific genes, such as conventional polymerase chain reaction (PCR) and real-time PCR, provide better sensitivity than conventional microbiological tests and higher specificity than the traditional serological methods. Genetic loci containing a variable number of tandem repeats (VNTRs), multilocus sequence typing (MLST) and multilocus variable number of tandem repeats analysis (MLVA) can be used for molecular typing of *Brucella* strains.

Vaccination and Treatment

Animals

The details of vaccines commonly used in animals are provided below.

- Live attenuated vaccines.
- Killed vaccines: *B. abortus* 45/20 and *B. melitensis* H38.

Cattle

- In cattle, *B. abortus* strain 19 (S19) vaccine is still in use in many countries for the prevention of brucellosis by induction of antibodies to the O-side chain of LPS. A major problem associated with this vaccine is that vaccinated animals cannot be differentiated from infected animals by current serological tests and the vaccine may also induce abortions in pregnant animals.
- *B. abortus* strain RB51 (SRB51) is a rough mutant derived from the standard smooth virulent strain 2308 of *B. abortus* (deficient in the O-side chain). SRB51 has attenuated virulence and has been widely used as an alternative to the S19 vaccine in cattle. Unlike S19, it does not induce antibodies to the O-side chain which enables differentiation among vaccinated and naturally infected animals [6].

Sheep and Goats

- *B. melitensis* strain Rev1 has been used for control of ovine and caprine brucellosis but it is associated with a considerable degree of virulence and may induce abortions when administered during pregnancy.

Note: In animals, treatment of brucellosis is not advisable, so culling of the infected animal is suggested by most veterinary experts.

Humans

- **Vaccines:** Live human vaccines *B. abortus* strain 19-BA and strain104M were used in the former Soviet Union (USSR) and China, respectively, but tend to be reactogenic and of limited efficacy.
- **Treatment:** The intracellular localisation of *Brucella* and its ability to adapt to the environmental conditions encountered in its replicative niche (e.g. macrophage) usually result in treatment failure and high relapse rates. The joint Food and Agriculture Organization (FAO)/World Health Organization (WHO) expert committee on brucellosis recommends treatment of adult acute brucellosis with rifampicin (600–900 mg/day orally) plus doxycycline (200 mg/day orally) for 6 weeks.

Prevention and Control

Animals

Vaccination alone will not eradicate brucellosis, as the immunity produced by vaccines is not absolute and can be circumvented with an increased level of infection. Therefore, vaccination policy is more likely to succeed if it is combined with good animal husbandry management measures. Some important measures are as follows.

- Proper biosecurity of farms with regular screening of herds. Positive cases must be removed from the herd by following the 'test and segregate/slaughter' policy.
- Careful selection of replacement animals with proper quarantine procedures.
- The preponderance of natural bull service in rural areas, especially in buffaloes, is an important factor in the maintenance and spread of infection. Hence, proper screening of bulls or use of artificial insemination (AI) technology can be employed to avoid sexual transmission.
- Surveillance programmes to control the disease in the domestic and wild animal reservoirs should be carried out.
- Proper disposal of contaminated materials (aborted foetuses and genital discharge) as per the guidelines.

Humans

The One Health approach including interdisciplinary co-ordination, surveillance and political commitment is important in addressing the problem of brucellosis in endemic regions. Some important measures include the following.

- Proper storage and consumption of animal foods, especially unpasteurised milk and meat products.
- Health education of at-risk groups through community participation.

- Encourage the use of personal protective equipment during hazardous activities (especially for risk groups like veterinarians, laboratory workers, slaughter workers, etc.).
- Strict use of BSL-3 cabinets while handling live cultures.

References

1 El-Sayed, A. and Awad, W. (2018). Brucellosis: evolution and expected comeback. *International Journal of Veterinary Science and Medicine* 6: S31–S35.

2 Gotuzzo, E. and Carillo, C. (2004). *Brucella*. In: *Infectious Diseases*, 3e (eds. S.L. Gorbach, J.G. Bartlett and N.R. Blacklow), 1837–1845. Philadelphia: Lippincott Williams & Wilkins.

3 Franco, M.P., Mulder, M., Gilman, R.H., and Smits, H.L. (2007). Human brucellosis. *Lancet Infectious Diseases* 7 (12): 775–786.

4 de Figueiredo, P., Ficht, T.A., Rice-Ficht, A. et al. (2015). Pathogenesis and immunobiology of brucellosis: review of Brucella–host interactions. *American Journal of Pathology* 185 (6): 1505–1517.

5 Banai, M. and Corbel, M. (2010). Taxonomy of Brucella. *Open Veterinary Science Journal* 4 (1): 85–101.

6 Kianmehr, Z., Ardestani, S.K., Soleimanjahi, H. et al. (2015). Comparison of biological and immunological characterization of lipopolysaccharides from *Brucella abortus* RB51 and S19. *Jundishapur Journal of Microbiology* 8 (11): e24853.

3

Cat-Scratch Disease

Aetiology

Cat-scratch disease (CSD) is a zoonotic infection caused by the fastidious Gram-negative bacillus *Bartonella henselae*. The organism is found worldwide in bacteraemic cats. The disease is also known as cat-scratch fever and Teeny disease.

Historical Context

Cat-scratch disease was first recognised by Parinaud in 1889 in three patients with granulomatous conjunctivitis, preauricular lymphadenopathy and chronic fever. These symptoms were initially known as 'Parinaud's oculoglandular syndrome' and subsequently reported with the history of cat exposure in some patients with this syndrome [1, 2]. The association between CSD and cats was first described by Robert Debré in 1931; however, his team could not publish any data until 1950 [3]. It was not until 1992 that *B. henselae* (previously known as *Rochalimaea henselae*) was identified as the causative agent of CSD [4, 5].

Disease Transmission

Cats are the principal reservoir species for *B. henselae*. The organism is maintained and spread among cats by the cat flea (*Ctenocephalides felis*). Cats can become infected with *B. henselae* from flea bites and flea dirt (droppings) getting into their wounds. By scratching and biting at the fleas and flea bite areas, cats pick up the contaminated flea dirt under their nails and between teeth. Cats can also become infected while fighting with other infected cats.

Transmission of the pathogen to humans occurs via scratches and bites from infected cats and by contact of cat saliva with an open wound. However, the role of the cat flea in cat-to-human transmission remains questionable.

Disease in Cats

Around 40% of cats harbour *B. henselae* at some stage of their lives without showing any signs of illness [6].

Textbook of Zoonoses, First Edition. Jasbir Singh Bedi, Deepthi Vijay, and Pankaj Dhaka.

Disease in Humans

Cat-scratch disease is a systemic infectious disease and often manifest as a self-limited condition. Most patients remain afebrile and are not systemically ill. The predominant clinical feature of CSD is lymphadenopathy proximal to the site of a cat scratch or bite. A small localised papule is usually first seen at the site of inoculation after 3–10 days. Several weeks after exposure, mild local infection is followed by tender regional lymphadenopathy and then low-grade fever, malaise, headache and myalgias. Lymphadenitis can persist for months; with some patients, the lymph node enlargement occurs for as long as 12–24 months.

Approximately 10% of CSD patients develop extranodal manifestations, presumed to be the consequence of haematogenous spread of the infection, known as 'atypical CSD'. This may include serious manifestations, such as neuroretinitis, Parinaud oculoglandular syndrome, osteomyelitis, encephalitis and/or endocarditis [4, 5]. In immunocompromising conditions, such as AIDS, *B. henselae* infection can be severe and may develop vascular proliferative lesions (bacillary angiomatosis and bacillary peliosis).

Note:
The common ocular complication caused by *Bartonella* infection is Parinaud oculoglandular syndrome, which affects approximately 2–5% of symptomatic patients [7]. The syndrome is self-limiting conjunctivitis associated with preauricular lymphadenopathy. Other ocular manifestations mainly dominated by neuroretinitis and retinitis have also been described.

Diagnosis in Humans

Isolation of the Pathogen

The culture of *Bartonella* spp. remains tedious. Many laboratories continue to rely on standard blood agar plate cultures (5% rabbit blood heart infusion-Trypticase^{TM} agar or chocolate agar) for the isolation of *Bartonella* spp. (however, this method has questionable sensitivity). Bartonella-Alphaproteobacteria growth medium (BAPGM), a new insect-based liquid culture medium, has been found to support the growth of at least seven *Bartonella* species [8].

Serological and Molecular Assays

As *B. henselae* is difficult to culture, serological examinations are always performed to diagnose CSD in combination with the history of exposure to cats and clinical manifestations. Two important serological tests for the diagnosis of CSD are:

- indirect fluorescent antibody test (IFA)
- enzyme immunoassay (EIA).

Molecular tools like polymerase chain reaction (PCR) assays can also be performed on tissue or pus samples obtained from affected lymph nodes to detect the pathogen.

Immunohistochemistry and Warthin–Starry Silver Staining

The immunohistochemistry (IHC) and Warthin–Starry silver stain (WS) are considered important diagnostic tools for CSD in combination with morphological characteristics [9].

Note:
In the process of Warthin–Starry silver staining, the cell wall of *B. henselae* can absorb silver ions, which are reduced to metal silver through the chromogenic agent and the bacteria appear black.

Treatment

Cat-scratch disease is a self-limited condition and antibiotics are generally reserved for those with a severe form of infection. Immunocompromised patients affected with CSD may require antibiotic therapy (such as erythromycin or doxycycline) to avoid serious outcomes [6].

Prevention and Control

Important prevention and control strategies include the following.

- Be alert to a cat scratch or bite.
- Do not allow cats to lick your wounds.
- In case of a bite or scratch accident, wash the area with soap and running water or any other effective disinfectant.
- Contact your physician if you develop any symptoms of CSD.

References

1. Henry, M. (1952). Leptothricosis conjunctivae (Parinaud's conjunctivitis): report of 13 cases; relationship to cat-scratch disease. *Transactions of the Pacific Coast Oto-Ophthalmological Society Annual Meeting*, 33, pp. 173–196.
2. Cassady, J.V. and Culbertson, C.S. (1953). Cat-scratch disease and Parinaud's oculoglandular syndrome. *AMA Archives of Ophthalmology 50* (1): 68–74.
3. Debré, R. and Job, J.C. (1954). La maladie des griffes du chat (cat scratch fever). *Acta Paediatrica 43* (4): 386–389.
4. Gandhi, T.N., Slater, L.N., and Welch, D.F. (2015). *Bartonella*, including cat-scratch disease. In: *Mandell, Douglas, and Bennett's Principles and Practice of Infectious Diseases*, 8e (eds. J.E. Bennett, R. Dolin and M.J. Balser), 2649–2663. Philadelphia, PA: Elsevier Saunders.
5. Giladi, M. and Ephros, M. (2015). Bartonella infections, including cat-scratch disease. In: *Harrison's Principles of Internal Medicine*, 19e (eds. D.L. Kasper, A.S. Fauci, S.L. Hauser, et al.), 1078–1083. New York: McGraw Hill.
6. Centers for Disease Control and Prevention (2020). Cat-scratch disease. www.cdc.gov/healthypets/diseases/cat-scratch.html
7. Carithers, H.A. (1985). Cat-scratch disease: an overview based on a study of 1,200 patients. *American Journal of Diseases of Children* 139 (11): 1124–1133.
8. Maggi, R.G., Duncan, A.W., and Breitschwerdt, E.B. (2005). Novel chemically modified liquid medium that will support the growth of seven Bartonella species. *Journal of Clinical Microbiology 43* (6): 2651–2655.
9. Peng, J., Fan, Z., Zheng, H. et al. (2020). Combined application of immunohistochemistry and Warthin-Starry silver stain on the pathologic diagnosis of cat scratch disease. *Applied Immunohistochemistry and Molecular Morphology 28* (10): 781–785.

4

Glanders

Aetiology and Pathogen Characteristics

Glanders is a highly contagious and often fatal zoonotic disease, primarily affecting solipeds (horses, mules and donkeys). It is a World Organization for Animal Health (OIE) notifiable disease of Equidae. It is caused by the bacterium *Burkholderia mallei*, which is classified as a 'Category B' biological agent by the CDC. The organism is a Gram-negative, facultative intracellular and non-spore-forming coccobacillus. It is closely related to *Burkholderia pseudomallei*, the causative agent of melioidosis. Unlike *B. pseudomallei*, *B. mallei* has no flagella and is therefore non-motile. A capsule-like coat has been demonstrated in the organism by electron microscopy [1].

In the past, *B. mallei* has been reported throughout the world, but at present glanders has been eradicated from many countries, except for some regions in Africa, Asia, Middle East, Central and South America [2]. *B. mallei* is highly infectious as it involves an aerosol route of transmission, and infection requires few organisms, which make it a potential candidate for intentional release as a biological threat agent.

Burkholderia mallei is unique in the *Burkholderia* family because it does not survive in soil, but needs an animal host for survival [1]. The organism is destroyed through heating to 55 °C for 10 minutes. The bacterium is sensitive to sunlight and can be inactivated within 24 hours of direct exposure, and is also susceptible to common disinfectants such as iodine, benzalkonium chloride (1/2000), sodium hypochlorite (500 ppm available chlorine), 70% ethanol and 2% glutaraldehyde [1].

Historical Overview

Glanders is one of the oldest known diseases and was first described by Aristotle. The organism was first isolated by Loeffler and Schutz in Germany in 1882 from the liver and spleen of an infected horse.

Several countries have studied glanders as a bioweapon, and it might have been the first biological weapon used in the twentieth century (including World War I and II) [3]. In the recent past, the former Soviet Union reportedly weaponised *B. mallei* and deployed it in Afghanistan during the 1980s. The inhalation route remains an important concern for the use of *B. mallei* as biological weapon, as the organism can be aerosolised easily.

Textbook of Zoonoses, First Edition. Jasbir Singh Bedi, Deepthi Vijay, and Pankaj Dhaka.

Pathogenesis and Virulence Factors

Burkholderia mallei is a facultative intracellular pathogen that establishes itself in host macrophages after respiratory or subcutaneous exposure. The infection can manifest in an acute phase, followed by dissemination to major organ systems in the chronic phase, sepsis and death. The organism has an extensive set of mechanisms for invasion and modulation of host cell environments. The key mechanisms of *B. mallei* pathogenicity are encoded in virulence factors and proteins that control and promote pathogenic internalisation, survival and replication within host cells. Some of the important virulence factors and their relative importance in animal models of glanders are listed below [2].

- **Capsule:** Required for optimal survival and replication in macrophages. The capsule contributes to survival in serum by reducing C3b-mediated opsonisation and phagocytosis.
- **Quorum sensing:** *B. mallei* encodes two *lux*I homologues and four *lux*R homologues which help in the quorum sensing process.
- **LPS O-antigen:** *B. mallei* O-antigen confers resistance against macrophage killing and promotes survival in serum by preventing killing by the alternative pathway of the complement system.
- **Type III secretion system (T3SS) and Type VI secretion system (T6SS):** The *B. mallei* T3SSs are similar to the T3SSs from *Salmonella* and *Shigella*. The T3SS and T6SS modulate the intracellular behaviour of the pathogen.

Transmission Cycle

In Animals

The most common sources of infection appear to be ingestion of food or water contaminated through discharges from the respiratory tract or ulcerated skin lesions of the carrier. Chronically infected or subclinical carrier animals can shed the pathogen intermittently or constantly into food and water sources. Other major routes of transmission are contamination of skin abrasions or mucous membranes or inhalation of contaminated aerosols.

In Humans

The disease is transmissible from animals to humans via contact with tissues or body fluids of infected animals. Naturally acquired human cases can typically occur among persons with prolonged contact with solipeds, such as veterinarians or farmers, or those working in the laboratory setting without proper biosafety measures. Human-to-human transmission is rare [4].

Disease in Animals

Clinically, *B. mallei*-infected solipeds can present with either a chronic (horses) or an acute (mules and donkeys) form. The clinical manifestations in different species are detailed below.

- In horses, *B. mallei* infection presents as either a nasal-pulmonary form (glanders) or a cutaneous form (farcy).
  - **Nasal-pulmonary form (glanders):** The lesions in the nasal cavity start as pyogranulomatous nodules in the submucosa which subsequently ulcerate and release copious amounts of

exudate containing *B. mallei* into the nasal cavity. Finally, ulcerative lesions in mucosa heal and are replaced by typical stellate (star-shaped), fibrous scars. In some cases, the lungs also contain numerous small grey miliary nodules (2–10 mm) resembling millet seeds which usually distribute randomly in one or more pulmonary lobes through the haematogenous route.
  - **Cutaneous form (farcy):** Cutaneous lesions, often referred to as equine farcy, are the result of severe suppurative lymphangitis which is characterised by nodular thickening of extended segments of lymph vessels in the subcutaneous tissue of the legs and ventral abdomen. Eventually, the affected lymph vessels rupture and release large amounts of purulent exudate through sinuses to the surface of the skin.
- In donkeys and mules, the disease generally takes an acute form with high fever and respiratory signs (swollen nostrils, dyspnoea, pneumonia) and death occurs within a few days.
- **Other animals:** Naturally infected dromedary camels can exhibit similar clinical signs as in equids, including fever, lethargy, emaciation, nodules and ulcers in the nasal passages, with severe mucopurulent discharge. Carnivores may become infected by eating infected meat and may exhibit nodules and ulcers in the nasal passages and on the conjunctivae, as well as deeper in the respiratory tract. Cattle and pigs are resistant to natural infection [5].

Disease in Humans

After an incubation period of 10–14 days, glanders can present with fever and any of four clinical manifestations.

Localised Infection

This includes localised cutaneous and/or localised mucous membrane infection.

- Localised cutaneous infection.
  - Usually results in a cutaneous nodule at the site of inoculation.
  - Lymphangitis is common, with cord-like induration of the lymphatic channels subcutaneously. The nodules often break down and ulcerate.
  - Fever and other symptoms (rigours, fatigue, headache, myalgias) may or may not be present.
- Localised mucous membrane infection.
  - Depending on the site of inoculation, this may affect the eyes, nose or oral cavity.
  - Ulcerating granulomatous reactions can occur.
  - Generally, mucopurulent nasal or ocular discharges are present.
  - Fever and other symptoms may or may not be present.

Pulmonary Form

This is mainly characterised by pneumonia, pulmonary abscess and pleural effusion. Fever and other symptoms (rigors, fatigue, headache, myalgias) are usually present.

Septicemic Form

This may occur at any point in the illness. The signs and symptoms are consistent with a typical sepsis syndrome and multiple abscesses involving the spleen, liver and lungs may occur. Glanders has a 95% case fatality rate in untreated septicemic infections and a 50% case fatality rate in treated individuals, even if diagnosed early [6].

Chronic Form

If the infection becomes chronic, multiple abscesses may develop in the muscles and skin of arms, legs, lungs, spleen and/or liver.

Laboratory Diagnosis

Isolation of the Bacteria

Burkholderia mallei can be isolated from clinical samples (e.g. blood, sputum, urine, skin lesions) by using sheep blood agar or Trypticase™ soy agar. The organism grows aerobically and prefers media containing glycerol. It grows well but slowly, with a recommended 72 hours of culture incubation.

Diagnostic Tests

Serology

The complement fixation test is considered a reliable serological method for diagnosis in equids. It delivers a positive result within 1 week post infection and can also recognise sera from exacerbated chronic cases [1]. The immunoblot assay and rose Bengal plate agglutination test can also be used in the diagnosis of glanders in equines. The major limitation of serological tests is cross-reactivity to other species of *Burkholderia*, including *B. pseudomallei*.

Mallein Test

The mallein test is a delayed-type hypersensitivity test against *B. mallei* on the skin. Mallein is a water-soluble protein fraction of the organism which is injected intradermo-palpebrally in animals. In infected animals, the eyelid swells markedly within 1–2 days. (*Note*: The mallein test is not used in humans.)

Molecular Diagnosis

Polymerase chain reaction (PCR) and real-time PCR assays are commonly used to target the specific genes of the organism. Other molecular tools such as PCR-derived restriction length polymorphism, gene sequencing, pulsed-field gel electrophoresis (PFGE), variable number tandem repeat polymorphism (VNTR) and multilocus sequence typing (MLST) can also be used to further characterise the pathogen.

Treatment

Most national legislations (e.g. Glanders and Farcy Act of 1899 in India) call for the detection and destruction of glanderous animals. Since human cases of glanders are rare, there is limited information about antibiotic treatment in humans. Sulfadiazine has been found effective in experimental animals and humans. The disease may relapse or recur, and long-term follow-up (minimum of 5 years) is recommended [7].

Prevention and Control

In humans and animals, there is currently no effective vaccine available for glanders. Therefore, prevention and control of glanders in animals requires a surveillance programme involving early detection, testing of suspect cases, screening of apparently healthy equids and humane elimination of reactors. Stable hygiene and manure management are imperative to contain the infection.

In humans, glanders is usually an occupational hazard, affecting individuals who have close contact with infected animals (e.g. farmers, groomers, veterinarians, laboratory personnel, etc.). In endemic regions, prevention of the disease in humans involves rapid identification and elimination of the infection in the animal population of that region. The laboratory manipulations should be performed with the appropriate biosafety level and with proper personal protective equipment.

References

1 World Organisation of Animal Health (2018). Glanders and melioidosis. www.oie.int/fileadmin/Home/eng/Health_standards/tahm/3.05.11_GLANDERS.pdf

2 Galyov, E.E., Brett, P.J., and DeShazer, D. (2010). Molecular insights into *Burkholderia pseudomallei* and *Burkholderia mallei* pathogenesis. *Annual Review of Microbiology 64*: 495–517.

3 Bossi, P., Tegnell, A., Baka, A. et al. (2004). Bichat guidelines for the clinical management of glanders and melioidosis and bioterrorism-related glanders and melioidosis. *Eurosurveillance 9* (12): E17–E18.

4 Van Zandt, K.E., Greer, M.T., and Gelhaus, H.C. (2013). Glanders: an overview of infection in humans. *Orphanet Journal of Rare Diseases 8* (1): 131.

5 Wittig, M.B., Wohlsein, P., Hagen, R.M. et al. (2006). Glanders – a comprehensive review. *Deutsche Tierarztliche Wochenschrift 113* (9): 323–330.

6 Estes, D.M., Dow, S.W., Schweizer, H.P., and Torres, A.G. (2010). Present and future therapeutic strategies for melioidosis and glanders. *Expert Review of Anti-Infective Therapy 8* (3): 325–338.

7 Centers for Disease Control and Prevention (2017). Glanders: treatment. www.cdc.gov/glanders/treatment/index.html

5

Leptospirosis

Leptospirosis is considered the most widespread zoonosis in the world due to its extensive host range [1]. The disease is endemic in many tropical regions of the world and causes epidemics after heavy rainfall and flooding. It is also considered an important occupational zoonosis in many risk groups (e.g. swimmers, farmers, fish handlers, sports persons, sewer workers, etc.). Several pathogenic species of the genus *Leptospira* can cause a wide range of clinical manifestations, from a mild, flu-like illness to a severe form of the disease (which is also known as Weil's disease) with jaundice and multiorgan involvement including acute kidney injury, pulmonary haemorrhage and adult respiratory distress syndrome [1].

Synonyms: Weil's disease, swine herder's disease, rice-field fever, cane-cutter fever, swamp fever, mud fever, autumn fever, seven-day fever, Fort Bragg disease.

Historical Overview

- **1886:** German physician Adolph Weil described the disease as infectious jaundice. It is also called Weil's disease.
- **1907:** Arthur Stimson first demonstrated leptospires by using Levaditi silver deposition staining in kidney tissue sections of a patient who died of yellow fever. He called the organism *Spirocheta interrogans* because the bacterium resembled a question mark.
- **1915:** The aetiology of leptospirosis was demonstrated independently in Japan and Germany by two different research groups.
- **1917:** Inada, Ido and colleagues observed and cultured spirochetes from the kidneys and urine of different species of house and wild rats.
- **1918:** The genus name *Leptospira* was first proposed by Noguchi to differentiate the Weil's disease spirochete from others.
- **1942:** Soldiers contracted the disease by swimming in contaminated ponds at Fort Bragg, North Carolina; therefore, it is also known as Fort Bragg disease.

Aetiological Agent and Characteristics

Leptospires (Greek *leptos* means fine or slender) are Gram-negative tightly coiled spirochetes. The cells have pointed ends, either or both of which are usually bent into a distinctive hook. The bacteria are obligate aerobes with an optimum growth temperature of 28–30 °C.

Textbook of Zoonoses, First Edition. Jasbir Singh Bedi, Deepthi Vijay, and Pankaj Dhaka.

The genus *Leptospira* can be divided into two species.

- *Leptospira interrogans* comprising all pathogenic strains.
- *Leptospira biflexa* containing the saprophytic strains isolated from the environment.

Both of the species, *L. interrogans* and *L. biflexa*, are divided into numerous serovars defined by agglutination after cross-absorption with homologous antigens. Within the species *L. interrogans*, over 250 serovars have been recognised, whereas more than 60 serovars of *L. biflexa* have been recorded [1].

Disease Transmission and Risk Factors

Leptospirosis is presumed to be the most widespread zoonosis in the world. The source of infection in humans is either direct or indirect contact with the urine of infected animals. Animals can be the maintenance hosts or accidental (incidental) hosts for the organism. A maintenance host is defined as a species in which infection is persistent and is usually transferred from animal to animal by direct contact. The disease is maintained in nature by chronic infection of the renal tubules of maintenance hosts. Rats and mice are regarded as the most common maintenance hosts for leptospire infections, where the infection remains mostly asymptomatic with the bacteria subsequently cleared from all organs except the kidneys [2]. Different rodent species may be reservoirs of distinct serovars, but rats are generally maintenance hosts for serovars of the serogroups *icterohaemorrhagiae* and *ballum*, and mice serve as maintenance hosts for serogroup *ballum*.

Rats and mice may transfer the infection to domestic farm animals, dogs and humans. The extent to which infection is transmitted depends on many external environmental factors, including climate, population density and the degree of contact between maintenance and accidental hosts. Some domestic animals also serve as maintenance hosts for some of the serovars as described below [3].

- Dairy cattle may harbour serovars *hardjo*, *pomona* and *grippotyphosa*.
- Pigs may harbour *pomona*, *tarassovi* or *bratislava*.
- Sheep may harbour *hardjo* and *pomona*.
- Dogs may harbour *canicola*.

Variations in maintenance hosts and the serovars they carry occur throughout the world. Therefore, knowledge of the prevalent serovars and their maintenance hosts is essential to understand the epidemiology and subsequent control measures of the disease in any region. An overview of transmission of leptospirosis in animals and humans is given in Figure 5.1.

Risk Factors for Leptospirosis

The incidence of the disease is significantly higher in tropical countries than in temperate regions [4]. This is mainly due to the longer survival of the pathogen in warm, humid conditions. Further, most tropical countries have large agriculture-based communities, thereby providing greater exposure of the human population to infected animals owing to their higher proximity to livestock. In addition, climatic changes related to flooding, poor hygiene and sanitation practices and a high population of maintenance hosts (e.g. rats) are also important determinants of infection in tropical countries.

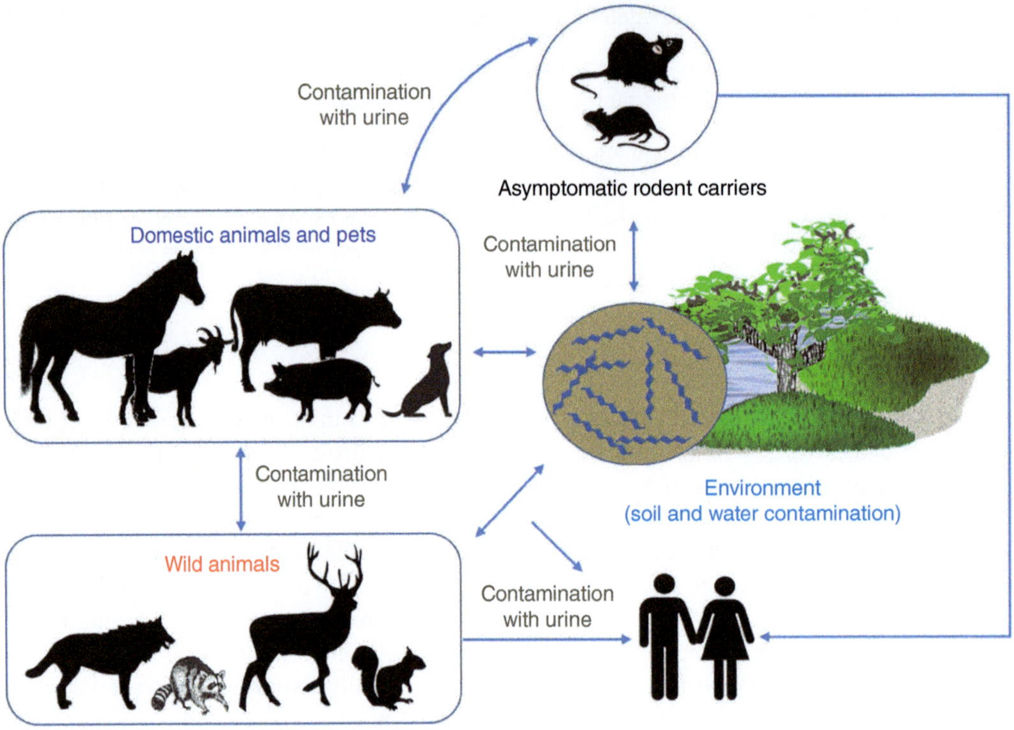

Figure 5.1 An overview of the transmission cycle of leptospirosis in animals and humans.

Human infections may acquire through occupational or recreational exposures. Direct contact with infected animals accounts for most of the infection in farmers, veterinarians, abattoir workers, meat inspectors, rodent control workers and other occupations which require frequent contact with animals. Indirect contact is an important transmission factor for sewer workers, miners, soldiers, septic tank cleaners, fish farmers, gamekeepers, canal workers, rice field workers, banana farmers and sugar cane cutters. Pets, mainly dogs, can also be an important source of infection to humans. In some instances, shedding of leptospires in the urine may persist for as long as 3 months after infection as a result of inadequate or lack of treatment [5]. It has been reported that leptospires can survive for up to 152 days in fresh water through cellular aggregation and therefore water sanitation and hygiene are important factors in the prevention and control of leptospirosis transmission [6].

Pathogenesis

The infection is acquired through contact with infected animals or their urine/body tissues. *Leptospira* invades the body through non-intact skin (e.g. cuts, abrasions, etc.) or mucous membranes (including conjunctiva). The pathogen can also be acquired by ingestion of contaminated food and water. The ability of leptospires to survive in moist environments makes them a high-risk agent for infection following contact with contaminated water sources.

The pathogenesis of leptospirosis involves several virulence factors, including lipopolysaccharides (LPS), hemolysins, outer membrane proteins (OMPs) and other surface proteins, as well as adhesion molecules. The ability of hemolysins to lyse erythrocytes and other cell membranes makes them potential virulence factors.

Once within the body, the bacteria spread through the lymphatics and then into the bloodstream. Later, the infection can spread to the entire body and the pathogen tends to settle in the liver and kidneys. Leptospires can persist in some of the anatomically localised and immunologically privileged sites. Immune privilege is a special immunological status of an organ or tissue for which the threshold of tolerance has been increased to reduce the chances of inflammatory injury. The most significant site of persistence is the renal tubule. Leptospires appear in the kidney 2–4 weeks after acute infection and attach to an interdigitated area in the brush border of the proximal renal tubular epithelium. The *in vitro* attachment of virulent leptospires to renal epithelial cells is enhanced by subagglutinating concentrations of homologous antibodies [7]. The animal may excrete leptospires intermittently or regularly for months or years, or a lifetime. However, humans do not remain carriers for long, and the urine is free of leptospires at the time of clinical recovery [8].

Disease in Animals

Cattle

Cattle are important maintenance hosts of serovars *hardjo* and *pomona*. After infection, leptospires localise in the kidneys and are excreted intermittently in the urine. The important manifestations are stillbirths or abortions (mainly in the last trimester), mastitis (with blood clots in milk) and/or 'milk drop syndrome'. The milk drop syndrome is distinguished by a loss or drop in milk production along with the udder appearing as if milking has already been done [9]. Some serovars (mainly *pomona*) can result in severe disease in calves in the form of acute leptospirosis which may be characterised by fever, anorexia, dyspnoea from pulmonary congestion, icterus, haemoglobinuria (red water of calves) and haemolytic anaemia.

Dogs

The disease in dogs is also known as canine typhus, Stuttgart disease and infectious jaundice (haemolytic icterus). Dogs act as maintenance hosts for *L. canicola*. It is difficult to diagnose the infection with host-adapted serovars because the infection generally produces only mild clinical signs. For this reason, it is believed that leptospiral infections are far more common than clinically evident. Predictably, the most severe cases of the disease are those resulting from infection with non-host-adapted serovars.

Cases of leptospirosis in dogs share many common features, and the pathogenic serovars tend to produce leptospiraemia and vasculitis. The organ system involvement has been thought to be serovar specific. For example, infection with serovars *icterohaemorrhagiae* or *canicola* has been associated with coagulopathies, hepatic disease and renal failure, whereas infection with other emerging serovars has been associated with acute renal failure (ARF) rather than hepatic disease or coagulopathies [10].

Horses

The mild form of equine leptospirosis is characterised by mild fever, loss of appetite and lethargy. The severe manifestations are jaundice and haemorrhages on the mucosa whereas the pathogenic serovars may also cause placentitis, abortions and stillbirths in pregnant mares [11]. Recurrent uveitis (moon blindness) has been observed as a common immunological reaction due to antigenic cross-reactivity between leptospiral protein and protein of equine cornea [12]. Renal failure is more common in foals than old horses. Leptospiral abortions in the late stage of gestation, with no apparent clinical signs, are also common. Infected mares shed leptospires in the urine for prolonged periods and can transmit the infection.

Disease in Humans

Leptospirosis has been described as a zoonosis of protean manifestations. The incubation period of the disease ranges from 2 days to 4 weeks [13]. The clinical presentation of leptospirosis is biphasic, with the acute or septicemic phase lasting about a week, followed by the immune phase, characterised by antibody production and excretion of leptospires in the urine. Most of the complications of leptospirosis are associated with the localisation of leptospires within the tissues during the immune phase and thus occur during the second week of the illness [14].

Anicteric Leptospirosis

The majority of infections caused by leptospires are either subclinical or of mild severity. A smaller proportion of infections present with a febrile illness of sudden onset with other symptoms including chills, headache, myalgia, abdominal pain, conjunctival suffusion and less often a skin rash. The fever may be biphasic and can recur after remission of 3–4 days. The headache is often severe (resembling that which occurs in dengue) with retro-orbital pain and photophobia. This anicteric syndrome usually lasts for about a week, and its resolution coincides with the appearance of antibodies.

Icteric Leptospirosis

Icteric leptospirosis is a much more severe form of the disease. Between 5% and 10% of all patients with leptospirosis have the icteric form. Severe cases often present late in the course of the disease, and this contributes to the high mortality rate (range: 5–15%). The severe manifestations during this phase include renal failure, jaundice, haemorrhage and respiratory distress. The icteric phase may also involve the heart, central nervous system (CNS) and muscles. The jaundice occurring in leptospirosis is not associated with hepatocellular necrosis, and the liver function returns to normal after recovery from infection. The complications of severe leptospirosis are due to the multisystemic nature of the disease. Leptospirosis is a common cause of ARF and ocular manifestations have also been reported in many cases. Conjunctival suffusion is seen in the majority of patients. Conjunctival suffusion in the presence of scleral icterus is said to be pathognomonic of Weil's disease. The infection can be transmitted across the placenta during pregnancy and it may cause foetal loss and miscarriage (usually within the first few months of pregnancy), stillbirth and congenital infection [15].

Laboratory Diagnosis

Staining techniques such as Warthin– Starry silver stain and Fontana stain can be used on clinical samples and the organism can be visualised under dark-field microscopy. However, the limitations of these methods involve poor staining of pathogen, and dark-field microscopy is relatively unreliable due to possible errors caused by *Leptospira*-like artefacts.

Culture Media

Leptospires are fastidious organisms and need the addition of animal protein in the form of fresh rabbit serum or bovine serum albumin 'fraction V' for their growth. In the past, several liquid media containing rabbit serum were described by Fletcher, Korthoff, Noguchi and Stuart for the growth of leptospires. The most widely used medium in current practice is based on the oleic acid-albumin medium, i.e. EMJH (Johnson and Harris medium–modification of Ellinghuasen McCollough).

The growth of leptospires is often slow on primary isolation, and the cultures should be retained for up to 13 weeks before being discarded. However, pure subcultures in liquid media usually grow within 10–14 days.

Serodiagnosis

Most leptospirosis cases are diagnosed by serology. The microscopic agglutination test (MAT) is considered the reference method for serological diagnosis of leptospirosis. In this method, the patient sera react with live antigen suspensions of leptospiral serovars. After proper incubation, the serum-antigen mixtures are examined microscopically for agglutination and the titers are determined. The MAT is read by dark-field microscopy where the endpoint is the highest dilution of serum at which 50% agglutination occurs. However, the complexity of performance and interpretation and the continuous risk of cross-contamination of the antigen cultures remain major limitations of MAT. The live cultures of all serovars required for use as antigens must be maintained by repeated weekly subculturing of strains which can also pose hazards to laboratory workers.

Other serological tests include complement fixation test, sensitised erythrocyte lysis, macroscopic slide agglutination, immunofluorescence assay, indirect haemagglutination, ELISA, Dot-ELISA, IgM dipstick, counter immunoelectrophoresis and latex agglutination test.

Molecular Diagnosis

Leptospiral DNA can be detected from clinical material by dot-blotting, *in situ* hybridisation and PCR targeting specific genes. Further, characterisation of the pathogen by molecular typing includes digestion of chromosomal DNA by restriction endonucleases (REA), restriction fragment length polymorphism (RFLP), ribotyping, pulse-field gel electrophoresis (PFGE) and other PCR-based approaches.

Vaccination and Treatment

Vaccination

It is important to ensure that pets are vaccinated against leptospirosis. Always remember that vaccine does not provide 100% protection, as there are many strains (types) of leptospires and the vaccine does not provide immunity against all strains. In humans, vaccination of at-risk populations remains limited to some parts of the world where vaccines contain mono- or polyvalent inactivated whole-cell leptospires as per the endemicity of the strains.

Treatment

The treatment of leptospirosis depends on the severity. The mild form of leptospirosis is rarely fatal, but the severe form (or Weil's disease) is associated with high mortality rates. Patients with icteric leptospirosis usually need intensive care unit admission as multiple organs can be involved and decompensation can occur rapidly.

Prevention and Control

The important prevention and control methods of leptospirosis consist of source (rodent) reduction, environment and water sanitation and hygienic personal practices. Understanding the eco-epidemiological and cultural characteristics of communities where leptospirosis is a problem is an essential prerequisite for evolving effective control measures.

Leptospira serovars are maintained by subclinical infections in both wild and domestic animals, which thereby serve as a source of infection and disease for incidental hosts, both animals and humans. There is no human vaccine suitable for worldwide use. Therefore, prevention and control should target the maintenance hosts of the infection. Some of the important considerations are as follows.

- Control of rodents (rats, mice, other animal pests) is highly important in animal farms and homes.
- Pet owners should also take steps to prevent themselves and others from becoming infected with the disease due to an infected pet. The primary mode of transmission of leptospirosis from pets to humans is through direct or indirect contact with contaminated animal tissues, organs or urine.
- Use proper antibacterial cleaning solutions during cleaning of surfaces that may be contaminated with urine from an infected pet.
- Proper use of personal protective equipments (PPE) (e.g. gloves and boots) by people who have a high risk of occupational exposure (veterinarians, farm workers, sewer workers, etc.).
- Always wash hands after handling pets or any substance that might have been exposed to the infected animal, animal tissues/products or contaminated surfaces.

References

1 Evangelista, K.V. and Coburn, J. (2010). Leptospira as an emerging pathogen: a review of its biology, pathogenesis and host immune responses. *Future Microbiology* 5 (9): 1413–1425.
2 Athanazio, D.A., Silva, E.F., Santos, C.S. et al. (2008). Rattus norvegicus as a model for persistent renal colonization by pathogenic *Leptospira interrogans*. *Acta Tropica* 105 (2): 176–180.
3 Bolin, C. (2000). Leptospirosis. In: *Emerging Diseases of Animals* (eds. C. Brown and C. Bolin), 185–200. Washington, DC: ASM Press.
4 Hartskeerl, R.A. (2006). Leptospirosis: current status and future trends. *Indian Journal of Medical Microbiology* 24 (4): 309.
5 Centers for Disease Control and Prevention (2015). Leptospirosis: prevention in pets. www.cdc.gov/leptospirosis/pets/prevention/index.html
6 Trueba, G., Zapata, S., Madrid, K. et al. (2004). Cell aggregation: a mechanism of pathogenic Leptospira to survive in fresh water. *International Microbiology* 7 (1): 35–40.

7 Ballard, S.A., Williamson, M., Adler, B. et al. (1986). Interactions of virulent and avirulent leptospires with primary cultures of renal epithelial cells. *Journal of Medical Microbiology 21* (1): 59–67.

8 Rao, R.S., Gupta, N., Bhalla, P., and Agarwal, S.K. (2003). Leptospirosis in India and the rest of the world. *Brazilian Journal of Infectious Diseases* 7 (3): 178–193.

9 Ellis, W.A., O'Brien, J.J., Cassells, J.A. et al. (1985). Excretion of *Leptospira interrogans* serovar hardjo following calving or abortion. *Research in Veterinary Science 39* (3): 296–298.

10 Goldstein, R.E., Lin, R.C., Langston, C.E. et al. (2006). Influence of infecting serogroup on clinical features of leptospirosis in dogs. *Journal of Veterinary Internal Medicine* 20 (3): 489–494.

11 Timoney, J.F., Kalimuthusamy, N., Velineni, S. et al. (2011). A unique genotype of *Leptospira interrogans* serovar Pomona type kennewicki is associated with equine abortion. *Veterinary Microbiology* 150 (3–4): 349–353.

12 Verma, A., Kumar, P., Babb, K. et al. (2010). Cross-reactivity of antibodies against leptospiral recurrent uveitis-associated proteins A and B (LruA and LruB) with eye proteins. *PLoS Neglected Tropical Diseases* 4 (8): e778.

13 Centers for Disease Control and Prevention (2017). Leptospirosis: signs and symptoms. www.cdc.gov/leptospirosis/symptoms/index.html

14 Levett, P.N. (2001). Leptospirosis. *Clinical Microbiology Reviews* 14: 296–326.

15 Koe, S.L.L., Tan, K.T., and Tan, T.C. (2014). Leptospirosis in pregnancy with pathological fetal cardiotocography changes. *Singapore Medical Journal* 55 (2): e20.

6

Lyme Disease (or Lyme Borreliosis)

Aetiology

Lyme disease is a tick-borne zoonosis caused by several genospecies of the spirochete *Borrelia burgdorferi* sensu lato complex. Lyme disease is the most common vector-borne disease in Europe and the United States. Most human infections are caused by three genospecies: *B. burgdorferi* sensu stricto, *B. afzelii* and *B. garinii*. Among these, *B. burgdorferi* sensu stricto is the main causative agent of Lyme disease in North America. In Europe and Asia, in addition to *B. burgdorferi* sensu stricto, *B. afzelii*, *B. garinii* and other related species are associated with Lyme disease [1].

Historical Context

The word 'Lyme' is derived from a small coastal town of Lyme in Connecticut. In 1975, a woman brought an unusual cluster of paediatric arthritis cases to the attention of Yale researchers. In 1977, the Yale researchers identified and named the clusters as 'Lyme arthritis'. In 1979, the name was changed to 'Lyme disease', when symptoms such as neurological problems and severe fatigue were linked to the disease. In 1982, the cause of the disease was discovered by Dr Willy Burgdorfer. Dr Burgdorfer published a paper on the infectious agent of Lyme disease and earned the right to have his name placed on the Lyme disease spirochete, now known as *Borrelia burgdorferi*. The discovery of *B. burgdorferi* as the causative agent of Lyme disease prompted further development of epidemiological research on the disease.

Epidemiology and Disease Transmission

The organism normally cycles among small mammals and birds, where it is transmitted by multiple species of *Ixodes* ticks. *Ixodes scapularis* (black-legged or deer tick) is considered the principal vector in the United States whereas *I. ricinus* and *I. persulcatus* are the principal vectors in Europe and Asia, respectively. The important reservoir hosts of the pathogen are mice, shrews, other small mammals and various species of birds. Adult ticks feed preferentially on deer, which are immune to *B. burgdorferi* but play an important role in the ecology of disease by transporting ticks and supporting the tick population [2].

There is a complex interaction of multiple factors in determining the epidemiology of Lyme disease in humans. These include the genospecies of *B. burgdorferi* and its distribution in nature, the

Textbook of Zoonoses, First Edition. Jasbir Singh Bedi, Deepthi Vijay, and Pankaj Dhaka.

abundance and feeding habits of the vector tick species, the reservoir host involved and the demographic and behavioural characteristics of the exposed human population. The emergence of Lyme disease has been attributed to the population recovery of deer, which are not competent hosts for transmitting *B. burgdorferi* to ticks but are nonetheless important reproductive hosts for adult ticks [3]. The increase in deer during the early twentieth century is thought to have allowed the tick population to grow and spread from small remnant populations, and this probably contributed significantly to the initial rise in Lyme disease cases [4]. The emergence of Lyme disease in the northeast United States in 1970 was thought to be due to expansion of the tick population associated with reforestation and expansion of the deer population as a key host for the tick life cycle. In addition, other factors such as climate change, shifting land-use patterns and relative abundance and distribution of reservoir hosts allow the geographic range of the tick vector to keep expanding [1].

Transmission Cycle

The life cycle of *I. scapularis* generally lasts 2 years, during which the tick takes three blood meals, one each as larvae, nymph and adult. The tick vector species may differ from region to region. The pathogen *B. burgdorferi* lives in the midgut of ticks. As the tick becomes engorged with blood during feeding, bacteria replicate and migrate to the tick's salivary glands, from which the organism can be injected into the host. The salient features of the transmission cycle are as follows [4].

- Ticks are uninfected when they hatch from the eggs; they acquire *B. burgdorferi* by feeding on infected reservoir hosts, principally mice, shrews, other small mammals and various species of birds. The abundance of small mammals is considered a key determinant of the density of infected nymphs.
- Infected ticks can transmit the pathogen during subsequent feeding to new reservoir hosts, thereby perpetuating the natural cycle.
- The ticks feed preferentially on deer, which support the tick but not the spirochete (not a reservoir of infection). These hosts provide the ticks with a bountiful supply of food (i.e. blood meals), enabling the ticks to live, reproduce and infect humans.
- Unlike reservoir hosts, humans are incidental or dead-end hosts that do not sustain large numbers of spirochetes in their tissues.

The transmission of the disease is most likely during the nymph stage since nymphs are abundant in the spring and early summer and are small and difficult to detect with the naked eye. Correspondingly, the peak incidence of human cases is during the spring and summer months. Studies of the transmission of *B. burgdorferi* to humans are consistent with studies in animals indicating that transmission from infected nymphal ticks generally occurs only after 36–48 hours of attachment, and transmission from adult ticks occurs after an even longer period (≥48 hours) [5].

The risk factors for Lyme disease include occupational and recreational exposure to fields and woods in endemic areas, as well as outdoor activities such as gardening on residential properties near woodlands.

Among animals, dogs can be affected clinically with Lyme disease. The most common sign of Lyme disease in dogs is arthritis, which causes sudden lameness, pain and sometimes swelling in one or more joints. Other signs that may be seen include fever, lack of appetite, dehydration, inactivity and swollen lymph nodes. In severe cases, the infection can cause kidney failure and death, although such a severe form is not common in dogs.

Pathogenesis and Disease in Humans

In humans, the infection begins at the site of the tick bite, which may be demarcated by erythema migrans (EM) or bull's eye rash, and generally accompanied by flu-like symptoms. The spirochetes migrate from the lesion via the vasculature and lymphatics and can invade distal sites to manifest clinical signs in the skin, joints, heart, nervous system, endocrine glands and gastrointestinal tract. Lyme disease is also called the 'great imitator' as it can cause debilitating illness that mimics varying conditions such as multiple sclerosis and cancer. The presentation of the disease can vary considerably between patients from different geographic regions [6].

There are three stages of *B. burgdorferi* infection: early localised, early disseminated and late disseminated. The symptoms of Lyme disease can be considered mostly due to the innate and adaptive immune response of the host to the infection. For example, early Lyme disease is characterised by high levels of immune mediators, which may be beneficial in clearing the infection but also can cause symptoms such as fever and malaise. In patients with prolonged and persistent symptoms, the host immune response may become dysregulated through inflammatory or secondary autoimmune pathways or non-specific immune activation. Other systems, such as central neural pathways and networks, may also be disrupted and have a significant impact on symptoms [5, 6]. Immunological processes and genetic predisposition also play an important role in the pathogenesis of the disease.

Clinical Signs in Humans

Typical symptoms following bite from an infected tick can include erythema migrans, fever, headache, lymphadenopathy, arthralgia, myalgia and fatigue. The erythema migrans, a localised skin lesion, is considered the most common and earliest clinical manifestation of Lyme disease, which is present in 70–80% of patients. The lesion typically occurs within 1–2 weeks following a tick bite and is defined as a gradually expanding annular lesion of more than 5 cm in diameter. Although reputed to have a bull's-eye appearance, approximately two-thirds of single erythema migrans lesions either are uniformly erythematous or have enhanced central erythema without clearing around it [7]. If the infection is not treated, the bacteria might spread haematogenously and cause early disseminated Lyme disease, which can manifest as multiple erythema migrans skin lesions, facial palsy, meningitis or endocarditis. Recurrent large-joint arthritis is the hallmark of late disseminated disease. Although rare, late neurological Lyme disease symptoms might include peripheral neuropathy, encephalopathy or encephalomyelitis. Chronic Lyme borreliosis with joint involvement is characterised by persistent joint oedema or recurrent inflammatory episodes.

Diagnosis

Clinical diagnosis of Lyme disease is typically made by recognition of the erythema migrans skin lesion. The direct detection of *B. burgdorferi* by PCR or culture remains challenging due to the transient presence of spirochetes in small numbers in the bloodstream of infected patients [1]. Due to the slow-growing nature of *B. burgdorferi*, current culture methods are labour intensive with poor sensitivity. Molecular diagnosis of the nucleic acid of the pathogen by PCR can provide specific evidence in a variety of samples, including synovial fluid, skin biopsy, tissue, blood and cerebrospinal fluid (CSF). However, its clinical utility is limited by low sensitivity (particularly for blood and CSF samples) and its potential for contamination. Therefore, most diagnostic test development has focused on indirect detection of infection by assessing the antibody response of the patient. Two-tier serological testing for antibodies to *B. burgdorferi* is recommended, where a quantitative test, usually an enzyme-linked immunosorbent assay (ELISA), is performed to quantify the antibodies against *B. burgdorferi* and, if results are positive or equivocal, a Western blot test can be performed as confirmation [6].

Treatment

Prompt diagnosis and proper treatment of early Lyme disease cases are essential to prevent serious complications. Early treatment of Lyme disease with appropriate antibiotics usually leads to a full recovery. Treatment with doxycycline, amoxicillin or cefuroxime is considered safe and highly efficacious for early Lyme disease cases [5].

Most of the time, early Lyme disease cases can be cured with appropriate antibiotic treatment; however, patients can sometimes have symptoms of pain, fatigue or neurological signs that can last for more than 6 months after they finish treatment. This condition is called post-treatment Lyme disease syndrome (PTLDS). It has been reported that *B. burgdorferi* can trigger an 'autoimmune' response causing symptoms that last well after resolution of the infection. Autoimmune responses are known to occur following other infections also, for example, campylobacteriosis (Guillain–Barré syndrome), chlamydia (Reiter syndrome), strep throat (rheumatic heart disease), etc. However, the association between PTLDS and persistent *B. burgdorferi* infection is still unclear and it has also been hypothesised that the symptoms of PTLDS may be due to other causes unrelated to the patient's *B. burgdorferi* infection [7].

Prevention and Control

The transmission of vector-borne zoonotic diseases like Lyme disease to humans depends on multiple species interactions that influence host and vector abundance and infection prevalence. Vaccines are not much in use for Lyme disease due to poor sales and complaints related to adverse events. However, vaccination is recommended for dogs living in Lyme-endemic areas or those who spend a lot of time in the woods. Vaccinated dogs can still become infected with *B. burgdorferi* due to exposure to a different strain than what was included in the vaccine, or due to insufficient antibody production levels. Avoidance of tick-infested areas is the best way to prevent Lyme disease, but occupational and recreational activities and the proximity of residential areas to woodlands often make such directives impractical.

Some considerations that should be taken into account include the following [8].

- Tick bites can be prevented by the application of insect repellents that contain N,N-diethyl-metatoluamide (DEET) in concentrations of at least 20% or covering skin with long trousers and shirts. Bathing within 2 hours after exposure may also be effective because ticks take longer than 2 hours to fully attach.
- Regular checking of clothes and body surface for ticks, and removing them properly is recommended.
- Always wear protective clothing (long-sleeved clothes, hunter boots, etc.) while going for outdoor activities like hunting.

- Tick abundance around homes and recreational areas can be reduced by spraying with acaricides, removing leaf litter and creating buffer zones of wood chips or gravel between forests and lawns.
- Keep pet dogs clean and away from ticks. Dogs are not a direct source of infection to people but a carrier tick could be brought into the house on a pet dog's fur.
- Education and awareness of the population at risk can play an important role in disease prevention.

References

1 Steere, A.C. (2001). Lyme disease. *New England Journal of Medicine 345* (2): 115–125.

2 Nelson, C.A., Saha, S., Kugeler, K.J. et al. (2015). Incidence of clinician-diagnosed Lyme disease, United States, 2005–2010. *Emerging Infectious Diseases 21* (9): –1625.

3 Barbour, A.G. and Fish, D. (1993). The biological and social phenomenon of Lyme disease. *Science* 260: 1610–1616.

4 Levi, T., Kilpatrick, A.M., Mangel, M., and Wilmers, C.C. (2012). Deer, predators, and the emergence of Lyme disease. *Proceedings of the National Academy of Sciences 109* (27): 10942–10947.

5 Bamm, V.V., Ko, J.T., Mainprize, I.L. et al. (2019). Lyme disease frontiers: reconciling borrelia biology and clinical conundrums. *Pathogens 8* (4): 299.

6 Aguero-Rosenfeld, M.E., Wang, G., Schwartz, I., and Wormser, G.P. (2005). Diagnosis of Lyme borreliosis. *Clinical Microbiology Reviews 18* (3): 484–509.

7 Wormser, G.P., Dattwyler, R.J., Shapiro, E.D. et al. (2006). The clinical assessment, treatment, and prevention of Lyme disease, human granulocytic anaplasmosis, and babesiosis: clinical practice guidelines by the Infectious Diseases Society of America. *Clinical Infectious Diseases 43* (9): 1089–1134.

8 Centers for Disease Control and Prevention (2021). Post-Treatment Lyme Disease Syndrome. www.cdc.gov/lyme/postlds/index.html

7

Plague

Plague (also known as black death) is a vector-borne illness caused by the bacterium *Yersinia pestis*. The disease is transmitted by fleas to a variety of rodents, which represent the natural reservoirs in a wide range of habitats around the world. Owing to its zoonotic nature, the disease can be transmitted from animals to humans and also from human to human (in the case of the pneumonic form).

Plague has affected the history of humankind through several pandemics that initially spread from Central Asia to Africa and Europe, and gradually plague has reached every continent during the last 150 years. In the twenty-first century, plague is endemic in many countries in the Americas, Asia and Africa [1]. More than 90% of cases are currently being reported from Africa, and the three most endemic countries are the Democratic Republic of Congo, Madagascar and Peru [2].

Aetiology and Pathogen Characteristics

The aetiological agent of plague is the Gram-negative, non-motile, facultative anaerobic coccobacillus bacterium *Y. pestis*. The genus *Yersinia* is a member of the family Enterobacteriaceae and consists of 11 species, including three that are pathogenic in humans: *Y. pestis*, *Y. pseudotuberculosis* and *Y. enterocolitica*. While *Y. enterocolitica* and *Y. pseudotuberculosis* cause a self-limiting gastrointestinal illness, *Y. pestis* is associated with severe, acute and rapidly progressing febrile illness with significant mortality rates. *Y. pestis* is considered as one of the most pathogenic bacteria for humans, and the pneumonic form of plague has the most severe manifestation with mortality rates approaching 100% in the absence of treatment [1]. Due to its extreme lethality and potential to be transmitted via the aerosol route, *Y. pestis* is categorised as a 'category A' agent by the Centers for Disease Control and Prevention (CDC). Unlike many bacterial pathogens, *Y. pestis* has only one serotype. It is generally thought that the high virulence of *Y. pestis* emerged from a clone of *Y. pseudotuberculosis* that acquired the ability to survive within the flea [3]

Historical Overview

- **1894:** The causative bacterium *Y. pestis* was discovered by Alexandre Yersin during a plague outbreak in Hong Kong.
- The disease has given rise to three pandemics in the past as described below.

Textbook of Zoonoses, First Edition. Jasbir Singh Bedi, Deepthi Vijay, and Pankaj Dhaka.

  - During the sixth to eighth centuries, the first pandemic ('Justinian plague') spread around the Mediterranean Sea.
  - During the fourteenth to eighteenth centuries, the second pandemic ('Black Death') started in Europe and recurred intermittently for more than 300 years, during which approximately 30% of Europe's population succumbed to this disease.
  - During the middle of the nineteenth century (1855), the third pandemic started in China and spread throughout the world.
- Each pandemic of plague was caused by a different biovar of *Y. pestis*, respectively antiqua (still found in Africa and Central Asia), medievalis (currently limited to Central Asia) and orientalis (worldwide in its distribution, differentiated by its ability to ferment glycerol and reduce nitrate) [4].

Pathogenesis and Virulence Factors

Humans become accidental hosts via contact with infected animals or a flea vector that has fed on an infected animal. Intradermal infection of humans via the flea results in bubonic plague, while primary septicemic plague arises from a deeper bite that inoculates bacteria directly into the bloodstream. The secondary pneumonic plague develops from the dissemination of *Y. pestis* into the lungs during the bubonic or septicemic plague. Individuals with secondary pneumonic plague can be involved in the person-to-person transmission of *Y. pestis*.

The dispersal of *Y. pestis* within the host is enhanced by a plasminogen activator (Pla) that has fibrinolytic activity. Other virulence factors include an array of *Yersinia* outer proteins (Yops) and the pH 6 antigen (PsaA protein), which are involved in cytotoxic processes, immune suppression or survival of *Y. pestis* within native host phagocytes during the initial stages of infection [5].

Upon entry into the host, *Y. pestis* begins to express the F1 capsular antigen (Caf1), thereby enabling it to resist phagocytosis and killing by potentially activated monocytes during the later course of infection. The Yersinia bactin siderophore system and other iron uptake systems enable *Y. pestis* to acquire this essential nutrient in blood or other environments where its availability is limited by host iron-binding molecules. Yersinia murine toxin is also associated with the signs and symptoms associated with septic shock, systemic inflammatory response syndrome and other serious conditions [5].

Transmission Cycle

Transmission in Animals

In nature, around 200 species of rodents and lagomorphs are associated with the epidemiology of plague [6]. Rodents are considered as amplifying hosts for plague and thus a source of infection for domestic animals.

Within its reservoir host, *Y. pestis* circulates via flea bites. Most infected fleas come from the domestic black rat, *Rattus rattus*, or the brown sewer rat, *Rattus norvegicus* [7]. The most common and efficient flea vector is *Xenopsylla cheopis*, which parasitises black rats living inside houses, but many other flea species can transmit plague. The 'blocked flea' model of the transmission of plague bacteria is the dominant paradigm for rat flea-borne transmission of *Y. pestis*. Under this scenario, rat fleas (*X. cheopis*) ingest a blood meal from a bacteraemic host, allowing *Y. pestis* to colonise the flea's gut. Then, following an extrinsic incubation period (typically 7–31 days), a blockage is formed of blood and multiplying *Y. pestis* in the flea's proventriculus [8]. This obstruction prevents subsequent blood meals from reaching the midgut. And as the flea begins to starve, it increases its feeding attempts. This voracious feeding, coupled with regurgitation into a bite wound of fresh blood and infective blockage material, results in high vectorial capacity (a measure of the number of secondary infections that arise from a focal infection).

In addition to the classic blocked flea model, owing to the rapid spread of *Y. pestis* in the plague epizootics (shorter than the extrinsic incubation period before blockage formation in fleas), an early phase transmission of *Y. pestis* by unblocked fleas has been proposed by many researchers [9].

Transmission in Humans

In humans, *Y. pestis* can be transmitted by flea bites (causing bubonic plague), respiratory droplets (causing pneumonic plague), consumption of uncooked contaminated meat (causing gastrointestinal plague) and contact with infected pets/domestic animals (causing conjunctivitis, skin plague or pneumonic plague) [10]. In addition to the rat flea, the human flea (*Pulex irritans*) is associated with interhuman transmission cases during modern plague outbreaks [11], although the human-to-human transmission of bubonic plague is rare. The pneumonic form can also trigger severe epidemics through person-to-person contact via droplets in the air. Bubonic or pneumonic plague can progress to the septicemic form through haematogenous spread.

An overview of the transmission cycle of plague in humans is shown in Figure 7.1

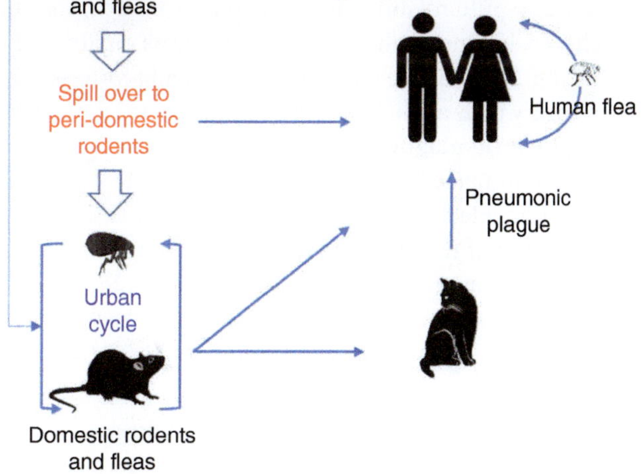

Figure 7.1 An overview of the sylvatic and urban cycle of plague in humans.

Disease in Animals and Humans

Animals

Many species of animals, such as rats, ground squirrels, prairie dogs, chipmunks, mice, voles and rabbits, can be affected by the plague. Wild carnivores can become infected by eating other infected animals. Cats are highly susceptible to plague and are a common source of *Y. pestis* infection in humans. Most cases of plague in cats present with submandibular lymphadenitis, which is clinically indistinguishable from abscesses due to other causes, such as bite wounds. Animals with the respiratory form of plague can transmit the disease to other animals or humans when they cough or sneeze (aerosol). Cats with pneumonic plague can pose a significant risk to owners, veterinarians and others who handle or come into close contact with them. Dogs infected with plague are less likely to develop clinical illnesses than cats [10].

Humans

The incubation period of plague in humans is 3–7 days. Patients typically experience a sudden onset of fever, chills, headaches, body aches, weakness, vomiting and nausea. Clinical plague infection can manifest in three forms which depend on the route of infection.

- **Bubonic form:** This is the most common form which results from the bite of an infected flea. Plague bacillus (*Y. pestis*) enters the bite site and travels through the lymphatic system to the nearest lymph node where it replicates itself. The lymph node draining the site of the flea bite becomes inflamed, tense and painful, and is called a 'bubo'. Buboes are commonly found in the groin, armpit or neck regions of the body. At advanced stages, the inflamed lymph nodes can turn into open sores filled with pus. Without treatment, the lethality rate can be 40–70% of cases. Bubonic plague can advance and spread to the lungs, resulting in a more severe form of plague called pneumonic plague. The infection can also rapidly disseminate to the spleen, liver and other organs, and can cause fatal septicemia.
- **Pneumonic plague:** The pneumonic form is considered the most virulent form of plague. The incubation period can be as short as 24 hours. It can be directly transmitted from person to person via inhalation of infected respiratory droplets and can also progress from bubonic plague through haematogenous spread to lungs. The signs and symptoms include cough with bloody mucus (sputum), difficulty in breathing, nausea, vomiting, high fever, headache, weakness and chest pain. Pneumonic plague can progress rapidly and may cause respiratory failure and shock within 2 days of infection. The pneumonic form is highly fatal unless treated early; however, recovery rates are high if detected and treated in time (within 24 hours of symptom onset) [12].
- **Septicemic plague:** This form occurs when the plague bacteria multiply in the bloodstream. The common signs and symptoms include fever, chills, weakness, abdominal pain, diarrhoea, vomiting, bleeding from natural orifices (mouth, nose, rectum) or under the skin, blackening and death of tissue (gangrene) in extremities (e.g. fingers, toes, nose) and shock. Without treatment, the case fatality rate is around 100% [12].

Laboratory Diagnosis

An important clue for suspecting plague is a history of contact with wild animals in natural plague foci or with other plague patients. If a patient develops a sudden high fever after close contact with dead animals (rodents or other wild animals) in a region where plague is endemic, bubonic plague (with regional lymph node swelling), pneumonic plague (with severe coughing and pneumonic signs) or septicemic plague (with sudden high fever and chills) should be suspected.

The common methods of diagnosis of plague are as follows.

- **Clinical diagnosis:** This can be carried out by targeting the clinical signs and history of the patient. The clinical symptoms and signs should always be correlated with typical epidemiological features, including a trip to or residence in an endemic area, exposure to plague patients or infected animals, and/or history of flea bites. Important clinical observations include fever, adenitis, buboes (in bubonic form), rusty sputum and respiratory distress (pneumonic plague).
- **Staining procedure:** Demonstration of the pathogen from the sample of bubo pus, blood or sputum, or lymph node specimen can be done by using bipolar staining with Wright/ Giemsa/ Gram/Wayson stain. Visualisation of the pathogen by bipolar staining as an ovoid, Gram-negative bipolar coccobacillus with a 'safety pin' appearance permits rapid presumptive diagnosis.
- **Isolation of pathogen:** The gold standard for plague diagnosis is the isolation and identification of the plague pathogen from clinical specimens. The pathogen can be cultivated on many routinely used media, including brain heart infusion broth, MacConkey agar and sheep blood agar. *Y. pestis* grows optimally at 26–28 °C but incubation at 37 °C is necessary for F1 antigen production. The colonies formed on the agar plate after 48 hours of incubation are small (about 1–2 mm in diameter), with a raised centre and flat periphery. Isolation of *Y. pestis* should be performed in a biosafety level 3 laboratory.
- **Immunological methods:** F1 antigen is typically used as a target to detect *Y. pestis* by various immunological methods. A passive haemagglutination test and F1 antigen haemagglutination inhibition test are conventionally employed for detecting F1 antigen. However, direct fluorescent antibody testing and enzyme-linked immunosorbent assays have also been reported for detecting F1 antibody or F1 antigen quantitatively [10].
- **Molecular detection:** Polymerase chain reaction (PCR) detection of *Y. pestis* in sputum, bubo aspirate or blood can be carried out by targeting suitable genes (e.g. *caf1*, *pla* gene or chromosomal fragments).

Treatment in Humans

The World Health Organization does not recommend vaccination for plague (except for high-risk groups such as laboratory personnel who are constantly exposed to the risk of contamination). Rapid diagnosis and treatment are essential to reduce the risk of complications and death due to the disease. Untreated pneumonic plague can be rapidly fatal with around a 100% case fatality rate, so early diagnosis and treatment are essential for survival and reduction of complications. Patients with pneumonic plague must be isolated to avoid respiratory transmission. Antibiotics and supportive therapy are effective against plague if patients are diagnosed in time. Streptomycin is considered the most effective antibiotic against *Y. pestis* and is the drug of choice for the treatment of plague, particularly the pneumonic form [13].

Prevention and Control

The pathogenic *Yersinia* spp. are closely related micro-organisms that have a wide range of transmission modalities (food-borne, vector-borne, air-borne) with varying pathogenic potential. *Y. pestis*, the causative agent of plague, is considered the deadliest of these species which is historically associated with large pandemics. Some important prevention and control measures for plague are listed below [13].

- **Flea control in reservoir:** Regular treatment of pet dogs and cats for flea control can be instigated as a preventive measure. During epidemics, the killing of rodents before vectors should be avoided as it can cause the fleas to jump to new hosts (including humans). Therefore, flea control should be the primary step during a plague epidemic.
- **Rodent control:** After proper vector control, controlling plague in wild rodents is an alternative method to prevent infection in domestic animals. Environmental and source reduction measures need to be instigated to reduce the rodent population.
- **Surveillance in animals.**
  - Investigating animal and flea species implicated in the plague cycle in the region.
  - Developing environmental management programmes to understand the natural transmission of the disease cycle and limit its spread.
  - Active long-term surveillance of animal foci, coupled with rapid response during animal outbreaks, can be helpful in the control of human plague outbreaks.
- **Surveillance in humans.**
  - Identify the most likely source of infection in the area where the human case(s) was reported. Typically, investigators should look for clustered areas with large numbers of small animal deaths.
  - Identify and monitor the close contacts of pneumonic plague patients and give them 7-days chemoprophylaxis. Chemoprophylaxis should also be given to household members of bubonic plague patients.
  - Routine hand-washing is recommended with soap and water or use of alcohol hand rub. Larger areas can be disinfected using 10% diluted household bleach.

References

1 Stenseth, N.C., Atshabar, B.B., Begon, M. et al. (2008). Plague: past, present, and future. *PLoS Medicine 5* (1): e3.

2 World Health Organization (2021). Plague. www.who.int/health-topics/plague#tab=tab_1

3 Achtman, M., Morelli, G., Zhu, P. et al. (2004). Microevolution and history of the plague bacillus, *Yersinia pestis*. *Proceedings of the National Academy of Sciences 101* (51): 17837–17842.

4 Oyston, P.C. and Williamson, D. (2011). Plague: infections of companion animals and opportunities for intervention. *Animals 1* (2): 242–255.

5 Li, B. and Yang, R. (2008). Interaction between *Yersinia pestis* and the host immune system. *Infection and Immunity 76* (5): 1804–1811.

6 Gratz, N.G. (1999). *Rodent Reservoirs and Flea Vectors of Natural Foci of Plague/Plague Manual: Epidemiology, Distribution, Surveillance and Control*, 63–96. Geneva: WHO.

7 Keim, P.S. and Wagner, D.M. (2009). Humans and evolutionary and ecological forces shaped the phylogeography of recently emerged diseases. *Nature Reviews Microbiology 7* (11): 813–821.

8 Eisen, R.J., Eisen, L., and Gage, K.L. (2009). Studies of vector competency and efficiency of North American fleas for *Yersinia pestis*: state of the field and future research needs. *Journal of Medical Entomology 46* (4): 737–744.

9 Eisen, R.J., Dennis, D.T., and Gage, K.L. (2015). The role of early-phase transmission in the spread of *Yersinia pestis*. *Journal of Medical Entomology 52* (6): 1183–1192.

10 Yang, R. (2018). Plague: recognition, treatment, and prevention. *Journal of Clinical Microbiology 56* (1): e01519–e01517.

11 Ratovonjato, J., Rajerison, M., Rahelinirina, S., and Boyer, S. (2014). *Yersinia pestis* in *Pulex irritans* fleas during plague outbreak, Madagascar. *Emerging Infectious Diseases 20* (8): 1414.

12 Poland, J.D. and Dennis, D.T. (1999). Treatment of plague. In: *Plague Manual: Epidemiology, Distribution, Surveillance and Control* (eds. D.T. Dennis, K. Gage, N.G. Poland, et al.), 55–62. https://apps.who.int/iris/bitstream/handle/10665/66010/WHO_CDS_CSR_EDC_99.2.pdf?sequence=1&isAllowed=y.

13 Centers for Disease Control and Prevention. (2018). Plague: information for veterinarians. www.cdc.gov/plague/healthcare/veterinarians.html

8

Q Fever

Q fever is a highly infectious zoonosis caused by *Coxiella burnetii*. The disease is considered a 'neglected zoonosis' and has been ranked as one of the 13 'global priority zoonoses' [1]. The other names for Q fever are coxiellosis, abattoir fever, Burnet rickettsiosis, goat flu, Nine Mile fever, Red River fever and Balkan grippe. The disease is notifiable under the category of 'multiple species diseases, infections and infestations' by the World Organisation for Animal Health (OIE). In the past, the Netherlands outbreak of Q fever (2007–2010) provided an insight into the serious threat to public health posed by this pathogen, where more than 4000 human cases were reported [2]. The source of the reported cases was traced back to dairy goat farms near densely populated areas, where the pathogen was spread via wind-borne route. The Dutch Government decided to cull more than 50 000 pregnant ewes and goats to halt the worst Q fever outbreak ever reported [2].

Historical Context

The first outbreak of this hitherto unknown disease was observed in 1935 and later described in 1937 by Edward Holbrook Derrick among the abattoir workers of Queensland, Australia. The 'Q' stands for 'Query' and was applied at a time when the causative agent was unknown, as it was chosen over suggestions of 'abattoir fever' and 'Queensland rickettsial fever' to avoid directing negative connotations at either the cattle industry or the state of Queensland, respectively. The pathogen was discovered in 1937 when Frank M. Burnet and Mavis Freeman isolated the bacterium from one of Derrick's patients. They injected guinea pigs with blood and urine of Derrick's patients and observed the presence of intracellular Gram-negative organisms, which were morphologically similar to *Rickettsia* spp. in stained spleen cells preparations, and so they named it *Rickettsia burnetii* [3].

Aetiological Agent and Epidemiological Characteristics

The causative agent of Q fever is *C. burnetii*, a Gram-negative obligate intracellular bacterium. The organism was earlier classified as *Rickettsia* but based on its 16s-RNA gene sequence, it has been reclassified in the phylum Proteobacteria, class γ-Proteobacteria, order Legionellales and family Coxiellaceae. The organism is considered highly infectious as the inhalation of a single organism may produce the disease. It is classified as a potential bioterrorism weapon under Category 'B' of the CDC [4].

Textbook of Zoonoses, First Edition. Jasbir Singh Bedi, Deepthi Vijay, and Pankaj Dhaka.

Coxiella burnetti is considered a ubiquitous zoonotic contaminant. The disease is endemic in more than 50 countries but rarely reported, and thus remains a largely 'neglected zoonosis' [5]. Among the extensive list of reservoir hosts, ruminants are the most commonly identified sources for human infection, with the highest rates among persons exposed to goats, sheep and cattle. However, recent reports have shown that pets, including cats, rabbits and dogs, can be potential sources of Q fever outbreaks, especially in urban settings [4].

The important epidemiological characteristics of the pathogen and associated risk factors are listed below.

Phase Variation in *C. burnetii*

The organism exhibits antigenic variation which is associated with a loss of virulence. In nature, *C. burnetii* exists in phase I form, wherein the lipopolysaccharides (LPS) remain an important virulence factor. The phase I phenotype expresses full-length LPS, while the LPS of the phase II phenotype lacks the O-antigenic region.

On culturing the pathogen in eggs or cell cultures, phase I (wild virulent form) shifts to mutant phase II (less virulent form) [6].

Immune Response

The immune response against *C. burnetii* is T-cell dependent, but does not lead to its elimination [7]. In addition, specific immunoglobulins are secreted following the infection, where IgG is mainly directed against phase II antigens and IgM is directed against both phase I and II antigens.

Developmental Cycle and Environmental Resistance

The pathogen undergo a biphasic development cycle during which it differentiates from a spore-like resistant small cell variant (SCV) into a replicating metabolically active intracellular large cell variant (LCV). Later, the LCV undergoes sporogenic differentiation to produce resistant spore-like forms, i.e. SCV. The SCV is a compact, small rod with a highly electron-dense centre of condensed nucleoid filaments. These are released on lysis of cells and can survive for a long duration in the environment. The SCV is considered as the persistent form in the host and the resistant form of *C. burnetii* in the environment [8]. The survival period of the pathogen in the soil has been reported to be up to 150 days [9]. These facts explain the wide spread of this bacterium in the environment and its capacity to infect animals and humans for a long period after they are excreted from an infected host.

Risk Factors of *C. burnetii* Infection in Animals, Humans and Environment

Ruminants are considered as major reservoirs and the disease in ruminants is generally known as coxiellosis. The abortion materials of infected ruminants are an important excretion route of *C. burnetii*. The contaminated placenta from aborted animals was found to harbour around 10^9 organisms per gram of tissue [10]. Shedding of the pathogen has also been detected from vaginal mucus, faeces and milk from infected animals [11]. *C. burnetii* is considered the most heat-resistant vegetative pathogen found in raw milk and is therefore used as the reference pathogen for milk pasteurisation [12]. The important risk factors for infection among animals and humans are described below.

Risk Factors in Animals

- Large herd size with intensive farming practices, poor ventilation and confined conditions can facilitate dispersal of the pathogen [13].
- Improper biosecurity measures at the farm: Improper quarantine of purchased animals can lead to the entry of infected animals into the herd. Access of stray dogs and wild birds to farm premises can lead to spillover of infection [14]. The improper disposal of biological wastes (placenta, aborted materials, dung) on the farm can be a source of contamination to nearby premises.
- Infrequent floor and farm equipment disinfection, as well as suboptimal personal and hand hygiene of farm workers, can be an important source of contamination.
- Some species of tick can act as a vector for *C. burnetii*. Therefore, tick infestation on animals or the presence of ticks in the environment can be a source of infection [15].

Risk Factors in Human

The occupational risk groups include farmers, veterinarians, abattoir workers, laboratory workers, farm tourists, etc. Human infection usually occurs through the aerosol route, mainly from the abortion materials or faeces of infected animals. Some of the important risk factors associated with Q fever in humans are listed below.

- Direct contact with infected animals without proper personal protective equipment (PPE).
- Aerosols generated during milking of infected animals.
- Aerosols generated while assisting in calving and handling the placenta of infected animals.
- Handling of contaminated manure.
- Petting infected animals and close vicinity to infected animal farms.
- Handling of the pathogen in laboratories without appropriate biosafety facilities and PPE.
- Risky culinary habits such as the consumption of unpasteurised milk and milk products.
- Improper hand and personal hygiene after handling animals.
- Contaminated blood transfusion, xenotransplantation and live cell therapy have also been associated with Q fever cases [16].

Environment-Related Factors

The SCV of the bacterium can survive for a prolonged duration in the environment. Many outbreaks have been associated with wind-borne transmission from farms, slaughter houses and meat-processing plants [17]. In addition, the growth of *C. burnetii* has been reported within amoebae which can also play an important role in the environmental persistence of the pathogen [18].

Transmission Cycle

In ruminants, the uterus and mammary glands of females serve as sites for persistent *C. burnetii* infection. Reactivation of the bacterium during pregnancy results in the shedding of high number of infectious agents into the environment during abortion or via birth fluids, placenta and foetal membranes. Contaminated aerosols generated from the desiccation of infected placentas, body fluids or dust from contaminated manure are important sources of infection for both animals and humans.

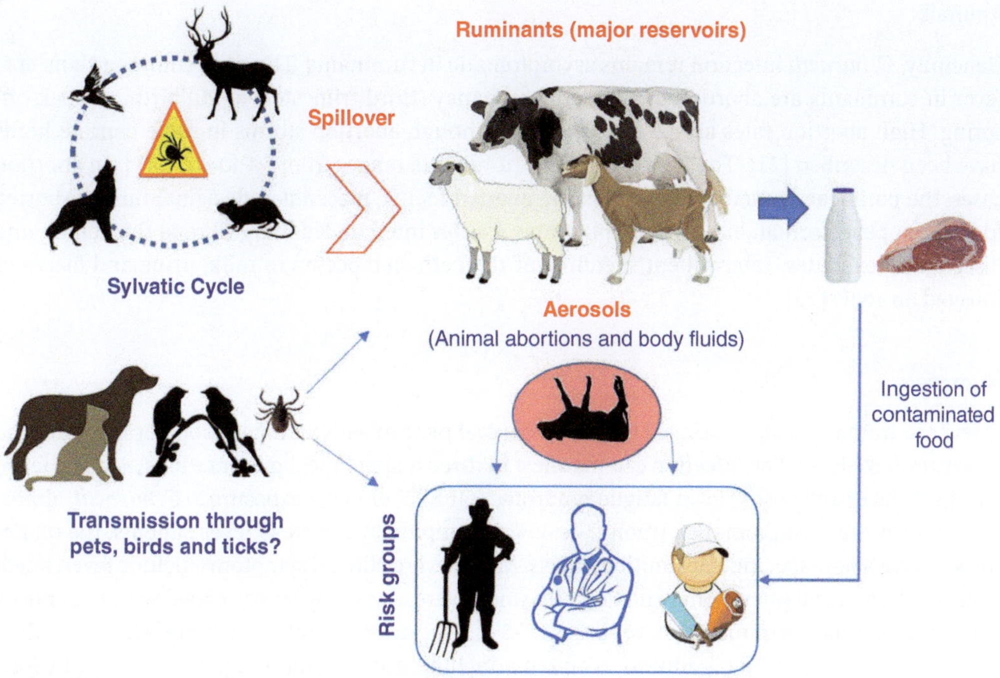

Figure 8.1 Major transmission routes of Q fever in humans. *Source:* Eric Isselée/Adobe Stock; BlackRiv/66 images/Pixabay.

The major transmission routes of Q fever in humans are represented in Figure 8.1. There are mainly two transmission cycles in nature for the circulation and transmission of *C. burnetii* as described below [19].

- **Wild cycle:** In this cycle, ticks and wild animals are involved in circulation of the pathogen. Infected ticks serve as vectors to maintain the wild cycle in nature, where they can transmit infection among wild vertebrates, especially rodents, lagomorphs and wild birds [20].
- **Domestic cycle:** In this cycle, ruminants and other pet animals such as dogs and cats are the main reservoirs of infection. Dogs may be infected by the consumption of placenta or milk from infected ruminants, or through the aerosol route [14].

The link between both wild and domestic cycles is inadequately understood, especially because the domestic cycle has been considered the main source of human infection [20].

Disease in Animals and Humans

In animals, the infection generally remains asymptomatic (except in pregnant ruminants). The clinical presentation of Q fever in humans may be acute, most often with pneumonia or hepatitis, or chronic manifestations including endocarditis. Variability in clinical expression may be caused by host factors, the extent of exposure or bacterial virulence factors. Details of the clinical presentation of Q fever in animals and humans are described below.

Animals

Generally, *C. burnetii* infection remains asymptomatic in ruminants. The most common signs of Q fever in ruminants are abortion during late pregnancy (third trimester) or stillbirth or weak offspring. High abortion rates are rarely observed, although abortion storms in some caprine herds have been described [21]. The abortion rate in ruminants ranges from 3% to 80% [19]. In abortion cases, the pathogen is excreted heavily in the aborted foetus, placenta and vaginal fluids. Aborted foetuses appear normal, but infected placentas exhibit intercotyledonary fibrous thickening and discoloured exudates. Intermittent shedding of the pathogen occurs in milk, urine and faeces of infected animals [19].

Humans

Q fever in humans is characterised by a wide clinical picture with an incubation period of around 20 days (14–39 days). The infection can manifest in three main clinical presentations: acute Q fever, chronic Q fever and post-Q fever fatigue syndrome (QFS). Following exposure to *C. burnetii*, almost 60% of cases are asymptomatic. Among the 40% of symptomatic acute Q fever patients, the majority will have a non-specific self-limiting illness. More severe clinical symptoms include fever, headache, chills, atypical pneumonia and hepatitis and severe cases may be associated with respiratory distress syndrome. In chronic Q fever cases (1–5%), long-term complications can become evident years after initial infection. Clinical symptoms include non-specific fatigue, fever, weight loss, night sweats, hepatosplenomegaly and endocarditis [18].

The post-QFS is another long-term presentation of Q fever that may last up to 10 years or longer [22]. Contrary to chronic Q fever, *C. burnetii* cannot be detected in QFS patients due to low or negligible antibody levels. Symptoms of QFS include prolonged fatigue, arthralgia, myalgia, blurred vision and enlarged painful lymph nodes.

In pregnant women, *C. burnetii* infection may lead to adverse pregnancy outcomes, especially when the acute Q fever remains untreated. Pregnancy outcomes include spontaneous abortion, intrauterine foetal death, premature delivery and low birth weight [23].

Diagnosis of Q Fever

The diagnosis of Q fever in animals and humans is a tedious and challenging task on account of asymptomatic cases in animals and non-specific clinical symptoms in humans that can obscure, complicate and delay the clinical diagnosis. It is important to rapidly diagnose infected animals and isolate them appropriately, which is critical for control of disease transmission among animals and humans.

Diagnosis in Animals

- **Staining of *C. burnetii*:** At the field or small laboratory level, different staining techniques can be used to identify the pathogen. In the case of an abortion suspected to be due to infectious origin, smears of placental cotyledon can be prepared. In addition, spleen, lung, liver and abomasal contents of the aborted foetus or vaginal discharge can also be used. These samples can be stained using different stains such as Stamp, Gimenez, Macchiavello, Giemsa and modified Koster stains. The limitations of these staining techniques include non-specificity and poor sensitivity [18].

- **Serological testing:** Among different serological tests, the complement fixation test (OIE recommended test) and enzyme-linked immunosorbent assay (ELISA) (EU recommended test) are commonly used.
- **Molecular diagnosis:** Polymerase chain reaction (PCR) techniques allow the direct identification of early acute cases of Q fever and *Coxiella* shedders, which is important for assessing the risk of transmission. Thus, a combination of PCR and serological tests such as ELISA is considered the best tool for diagnosis of Q fever and identification of flocks and animals shedding *C. burnetii* [24].

Diagnosis in Humans

The major diagnostic dilemma associated with Q fever diagnosis is the protean clinical manifestations. The initial flu-like symptoms can easily be overlooked or misdiagnosed, resulting in under-reporting of the disease. The European Union (EU) harmonised the 'Q fever case definition'. This includes *clinical* (any person with at least one of the following three symptoms: fever, pneumonia, hepatitis), *laboratory* (at least one of three diagnostic findings: isolation of *C. burnetii* from a clinical specimen, detection of *C. burnetii* nucleic acid in a clinical specimen, *C. burnetii* specific antibody response [IgG or IgM phase II]) and *epidemiological* (at least one of these epidemiological links: exposure to a common source, animal-to-human transmission) criteria [18].

Diagnosis of Acute Q Fever

A laboratory diagnosis of acute Q fever can be made based on serological results, but the requirement of a four-fold rise in phase II IgG antibody titre between acute and convalescent samples for a definitive diagnosis makes this primarily a retrospective diagnosis. Therefore, to diagnose the early stages of the disease, PCR in combination with serological testing is recommended [24]. The insertion sequence *IS 1111* gene is considered as the target of choice in PCR detection of *C. burnetii*. Notably, PCR-based technology is sensitive in the early stage of disease (acute cases). As the disease progresses, the neutralising antibodies clarify the infectious agent present in the patient's blood which makes the *C. burnetii* DNA undetectable in serum [24].

For serological screening, the indirect immunofluorescence assay (IFA) and ELISA are the most commonly used methods. Other methods include complement fixation and radioimmunoassay.

Diagnosis of Chronic Q Fever

Serological testing remains the method of choice for the diagnosis of chronic Q fever. In addition, patients with suspected chronic Q fever, with recurrent bacteraemia similar to early acute infection, can be diagnosed with PCR assay on whole blood or serum samples. PCR assays can also be performed on excised heart valve tissue, cerebrospinal fluid, pleural fluid, bone marrow, bone biopsies, liver biopsies, milk, placenta and foetal tissue [18].

Isolation of the Organism

For specific laboratory investigations and genotyping, it may be necessary to isolate the pathogen. *C. burnetii* can be directly isolated by inoculation of embryonated chicken eggs or by cell culture technique. Cell culture is a more cost-effective and time-efficient method compared to the use of embryonated eggs or animal inoculation. Continuous cell lines such as Vero and L929 cells can be used. However, the recent development of axenic medium for *C. burnetii*, i.e. acidified citrate cysteine medium 2 (ACCM2), has removed the experimental obstacles associated with *C. burnetii*'s obligate reliance on the eukaryotic host cell for growth. The colonies develop in ACCM2-agarose medium in 4–7 days when incubated in a 2.5% oxygen environment [25].

Genotyping Studies

The availability of complete genome sequences of *C. burnetii* allows the application of molecular methods to differentiate the isolates according to their environment, hosts and pathogenicity. Currently, sequence-based genotype methods are frequently used, such as multispacer sequence typing (MST), multiple-locus variable number of tandem repeats (VNTR) multiple-locus variable analysis (MLVA), *IS1111*-element positioning, infrequent restriction site-polymerase chain reaction (IRS-PCR) and single nucleotide polymorphism (SNP) [18].

Treatment in Animals and Humans

Animals

Vaccination is important to decrease the abortion rates and spread of the infection. Currently, only inactivated vaccines are available against *C. burnetii*. The phase I vaccine Coxevac® which contains inactivated (killed) *C. burnetii* is effective in decreasing abortion rates and bacterial load in vaginal mucus, faeces and milk in ruminants [19]. Once *C. burnetii* is confirmed as a cause of abortion in herd or flock, treatment of pregnant animals with tetracycline may reduce the risk of further abortions, but is unlikely to eliminate the problem [26].

Humans

In humans, studies on the Q fever vaccine were performed in Australia, where the vaccine Q-Vax® demonstrated high protective efficacy of 98% [27]. Since Q fever in humans is often an occupational hazard, vaccination should be considered primarily among exposed populations. In infected humans, the combination of doxycycline with hydroxychloroquine (for at least 18 months) is the treatment of choice for chronic Q fever, but therapy regimens may be individualised [28].

Prevention and Control Strategies

Q fever is a highly infectious zoonosis affecting both animals and humans. Prevention and control measures should be employed within the framework of the One Health approach. A combination of measures such as preventive vaccination, quarantine, testing and isolation of infected animals, manure management, removal of bio-risk material and control of other animal reservoirs and ticks can be used to prevent disease outbreaks. Some of the important points to be considered are as follows [18].

- To prevent and reduce animal and environmental contamination, the placenta and dead foetus must be destroyed as soon as possible away from farm premises. Prevent access of these contaminated bio-risk materials to domestic or wild carnivores that may disseminate the pathogen.

- High numbers of *C. burnetii* are excreted not only during an abortion but also during normal parturition of live healthy kids. Therefore, proper detection of shedders of *C. burnetii* is one of the critical points for control of its spread among other farm animals and farm workers.
- All the laboratory manipulations with live cultures or potentially infected/contaminated material must be performed at an appropriate biosafety and containment level (Class III or above).
- Only pasteurised milk and milk products should be consumed. Reducing exposure to raw milk, especially in the case of people at high risk (pregnant women, patients with cardiac pathology or immunosuppression) will contribute to lowering the risk of Q fever.
- It is important to create awareness about the disease among risk groups and to generate clinical curiosity among veterinarians for considering Q fever in the differential diagnosis and management of reproductive disorders and mastitis in livestock.

References

1 Grace, D., Mutua, F., Ochungo, P., et al. (2012). Mapping of poverty and likely zoonoses hotspots. Zoonoses Project 4. Report to the UK Department for International Development. Nairobi, Kenya. https://hdl.handle.net/10568/21161

2 Schneeberger, P.M., Wintenberger, C., Van der Hoek, W., and Stahl, J.P. (2014). Q fever in the Netherlands 2007–2010: what we learned from the largest outbreak ever. *Médecine et Maladies Infectieuses 44* (8): 339–353.

3 McDade, J.E. (1990). Historical aspects of Q fever. In: *Q Fever. Volume I: The Disease* (ed. T.J. Marrie). Boca Raton, FL: CRC.

4 Honarmand, H. (2012). Q Fever: an old but still a poorly understood disease. *Interdisciplinary Perspectives on Infectious Diseases* 2012: 131932.

5 Guatteo, R., Seegers, H., Taurel, A.F. et al. (2011). Prevalence of *Coxiella burnetii* infection in domestic ruminants: a critical review. *Veterinary Microbiology 149* (1–2): 1–16.

6 Voth, D.E. and Heinzen, R.A. (2009). *Coxiella* type IV secretion and cellular microbiology. *Current Opinion in Microbiology 12* (1): 74–80.

7 Honstettre, A., Ghigo, E., Moynault, A. et al. (2004). Lipopolysaccharide from *Coxiella burnetii* is involved in bacterial phagocytosis, filamentous actin reorganization, and inflammatory responses through Toll-like receptor 4. *Journal of Immunology 172* (6): 3695–3703.

8 Coleman, S.A., Fischer, E.R., Howe, D. et al. (2004). Temporal analysis of *Coxiella burnetii* morphological differentiation. *Journal of Bacteriology 186* (21): 7344–7352.

9 Welsh, H.H., Lennette, E.H., Abinanti, F.R. et al. (1959). Q fever studies. XXI. The recovery of *Coxiella burnetii* from the soil and surface water of premises harboring infected sheep. *American Journal of Hygiene 70* (1): 14–20.

10 Arricau-Bouvery, N., Souriau, A., Bodier, C. et al. (2005). Effect of vaccination with phase I and phase II *Coxiella burnetii* vaccines in pregnant goats. *Vaccine 23* (35): 4392–4402.

11 Freick, M., Enbergs, H., Walraph, J. et al. (2017). *Coxiella burnetii:* serological reactions and bacterial shedding in primiparous dairy cows in an endemically infected herd – impact on milk yield and fertility. *Reproduction in Domestic Animals 52* (1): 160–169.

12 Stewart, D., Shieh, Y.C., Tortorello, M. et al. (2015). Quantitation of viable *Coxiella burnetii* in milk using an integrated cell culture-polymerase chain reaction (ICC-PCR) assay. *Journal of Dairy Research 82* (4): 478–484.

13 McCaughey, C., Murray, L.J., McKenna, J.P. et al. (2010). *Coxiella burnetii* (Q fever) seroprevalence in cattle. *Epidemiology and Infection 138* (1): 21–27.

14 Porter, S.R., Czaplicki, G., Mainil, J. et al. (2011). Q Fever: current state of knowledge and perspectives of research of a neglected zoonosis. *International Journal of Microbiology* 2011: 248418.

15 Duron, O., Noël, V., Mccoy, K.D. et al. (2015). The recent evolution of a maternally-inherited endosymbiont of ticks led to the emergence of the Q fever pathogen, *Coxiella burnetii*. *PLoS Pathogens 11* (5): e1004892.

16 Robyn, M.P., Newman, A.P., Amato, M. et al. (2015). Q fever outbreak among travelers to Germany who received live cell therapy – United States and Canada, 2014. *Morbidity and Mortality Weekly Report 64* (38): 1071–1073.

17 Wilson, L.E., Couper, S., Prempeh, H. et al. (2010). Investigation of a Q fever outbreak in a scottish co-located slaughterhouse and cutting plant. *Zoonoses and Public Health 57* (7-8): 493–498.

18 Eldin, C., Melenotte, C., Mediannikov, O. et al. (2017). From Q fever to *Coxiella burnetii* infection: a paradigm change. *Clinical Microbiology Reviews 30* (1): 115–190.

19 Arricau-Bouvery, N. and Rodolakis, A. (2005). Is Q fever an emerging or re-emerging zoonosis? *Veterinary Research 36* (3): 327–349.

20 Lang, G.H. (1990). Coxiellosis (Q fever) in animals. *Q Fever 1*: 23–48.

21 Sanford, S.E., Josephson, G.K., and MacDonald, A. (1994). *Coxiella burnetii* (Q fever) abortion storms in goat herds after attendance at an annual fair. *Canadian Veterinary Journal 35* (6): 376.

22 Wildman, M.J., Smith, E.G., Groves, J. et al. (2002). Chronic fatigue following infection by *Coxiella burnetii* (Q fever): ten-year follow-up of the 1989 UK outbreak cohort. *QJM 95* (8): 527–538.

23 Carcopino, X., Raoult, D., Bretelle, F. et al. (2007). Managing Q fever during pregnancy: the benefits of long-term cotrimoxazole therapy. *Clinical Infectious Diseases 45* (5): 548–555.

24 Schneeberger, P.M., Hermans, M.H., van Hannen, E.J. et al. (2010). Real-time PCR with serum samples is indispensable for early diagnosis of acute Q fever. *Clinical and Vaccine Immunology 17* (2): 286–290.

25 Omsland, A. (2012). Axenic growth of *Coxiella burnetii*. In: *Coxiella burnetii: Recent Advances and New Perspectives in Research of the Q Fever Bacterium* (eds. R. Toman, R. Heinzen, J. Samuel and J. Mege), 215–229. Dordrecht: Springer.

26 Berri, M., Rousset, E., Champion, J.L. et al. (2007). Goats may experience reproductive failures and shed *Coxiella burnetii* at two successive parturitions after a Q fever infection. *Research in Veterinary Science 83* (1): 47–52.

27 Chiu, C.K. and Durrheim, D.N. (2007). A review of the efficacy of human Q fever vaccine registered in Australia. *New South Wales Public Health Bulletin 18* (8): 133–136.

28 Anderson, A., Bijlmer, H., Fournier, P.E. et al. (2013). Diagnosis and management of Q fever – United States, 2013: recommendations from CDC and the Q Fever Working Group. *Morbidity and Mortality Weekly Report. Recommendations and Reports 62* (3): 1–29.

9

Tularaemia

Tularaemia is an infectious zoonotic disease caused by the bacterium *Francisella tularensis*. The pathogen is widely distributed over the northern hemisphere, predominantly in North America, Scandinavia, Russia and Japan. The bacterium is highly virulent for humans and a range of animals such as rodents, hares and rabbits. Wildlife animals are the main reservoir for humans. Tularaemia is considered an occupational disease for humans, especially for hunters, butchers, agricultural and forest workers. Human infections mainly occur while treating and preparing hunted hares. Among pet animals, cats may transmit the disease to humans, while dogs are considered relatively resistant. Tularaemia is known by other names like rabbit fever, deerfly fever, lemming fever, meat cutter's disease, Ohara disease, Francis disease, etc.

Aetiology and Pathogen Characteristics

Francisella tularensis is an intracellular non-motile, aerobic, encapsulated Gram-negative coccobacillus. *F. tularensis* is one of two species in the genus *Francisella*, the only genus of the family Francisellaceae. *F. tularensis* has four subspecies: *tularensis* (type A, the most virulent and found in relatively dry environments of North America), *holarctica* (type B, most widespread subspecies), *mediasiatica* (present in central Asia, isolated in Kazakhstan and Turkmenistan) and *novicida* (the least virulent subspecies).

Francisella tularensis subspecies *tularensis* (type A) is one of the most infectious known human pathogens. The infective dose in humans is extremely low (i.e. 10 bacterial cells) when injected subcutaneously and 25 bacteria when transmitted via the aerosol route [1]. Because of its very high infectivity and relative stability in aerosols, the bacterium (*F. tularensis*) is classified as a Centers for Disease Control and Prevention (CDC) 'Category A' bioterrorism agent. In most countries, the highly virulent subspecies *tularensis* is classified as risk group 3 (high risk for the laboratory worker, but low community risk) while the other subspecies are risk group 2 (moderate risk for the laboratory worker, low community risk) [2].

The organism has been reported to remain viable for weeks to months in various sources, including the carcasses and hides of infected animals, grain dust, straw, water and soil. The live bacteria were found after 3 years in rabbit meat stored at −15 °C [3].

Textbook of Zoonoses, First Edition. Jasbir Singh Bedi, Deepthi Vijay, and Pankaj Dhaka.

Historical Overview

The name 'tularaemia' comes from the first isolation of the organism from sick rodents in Tulare County, California, in 1911. 'The bubo is usually about the size of a pea and the gland structure is generally replaced by a firm caseous mass' – this first description of tularaemia was published in 1911 in the paper 'A Plague-like Disease of Rodents' written by George McCoy. The first human cases were reported by Wherry and Lamb in 1914. In 1919, Edward Francis suggested the name of the pathogen as *Bacterium tularensis*. Historically, tularaemia was a public health problem in the former Soviet Union and the USA where extensive outbreaks occurred during and after the Second World War.

Pathogenesis and Virulence Factors

After acquisition, the bacteria replicate in the lymphoid tissues of the host. *F. tularensis* form a capsule that is responsible for serum resistance. In the host, they can survive inside macrophages. They can manipulate the host immune response by phase variation of their lipopolysaccharide (LPS). The LPS of *F. tularensis* differs from that of other Gram-negative bacteria and does not induce interleukin-1 release from mononuclear cells and poorly induces tumour necrosis factor. Like other intracellular pathogens, they modulate phagosome biogenesis, thereby preventing fusion with lysosomes and escape to the cytoplasm. During the acute phase of the disease, the bacteria multiply rapidly and the severity of the disease depends on the patient's ability to mobilise an immunological response which mainly depends on cell-mediated immunity. The disease normally induces life-long immunity in humans.

Transmission Cycle

Francisella tularensis spreads in the environment principally by various terrestrial and aquatic mammals such as ground squirrels, rabbits, hares, beavers, muskrats and rodents such as meadow voles and water voles. Wild rodents (e.g. voles) and lagomorphs have been reported to maintain *F. tularensis* subsp. *tularensis* and *F. tularensis* subsp. *holarctica* during interepidemic periods in some regions. However, lagomorphs and rodents can become severely ill and thus might only act as amplifying hosts for the organism. Tularaemia is believed to have reservoirs in the environment [1]. A wide range of arthropods has been identified in the transmission of tularaemia between mammalian hosts, such as ticks (*Amblyomma*, *Dermacentor*, *Haemaphysalis* and *Ixodes*), flies (*Chrysops* spp.) and mosquitoes (*Aedes* spp., *Culex* spp., *Anopheles* spp.) [1]. Some of these tick species may transmit the agent through the transovarial route and can act as a natural reservoir [4]. In endemic countries, the disease is seasonal and its incidence seems to be highest during late spring, summer and early autumn [5].

Transmission in Animals

Ticks are the important vectors of *F. tularensis* which can transfer the bacterium between rabbits, hares and rodents, and can serve as an interepizootic reservoir. Horseflies, mosquitoes, sucking lice and biting flies may also serve as vectors of the pathogen. Animals can be infected by eating undercooked animal tissues or other foods that have been contaminated by infected carcasses or their excretions.

Transmission in Humans

Hunters are the commonly infected occupational risk group for tularaemia. Veterinarians, paraveterinarians, farmers, foresters and wildlife specialists who have a high chance of contact with wildlife are also at increased risk for tularaemia. In humans, the common modes of transmission of *F. tularensis* are:

- through bites from an arthropod vector that has previously fed on an infected animal
- by direct contact with infected animals, infectious animal tissues and/or fluids. The exudates from skin lesions, blood and respiratory secretions may be infectious
- by ingestion of contaminated water or food. In contrast to *F. tularensis* (type A), *tularensis holarctica* (type B) is mainly associated with streams, ponds, lakes, rivers and semi-aquatic animals such as muskrats and beavers. This mode of transmission appears to be much more common in Europe than in the US. The isolates of subspecies *novicida* have also been linked to water-borne transmission in Australia, Spain and the USA [6]
- by inhaling dust or aerosols contaminated with *F. tularensis*. This can occur during farming or landscaping activities, especially when machinery (e.g. tractors or mowers) runs over infected animals or carcasses. Although rare, this type of exposure can result in pneumonic tularaemia (one of the most severe forms of the disease).

Tularaemia in Animals

More than 250 species of terrestrial and aquatic animals are known to be susceptible to infection by *Francisella tularensis* subsp. *tularensis* and/or subsp. *holarctica*. Common wild animal hosts include lagomorphs, various hares and jackrabbits, muskrats, beavers and a variety of rodents such as voles, field mice, squirrels and lemmings. These species also develop clinical signs in many cases. Among domesticated animals, tularaemia occurs in sheep, cats, rabbits, dogs, pigs, horses, ranched mink, pet rodents and other species. Cattle seem to be relatively resistant to illness. Outbreaks have also been reported among captive non-human primates [1].

Type A tularaemia (subsp. *tularensis*) is highly virulent in rabbits, sheep and other animals. The manifestations are likely to be associated with the susceptibility of the particular animal species. Tularaemia is probably underdiagnosed in cats and dogs because of the non-specific clinical signs [6]. The manifestations of the disease in important animal species are described below [7].

- **Rabbits, hares and rodents:** These species are highly susceptible and often die in large numbers during outbreaks.
- **Sheep:** Tularaemia in sheep is typically a seasonal disease that generally coincides with tick infestations. The clinical signs include fever, rigid gait, diarrhoea, frequent urination, weight loss and difficulty in breathing. Mortality is common among young animals, and pregnant ewes may abort.
- **Horses:** There are limited reports of clinical disease in horses; however, fever, dyspnoea, incoordination and depression have been observed in animals with extensive tick infestation.
- **Domestic cats:** Infected cats experience diseases ranging from non-clinical infection to sepsis and death. Clinical signs may include fever, depression, lymphadenopathy, abscesses, oral ulceration, gastroenteritis, hepatomegaly, splenomegaly, icterus, weight loss, pneumonia and sepsis.
- **Dogs:** Limited reports describe inapparent or mild clinical signs of tularaemia in dogs, although there is ample evidence of seroconversion.

Tularaemia in Humans

In humans, the incubation period is usually 3–5 days but may range from 1 to 21 days depending on the mode of infection and the infective dose [1]. The onset of disease is abrupt, with rapid development of fever, fatigue, body aches and headache. Without proper treatment, the disease can last for 2–3 weeks and is followed by a long phase of convalescence.

Several clinical forms of the disease result due to the agent's virulence and its route of entry as described below.

- **Ulceroglandular and glandular forms:** These forms follow bacterial inoculation via arthropod vector or by direct contact (touching infected animals or material contaminated with *F. tularensis*) with a sign of primary ulcer at the infection site. The ulceration progresses to necrosis and lymphadenopathy. The lymph nodes may suppurate, ulcerate and become sclerotic, followed by fever, chills, headache and lethargy. The ulceroglandular form of tularaemia is the most common (75–85% of reported cases) and complications such as pneumonia may be present with parenchymal infiltrates and pleural effusion.
- **Oropharyngeal form:** With chronic pharyngitis, following ingestion of contaminated water or food. Patients with oropharyngeal tularaemia may have sore throat, mouth ulcers, tonsillitis and swelling of cervical lymph glands.
- **Oculoglandular form:** With conjunctivitis and local lymphadenopathy, following conjunctival contamination or touching the eye with contaminated fingers while butchering an infected animal or possibly from infective dust. The symptoms include irritation and inflammation of the eye and swelling of lymph glands in front of the ear.
- **Pneumonic form:** With lung infection following inhalation of bacteria or systemic infection when other forms of tularaemia (e.g. ulceroglandular) are left untreated and the bacteria spread through the bloodstream to the lungs. This is considered the most serious form of tularaemia. The symptoms include cough, chest pain and difficulty in breathing.
- **Typhoidal form:** With severe systemic symptoms. This form can be the result of any entry route of the bacteria. It is characterised by any combination of the general symptoms.

The subspecies *tularensis* (type A) can lead to serious clinical manifestations and significant mortality if untreated. High fever is accompanied by progressive weakness, malaise, anorexia and loss of weight. Respiratory symptoms, including dry cough, sore throat and substernal pain, may occur whether or not the disease is acquired by inhalation. Gastrointestinal symptoms such as nausea, vomiting and diarrhoea are more likely to occur in type A than in type B tularaemia. It may occasionally lead to rhabdomyolysis and septic shock. In type B tularaemia, fever predominates and is accompanied by focal and generally milder symptoms than those of type A. However, it is frequently associated with suppurative complications and a considerable period of convalescence. *F. tularensis* subsp. *mediasiatica* is only rarely reported as a cause of human disease. Subspecies *novicida* has also been isolated from patients with various clinical manifestations in Canada, Australia and Spain [6].

Laboratory Diagnosis

Diagnosis of Tularaemia

As the disease is relatively rare and the symptoms non-specific, tularaemia can easily be misdiagnosed. Therefore, early diagnosis and treatment may be difficult in regions where tularaemia occurs rarely because the clinical expression of the disease is similar to a wide variety of other acute infectious diseases. When the epidemiology is suggestive, tularaemia should be considered in any case of fever of unknown origin. The diagnosis is mainly by laboratory confirmation of tularaemia by detecting the bacteria in a biological sample or by specific antibody response.

Bacterial Culture

Cultivation of the bacterium is rarely carried out for diagnosis as the bacteria are slow-growing and require a biosafety level-3 (BSL-3) laboratory. The direct isolation of bacteria is frequently achieved from ulcer scrapings, lymph node biopsies or sputum but the organism is rarely cultured directly from blood. *F. tularensis* can be isolated from nutrient-enriched specimens (e.g. tissues) on sheep blood agar, but cysteine-enriched media such as cysteine glucose blood agar are strongly recommended for subculture, as the organism will usually fail to thrive with continued passage on sheep blood agar. Enriched chocolate agar (cysteine heart agar supplemented with 9% heated sheep red blood cells [CHAB]) may also be used for isolation. Antibiotics should be added to suppress the contaminant flora. Incubation under 5% CO_2 supports the growth of *Francisella* spp. with an incubation period of at least 48 hours, which can be extended to 10 days based on growth visibility.

Molecular Methods

The polymerase chain reaction (PCR) can be a valuable diagnostic tool when organisms are non-cultivable or when culture is not recommended due to biosafety concerns. Molecular methods including 16S rRNA sequencing can be used to determine species and subspecies of the pathogen.

Serological Methods

Serological diagnoses are routinely used and are considered specific despite cross-reactions with *Brucella*, *Yersinia*, *Proteus*, *Legionella* and *Mycoplasma* species. Serological testing usually requires paired sera samples taken a minimum of 2 weeks apart. Early antibiotic treatment can suppress the production of antibodies and lead to a misdiagnosis. Some of the important serological methods are as follows.

- Microagglutination or tube agglutination is the standard serological test used for determining the presence of antibodies to *F. tularensis*.
- The slide agglutination test can be used for rapid confirmation of recovered isolates and immunohistochemical staining, using a monoclonal antibody directed against the LPS in formalin-fixed samples.
- Direct fluorescent antibody staining, using a fluorescein isothiocyanate (FITC)-labelled rabbit antibody directed against whole killed *F. tularensis* cells, is a rapid assay for identification of *F. tularensis* in the primary specimen or recovered cases.
- Enzyme-linked immunosorbent assay (ELISA)-based tests can be used to detect the bacteria in clinical samples, e.g. capture ELISA using monoclonal antibodies against *F. tularensis* LPS.

Vaccination and Treatment in Humans

Currently, there is no licensed vaccine against tularaemia. Until recently, a vaccine has been available to protect laboratory workers routinely working with *F. tularensis*. However, this vaccine is currently under review by the US Food and Drug Administration (FDA) [8].

Without treatment, the case fatality rate for infection with *F. tularensis* subsp. *tularensis* is 5–15%. Fatal cases due to the other *F. tularensis* subspecies are rare. The antibiotics of choice are aminoglycosides (i.e. streptomycin or gentamicin), fluoroquinolones (i.e. ciprofloxacin) and tetracyclines (i.e. doxycycline) [8].

Prevention and Control

Tularaemia is non-transmissible from human to human. There is currently no effective and safe vaccine available against *F. tularensis*. Cases of tularaemia require prompt identification and treatment to prevent fatal outcomes. Therefore, prevention from exposure, especially among occupationally at-risk groups (e.g. hunters, farmers, tourists, etc.), should be the priority. The common prevention measures consist of avoiding ingestion, breathing and inoculation of the bacteria.

- Use insect repellents (e.g. DEET, picaridin, oil of lemon eucalyptus, etc.) to avoid arthropod bites. Wear long trousers, long sleeves and long socks to keep ticks and deer flies off the skin.
- Remove attached ticks promptly with fine-tipped tweezers.
- Don't drink untreated surface water.
- While performing the mowing or landscape activities, take care not to mow over dead animals. It is advisable to use masks during these activities to reduce the risk of inhaling the bacteria in endemic areas.
- Use personal protective measures while hunting hares and rabbits.
- Use gloves while handling animals, especially rabbits, muskrats, prairie dogs and other rodents.
- Cook game meat thoroughly before eating.
- Avoid contact with dead animals and wash hands after contact with wild and domestic animals.
- Handling of biological samples potentially contaminated with *F. tularensis* should be performed in BSL-3 laboratories.
- It is important to conduct systematic surveys of the natural foci of tularaemia, which would increase the early detection of outbreaks in animals and humans.

References

1 World Health Organization (2007). Guidelines on tularaemia. www.cdc.gov/tularemia/resources/whotularemiamanual.pdf

2 World Health Organization (2004). *Laboratory Biosafety Manual*, 3e. Geneva: World Health Organization.

3 Center for Food Safety and Public Health (2017). Tularemia. www.cfsph.iastate.edu/Factsheets/pdfs/tularemia.pdf

4 Tärnvik, A., Priebe, H.S., and Grunow, R. (2004). Tularaemia in Europe: an epidemiological overview. *Scandinavian Journal of Infectious Diseases* 36 (5): 350–355.

5 Markey, B., Leonard, F., Archambault, M. et al. (2013). *Clinical Veterinary Microbiology*, 2e. Edinburgh: Mosby Elsevier.

6 Whipp, M.J., Davis, J.M., Lum, G. et al. (2003). Characterization of a novicida-like subspecies of *Francisella tularensis* isolated in Australia. *Journal of Medical Microbiology* 52 (9): 839–842.

7 American Veterinary Medical Association (2003). Tularemia facts. www.avma.org/tularemia-facts#transmission

8 Centers for Disease Control and Prevention (2018). Tularemia: prevention. www.cdc.gov/tularemia/prevention/index.html

10

Chlamydial Zoonoses

Chlamydiae are obligate intracellular Gram-negative bacterial pathogens that have a wide host spectrum. They are clinically important in both humans and veterinary medicine. The recently reclassified single genus *Chlamydia* includes a total of 14 species (*Chlamydia trachomatis*, *C. pneumoniae*, *C. psittaci*, *C. abortus*, *C. suis*, *C. pecorum*, *C. avium*, *C. caviae*, *C. muridarum*, *C. felis*, *C. gallinacea*, *C. serpentis*, *C. poikilothermis* and *C. buteonis*) [1, 2]. Out of these species, two (*C. trachomatis* and *C. pneumoniae*) are of human clinical importance and two (*C. psittaci* and *C. abortus*) are of zoonotic importance.

Species Affecting Humans

- ***Chlamydia trachomatis*:** This is the most frequent bacterial pathogen of sexually transmissible diseases (STD) and also causes trachoma (keratoconjunctivitis). Chronic and repeated infections may lead to irreversible damage, including tubal infertility in females and blindness (trachoma) after the eye infection. The complications, most importantly reactive arthritis, are presumably linked to the immunological response to the infection.
- ***Chlamydia pneumoniae*:** This is recognised as a pathogen of community-acquired pneumonia. It causes infection in the upper and lower respiratory tracts. Recurrent or long-term exposure to *C. pneumoniae* has been associated with asthma symptoms and chronic infection, which can lead to the development of obstruction of the respiratory tract in non-atopic bronchial asthma.

Species of Zoonotic Importance

Human psittacosis (also known as ornithosis or parrot disease) is an important zoonosis caused by *C. psittaci*. The pathogen is mostly associated with psittacine birds. The main hosts of *C. psittaci* are small ruminants but the organism can also infect cattle, pigs, horses and deer. Isolated cases of the zoonotic transmission of closely related *C. abortus* from sheep have also been documented, the latter linked to subsequent abortion in pregnant women who are exposed to the secretions of *C. abortus*-infected ewes [3].

Textbook of Zoonoses, First Edition. Jasbir Singh Bedi, Deepthi Vijay, and Pankaj Dhaka.

Historical Context

The first recognition of the zoonotic potential of chlamydial infections is linked with the description of the bacteria [4]. In 1879, Jacob Ritter described an epidemic of fatal respiratory disease in humans associated to contact with caged parrots and finches. At that time, the aetiological agent of this disease (later called psittacosis) was unclear and it was suspected to be of viral origin. After an outbreak occurred in Paris in 1892, the disease was named after the Greek word for a parrot, *psittakos* [5]. The chlamydial organisms were first described by Halberstaedter and von Prowazek in 1907, who identified intracytoplasmic inclusions containing large numbers of micro-organisms within cells derived from the conjunctival scrapings of human patients with trachoma. They thought that these organisms were protozoa and named them 'chlamydozoa' after the Greek word *chlamys* for a mantle, as the reddish elementary bodies (EBs) appeared to be embedded in a blue matrix or mantle.

A worldwide pandemic of human psittacosis between 1929 and 1930 resulted from the shipment of exotic birds from Argentina to Europe and North America. Almost simultaneously, the causative agent was first described in smears from infected human patients and birds in 1930 by Levinthal, Coles and Lillie as small, filterable bodies in infectious material called Levinthal–Coles–Lillie (LCL) bodies. The pathogen was isolated by Bedson and Western in 1930. Later on, Bedson suggested the biphasic development cycle of the organism in 1932. By 1966, it was clear that the Chlamydiae were not viruses but bacteria, as they possessed both DNA and RNA and had a developmental cycle different from the replication mechanisms of viruses. Chlamydiae also have a cell wall similar to that of Gram-negative bacteria, and possess ribosomes with susceptibility to antibiotics, a feature characteristic of prokaryotes [6].

Developmental Cycle and Pathogenesis

Chlamydiae are obligate intracellular Gram-negative bacteria that cause a broad spectrum of disease in humans, other mammals and birds. They undergo a unique biphasic developmental cycle characterised by two distinct morphological forms: EBs and reticulate bodies (RBs). The developmental cycle is briefly described below.

Elementary bodies are the small extracellular and metabolically less active infectious form of the bacteria (0.3 μm in diameter). The developmental cycle starts with the endocytosis of EBs by eukaryotic cells. The extracellular EBs are responsible for dissemination of the bacteria inside the infected tissue or to other hosts. Once internalised into a host cell, EBs remain in special vacuoles named inclusions and differentiate to intracellular, non-infectious, osmotically unstable, metabolically more active reticulate bodies (RBs) (~1 μm in diameter). These bodies undergo repeated cycles of binary fission before they redifferentiate to EBs, which are released and able to restart the cell cycle.

In adverse conditions, such as nutrient starvation, the developmental cycle is interrupted, resulting in the appearance of aberrant bodies (ABs), a stress-activated and persistent state in which they survive even treatment with antibiotics [7].

Survival Strategy of the Organism

The EB is characterized by its resistance to both physical and chemical factors in the extracellular environment, and by its lack of metabolic activity. This resistance is a consequence of the rigidity of the cell envelope, which is both osmotically stable and poorly permeable. Thus, the EB is adapted for prolonged extracellular survival, which in the case of animal pathogens is an important means to survive outside the natural host.

Pathogenesis

Chlamydiae have substantially reduced genomes that lack many metabolic enzymes, which makes these bacteria reliant on the host for many of their metabolic requirements. Approximately two-thirds of the predicted proteins are shared across species, which reflects genetic conservation and the evolutionary constraints imposed by their intracellular lifestyle and conserved developmental cycle. However, there is a region of high genomic diversity termed the 'plasticity zone', which encodes an array of virulence factors, including cytotoxin, membrane attack complex/perforin protein (MACPF) and phospholipase D, which might have a role in host tropism and niche specificity. In addition, most strains also carry a plasmid that contributes to virulence [8].

Mode of Transmission for Chlamydial Zoonoses

The two important zoonotic pathogens in the genus *Chlamydia* are *C. psittaci* and *C. abortus*. The important transmission factors of these pathogens are described below.

Transmission of *C. psittaci*

The organism is largely shed in respiratory exudate, especially through nasal secretions, and in the faeces of the birds. Among birds, *C. psittaci* is primarily spread by inhalation of desiccated droppings and secretions from infected birds or through ingestion of contaminated faeces. There is also evidence of transmission of the pathogen through eggs [9]. The predominant route by which *C. psittaci* is introduced into flocks seems to be through wild birds. Vertical transmission may happen at a low frequency in turkeys, chickens and ducks. *C. psittaci* might also be transmitted from bird to bird by blood-sucking ectoparasites such as lice, mites and flies or, less commonly, through bites or wounds.

In humans, contact with infected birds and their excretions is the common route of transmission. Mostly the infections result from exposure to pet psittacine birds so the disease is referred to as psittacosis. However, transmission has been documented from free-ranging birds, including doves, pigeons, birds of prey and shore birds. The primary route of infection is the inhalation of aerosols containing the bacterium which has been aerosolised from dried faeces or respiratory secretions of infected birds, but infection by ingestion can also occur. Other means of exposure include mouth-to-beak contact and the handling of infected birds' plumage and tissues.

The EBs of the pathogen are thought to be environmentally resistant. Thus, given the danger of human infection, avian strains of *C. psittaci* have been classified into 'risk group level 3' organisms. It is considered an important occupational hazard for individuals working with domestic poultry or wildfowl (e.g. poultry processing industry, pet bird market, etc.). Persons handling infected birds at the farm and personnel at slaughter houses are at risk. Human-to-human transmission is rare.

Transmission of *C. abortus*

The main source of transmission to naive ewes and susceptible humans results from the aborted materials of infected ewes. A large number of organisms can be detected in the vaginal discharges and placentas of aborted ewes and skin coats of dead lambs. When placental infection is low, it is not uncommon for the ewe to give birth to weak lambs that fail to survive beyond 24 hours or live healthy lambs. Such live lambs are also important sources of infection for naive animals and represent a significant zoonotic risk. Once an ewe has aborted as a result of ovine enzootic abortion, they are considered immune and will not abort as a result of the recurrent infection. However, this immunity is not sterile and some animals may shed organisms during the following periovulation period and at subsequent lambing. Venereal transmission by males is not thought to play an important role in the spread of infection, although direct intravaginal infection of ewes has been demonstrated. Vertical transmission of infection from ewe to lamb can occur, although it is currently unknown whether this plays any role in the epidemiology of this disease [10].

Disease in Birds, Animals and Humans

Avian Chlamydiosis (Psittacosis, Ornithosis)

Chlamydia psittaci infections are most commonly identified in psittacine birds (e.g. parrots, budgerigars, parakeets, cockatoos, cockatiels and macaws), where the disease is known as psittacosis. The term *ornithosis* is used to describe the disease in all non-psittacine species of birds. However, as the disease is essentially the same in all avian species, the term *avian chlamydiosis* may be used to describe all avian *C. psittaci* infections.

Chlamydia psittaci comprises eight known serovars, which can be distinguished with serovar-specific antibodies or by known sequence variations in the *omp*A gene. Six of the eight serovars (A–F) are associated with avian hosts. Serovars A and B are principally associated with psittacine birds and pigeons, respectively. Specific hosts have not been identified for serovars C and D, which represent a particular zoonotic risk for those working in the poultry industry. Serovar E was first isolated from human pneumonitis cases and has subsequently been identified in a wide variety of avian species. Serovar F consists of an isolate from a parakeet. The remaining two serovars, M56 and WC, were isolated from mammals.

Clinical Signs in Birds

The incubation period varies from 3 days to several weeks depending upon the species of bird, the virulence of the strain, stress factors, and the age and condition of the bird. *C. psittaci* may produce subclinical, subacute, acute or chronic infections. Acute avian chlamydiosis is a generalised infection affecting all major organs. Typical symptoms include respiratory distress, lethargy, anorexia, ruffled feathers, diarrhoea, ocular and nasal discharges, and reduced egg production. Chronically infected pigeons may show lameness, torticollis, opisthotonus, tremor and convulsions. Chickens show relatively less severe clinical signs of chlamydial infection but blindness, weight loss and a moderate increase in mortality rate may occur. In most cases, lesions are limited to the spleen, liver and air sacs. In subclinical infections, the infected birds do not develop any symptoms but act as carriers through intermittent shedding of the organism. Shedding of the pathogen can be activated by stress factors, such as transportation, rehousing, overcrowding, breeding, poor nutrition or concurrent disease.

Human Infection

Avian chlamydiosis is the most important zoonotic chlamydiosis. The disease is highly under-reported, as psittacosis is difficult to diagnose. The at-risk occupational groups affected by psittacosis include bird fanciers, owners of pet birds, pet shop employees, aviary workers, veterinarians, laboratory workers, employees in poultry slaughtering and processing plants, farmers and zoo workers.

Historically, in humans, the disease was called either psittacosis or ornithosis depending on the source of the infection, and it was assumed that ornithosis was a less severe form of the disease. Nowadays, this differentiation is no longer considered to be correct, and the disease is generally called chlamydiosis. The incubation period is between 1 and 2 weeks. Symptoms of clinical psittacosis vary in severity from mild influenza-like illness with fever, headache, joint and muscle pains, photophobia and sore throat, to severe atypical pneumonia with non-productive cough and difficult or painful breathing. *C. psittaci* can affect organs other than the respiratory system, resulting in myocarditis, endocarditis, hepatitis, encephalitis or meningitis. Renal and neurological complications may also occur. The very young and old, or immunosuppressed are most at risk from severe outcomes of the infection [11].

Ovine Enzootic Abortion

In Animals

Infection in animals is usually asymptomatic (except in abortion cases), although some behavioural changes or vaginal discharge may be observed in some animals. Ewes/does may deliver stillborn or weak offspring that fail to survive. Depending on the severity, the infection can cause abortion in as many as 80% of ewes in affected stocks and can lead to serious economic problems in the animal husbandry of affected areas [12]. The majority of infected placentas will have dark red cotyledons with creamy-yellow coloured exudate on the surface. An infectious vaginal discharge may be observed for several days following abortion, but otherwise the ewes/does are clinically normal and considered immune to further episodes of the disease [12]. Aborted lambs may appear normal or show a degree of subcutaneous oedema, with a 'pot-bellied' appearance. The ability of *C. abortus* to infect male genital tissues and affect the quality of semen in both bulls and rams implies its potential role in bovine and ovine infertility.

Human Infection

In contrast to *C. psittaci*, clinical infection with *C. abortus* is relatively rare in humans. Most cases of *C. abortus*-induced human abortion are directly associated with exposure to infected sheep or goats. In many cases, transmission probably occurs through the mouth following the handling of an infected ewe or lamb or contaminated clothing. Such spread may result from ingestion of contaminated food, smoking with unwashed hands or the undesirable practice of mouth-to-mouth resuscitation of weak lambs.

The biggest threat of human infection is to pregnant women, because of the ability of *C. abortus* to colonise the human placenta. The organism can cause spontaneous abortion during the first trimester of pregnancy, whereas later infection causes stillbirths or preterm labour. Infection in pregnant women also typically causes renal failure, hepatic dysfunction and disseminated intravascular coagulation, which in severe cases may result in death [13]. Therefore, if a woman with pregnancy complications is associated with agriculture activities and/or has contact with pregnant animals in her medical history, then *C. abortus* must be included in the differential diagnosis [11].

Diagnosis

For clinical diagnosis of zoonotic chlamydiosis in endemic regions, the specific history of contact with birds and animals is important. Clinical diagnoses in birds such as increase in white blood cell count, changes in liver enzyme activity, radiographs showing enlargement of liver and spleen, and inflammation of air sacs are indicative of infection with *Chlamydia*. Spontaneous abortions among sheep can raise suspicion for *C. abortus* infection.

For laboratory diagnosis, suitable staining procedures include the use of Macchiavello, Giemsa or modified Ziehl–Neelsen stains. Under high-power microscopy, positive samples with modified Ziehl–Neelsen staining reveal large numbers of small, coccoid EBs, stained red against a blue background of cellular debris.

In research settings, the pathogen can be isolated from clinical tissue samples (e.g. exudates and faeces of birds, placental membranes and cotyledons from the aborted animal, and patient's sputum, blood, pleural fluid or biopsy material in humans) by growing in embryonated hens' eggs (via the yolk sac route) or in cell culture (McCoy, HeLa, L929 and baby hamster kidney cells are commonly used). However, as isolation procedures are time-consuming, expensive and hazardous to laboratory personnel, they are restricted to specialised laboratories only.

The serological assays are mostly used for diagnosis; commercial kits based on enzyme-linked immunosorbent assay (ELISA), complement fixation test or fluorescent antibody technique can be used to detect the genus-specific chlamydial lipopolysaccharides (LPS). Antigen detection can be carried out by polymerase chain reaction (PCR) and the species level of differentiation can be determined by restriction fragment length polymorphism (RFLP) analysis of amplified PCR fragments.

Treatment

Chlamydiosis

There are no commercially available vaccines for avian chlamydiosis. Birds that recover from chlamydiosis are subject to reinfection, so it is important to eliminate the possibility of environmental contamination by thorough cleaning and disinfection. Doxycycline is the preferred drug for oral treatment. During treatment, it is often necessary to provide supportive care, such as intravenous fluid therapy and a warm, uncrowded environment.

In humans, *C. psittaci* is sensitive to both macrolides and tetracyclines but tetracyclines remain the drug of choice [14].

Ovine Enzootic Abortion

If ovine enzootic abortion is believed to be present in a flock of pregnant ewes, long-acting oxytetracycline may be given to reduce the severity of infection. Although this reduces the number of organisms shed, it does not eradicate infection and cannot reverse any pathological damage that has already occurred in a heavily infected placenta. However, it is more desirable to control infection through flock management and vaccination. Some of the commercial vaccines are available as inactivated preparations and live attenuated vaccines. All the vaccines confer good immunity against abortion, and significantly reduce the shedding of chlamydial organisms at parturition [11].

Prevention and Control

Avian Chlamydiosis

There is no vaccine to prevent psittacosis, so control of human psittacosis depends on control of the disease in avian hosts. Accordingly, a high standard of husbandry should be maintained in aviaries. Always try to buy pet birds only from a well-known reliable pet store. If you own pet birds or poultry, follow good precautions while handling and cleaning birds and cages. The important aspect of preventing psittacosis is to control the infection among pet birds. Some of the important precautions which can be implemented are as follows [14].

- Poultry/pet birds' cages should be cleaned and disinfected daily. *C. psittaci* is susceptible to most disinfectants and detergents. Avoid dry sweeping or vacuuming to minimise circulation of feathers and dust. It is advisable to use water or disinfectant to wet surfaces before cleaning cages or surfaces contaminated with bird droppings. Also, remember to thoroughly wash your hands with running water and soap after contact with birds or their droppings.
- Always position cages in such a way that food, feathers and droppings cannot spread between them.
- Avoid overcrowding of the birds.
- Isolate and treat infected birds.
- Persons at risk should be educated about the disease. It is important to use personal protective equipment (PPE), such as gloves and appropriate masks while handling infected birds or cleaning their cages.
- In poultry processing plants, the risk of infection can be reduced by heat treatment of birds before plucking, and by providing either local exhaust ventilation or mask respirators in evisceration areas.
- During necropsies of infected birds, the carcass should be wetted with detergent and water to prevent the aerosolisation of infectious particles, and the work should be carried out in an appropriate biosafety cabinet.
- In laboratories, the correct biocontainment facilities should be available and personnel must be fully trained in safety procedures.

Ovine Enzootic Abortion

After abortion, ewes should immediately be isolated. All dead lambs, placentas and bedding material must be safely disposed of. Lambing pens should be cleaned and disinfected to limit the risk of spread of contamination. It is also essential that hands are thoroughly washed after dealing with infective material.

To prevent human infection, pregnant women are advised not to work with sheep, particularly during the lambing period, and should avoid contact with all potential sources of infection. Similarly, immunocompromised people should also take care to avoid contact with potential sources of infection during lambing time. Basic standards of hygiene, such as handwashing before eating, drinking or smoking, and the use of disinfectants, should be maintained. As for other chlamydial infections, early diagnosis is important, as infection responds well to early treatment with antibiotics.

References

1 Sachse, K., Bavoil, P.M., Kaltenboeck, B. et al. (2015). Emendation of the family Chlamydiaceae: proposal of a single genus, Chlamydia, to include all currently recognized species. *Systematic and Applied Microbiology 38* (2): 99–103.

2 Polkinghorne, A. and Branley, J. (2020). New insights into chlamydial zoonoses. *Microbiology Australia 41* (1): 14–18.

3 Pospischil, A. (2002). Abortion in humans caused by *Chlamydophila abortus* (*Chlamydia psittaci* serovar 1). *Schweizer Archiv für Tierheilkunde* 144: 463–466.
4 Pospischil, A. (2009). From disease to etiology: historical aspects of Chlamydia-related diseases in animals and humans. *Drugs Today 45* (Suppl): 141–146.
5 Morange, A. (1895). De la psittacose ou infection spéciale déterminée par des perruches. Doctoral dissertation. Verlag nicht ermittelbar.
6 Moulder, J.W. (1966). The relation of the psittacosis group (Chlamydiae) to bacteria and viruses. *Annual Reviews in Microbiology 20* (1): 107–130.
7 Wyrick, P.B. (2010). *Chlamydia trachomatis* persistence in vitro: an overview. *Journal of Infectious Diseases 201* (Suppl. 2): S88–S95.
8 Elwell, C., Mirrashidi, K., and Engel, J. (2016). Chlamydia cell biology and pathogenesis. *Nature Reviews Microbiology 14* (6): 385.
9 Vanrompay, D., Ducatelle, R., and Haesebrouck, F. (1995). *Chlamydia psittaci* infections: a review with emphasis on avian chlamydiosis. *Veterinary Microbiology 45* (2–3): 93–119.
10 Essig, A. and Longbottom, D. (2015). Chlamydia abortus: new aspects of infectious abortion in sheep and potential risk for pregnant women. *Current Clinical Microbiology Reports 2* (1): 22–34.
11 Knittler, M.R. and Sachse, K. (2015). *Chlamydia psittaci:* update on an underestimated zoonotic agent. *Pathogens and Disease 73* (1): 1–15.
12 Conraths, F.J., Geue, L., Groschup, M.H. et al. (2004). Zoonoses in working-and wild animals and their significance in Germany. An overview. *Bundesgesundheitsblatt, Gesundheitsforschung, Gesundheitsschutz 47* (7): 633–646.
13 Pospischil, A., Thoma, R., Hilbe, M., and Grest, P. (2002). Abortion in woman caused by caprine *Chlamydophila abortus* (*Chlamydia psittaci* serovar 1). *Swiss Medical Weekly 132* (5–6): 64–66.
14 Centers for Disease Control and Prevention (2019). Psittacosis: diagnosis, treatment, and prevention. www.cdc.gov/pneumonia/atypical/psittacosis/hcp/diagnosis-treatment-prevention.html

11

Zoonotic Tuberculosis

Zoonotic tuberculosis has long been a neglected zoonosis that is predominantly caused by *Mycobacterium bovis* [1]. The organism belongs to a group of mycobacteria, together with *Mycobacterium tuberculosis* and others that derive from a common ancestor, forming *Mycobacterium tuberculosis* complex (MTBC) [2].

Mycobacterium bovis is capable of infecting a broad range of hosts, including ruminants (predominantly domestic cattle, where it is referred to as bovine tuberculosis), humans and other primates [1]. The wide host range makes bovine tuberculosis difficult to eliminate, especially where wildlife reservoirs are involved, e.g. badgers (*Meles meles*) in the United Kingdom [2].

Epidemiology

Tuberculosis (TB) is a major cause of human deaths worldwide, affecting more than 9 million people every year. Most cases of human tuberculosis are caused by the bacterial species – *Mycobacterium tuberculosis*. Among human tuberculosis cases, a considerable proportion is attributable to *M. bovis* infection, which is also termed zoonotic tuberculosis (or bovine tuberculosis).

In industrialised countries, animal tuberculosis control, elimination programmes and pasteurisation of dairy products have drastically reduced the incidence of disease in both cattle and humans. However, in developing countries, animal tuberculosis is widely distributed, control measures are not applied systematically and raw milk consumption still occurs in some communities. It has been estimated that zoonotic transmission of *M. bovis* is responsible for 10–15% of new human TB cases in developing countries [3]. In 2016, the World Health Organization (WHO) estimated that there were 1 470 000 new human cases of zoonotic TB, and 12 500 deaths were reported due to the disease. However, estimates of the global burden of zoonotic TB are imprecise due to the lack of routine surveillance data from the human and animal populations of many countries, and in particular from the countries where bovine tuberculosis is endemic and where laboratory capacities are limited.

Bovine tuberculosis affects the well-being of rural communities that rely on livestock for their livelihood. The disease has an important economic impact through reduced meat and milk production, as well as condemnation of carcasses (or affected parts) that are unfit for human consumption. The disease also creates a barrier to the international trade of animals and animal products. When it becomes endemic in wildlife populations, this threatens conservation efforts and wildlife can serve as the reservoir of infection for livestock and humans.

Textbook of Zoonoses, First Edition. Jasbir Singh Bedi, Deepthi Vijay, and Pankaj Dhaka.

Disease Transmission

In Animals

The widespread distribution of *M. bovis* in the domestic and wild animal populations represents a large reservoir of this micro-organism. There are numerous ways in which tuberculosis spreads to farm animals, including horizontal spread by inhalation and ingestion of *M. bovis* directly from infected animals or indirectly from contaminated pastures, water or fomites. Since transmission between cattle occurs predominantly through aerosol inhalation, the transmission rate is increased by risk factors such as high herd density, intensive farming, poor ventilation, poor farm biosecurity, etc. Other factors such as the long survival period of the microbe in manure and soil, and close contact between animals (e.g. around water sources) also increase the risk of infection. Transmission from cows to suckling calves through infected milk has also been documented [2].

Wild animal TB represents an important reservoir of infection and poses a serious threat to control and elimination programmes [4]. Spread from infected to susceptible animals is likely to occur when wild and domesticated animals share pasture or territory. There are well-documented examples of such spread, including infection in badgers (*Meles meles*) in the United Kingdom and opossums (*Trichosurus vulpecula*) in New Zealand.

In Humans

The disease is considered an occupational hazard for at-risk groups who have continuous exposure to livestock, such as veterinarians, farmers and abattoir workers. The disease in humans primarily occurs through close contact with infected cattle, consumption of improperly cooked beef or drinking of unpasteurised milk and milk products. The main transmission route of *M. bovis* to people is through the consumption of contaminated raw milk and other dairy products. Direct airborne transmission of *M. bovis* has also been reported from infected animals or animal products to people, as well as between people [2]. Infection risks have also been linked to local cultural practices (e.g. consumption of fresh blood) [5]. There is evidence that human patients can transmit bovine tuberculosis to animals, and human-to-human transmission is also possible [4].

Pathogenesis

Tuberculosis, including bovine disease, is primarily an infection of the respiratory system. The tubercle bacilli that are inhaled usually lodge in the alveolar spaces where they are ingested by macrophages. Following ingestion of the bacillus, lysosomes fuse with the phagosome to form a phagolysosome, and phagocytes attempt to destroy the bacillus. Virulent bacilli can escape destruction and survive inside a mononuclear macrophage by inhibiting phagosome fusion with preformed lysosomes, thereby limiting acidification of the phagolysosome.

The pathogenicity of *M. tuberculosis* complex is a multifactorial phenomenon that requires the participation of the cumulative effect of several glycolipid complexes such as lipoarabinomannan that may interfere with phagosome maturation. Another glycolipid, trehalose-6,6′ dimycolate, is associated with virulence and cord formation in a liquid culture medium. Other glycolipids such as phosphatidylinositol mannoside are present in the cell walls of the bacilli.

Protective immunity against mycobacterial infections is dependent on the activation of cell-mediated immune responses. Inflammatory cytokines, i.e. interleukin (IL)-1, IL-2 and tumour necrosis factor α (TNF-α), produced by mononuclear cells sensitised by mycobacterial antigens recruit natural killer T-cells, CD4 T-cells, CD8 T-cells, and γδ T-cells. These cells produce cytokines that recruit additional cells to the site of infection, resulting in the formation of granulomas. Granuloma formation is an attempt by the host to localise the disease process. However, in cases in which the host response is unable to destroy the bacillus due to conditions that compromise immune function, such as old age, stress or human immunodeficiency virus (HIV), reactivation may occur, resulting in the release of bacilli and transmission of infection. Grossly visible lesions in bovines and humans are characterised by a caseous, necrotic centre surrounded by a zone of epithelioid cells, multinucleated giant cells, lymphocytes and a fibrous capsule [6].

Disease in Animals

Tuberculosis is usually a chronic and debilitating disease in cattle, but acute and rapidly progressive cases are also possible. The infection can remain latent for years and later reactivate in infected animals. The onset of disease is typically insidious, initially with few or no signs of illness. Common clinical signs in cattle include weight loss (emaciation may become severe in terminal stages), inappetence, low-grade fluctuating fever, lymphadenopathy and respiratory involvement with moist, intermittent cough that worsens in the morning, or during cold weather or exercise. Dyspnoea or tachypnoea may also be seen, and involvement of the gastrointestinal tract can result in intermittent diarrhoea or constipation. The superficial lymph nodes can be palpably enlarged, and sometimes rupture and drain. The retropharyngeal lymph node is often affected in this species. Other reported symptoms include ocular disease (e.g. anterior uveitis, choroidal infiltrates, subretinal exudates), repeated abortions and infertility caused by lesions in the uterus.

Disease in Humans

In humans, it is not possible to clinically differentiate between infections caused by *M. tuberculosis* and *M. bovis*. In countries where bovine tuberculosis is uncontrolled, most human cases occur in young persons resulting from drinking or handling contaminated milk. Zoonotic tuberculosis mainly involves the respiratory system but it often affects extrapulmonary sites also, including lymph nodes and other organs (e.g. bones, intestine, brain, etc.). The disease usually has a prolonged course and symptoms may take months or years to appear. The usual clinical signs include weakness, loss of appetite, weight loss, fluctuating fever, intermittent hacking cough, diarrhoea, chronic skin TB (lupus vulgaris), and large prominent lymph nodes (e.g. cervical lymphadenopathy). Such cases, however, may also be caused by *M. tuberculosis* [4]. In some cases, the bacteria can lie dormant in the host without causing any clinical forms of the disease.

Diagnosis

In Animals

Some of the important diagnostic methods which are used in animals are described below.

- **Clinical diagnosis:** The symptoms of bovine tuberculosis usually take months to develop. Bovine tuberculosis is usually a chronic debilitating disease in cattle where the common symptoms include progressive emaciation, a low-grade fluctuating fever, weakness and inappetence. Animals with pulmonary involvement usually have moist cough. In some animals, the retropharyngeal or other lymph nodes enlarge. Infections can remain dormant for years and reactivate during periods of stress or in old age. Therefore, bovine tuberculosis can be difficult to diagnose based only on the clinical signs.

- **Postmortem diagnosis:** Inspection of carcasses for evidence of bovine TB has been increasingly regarded as a control point in the prevention of human cases of TB caused by *M. bovis*. The disease is characterised by the formation of granulomas where bacteria are located. These granulomas are usually yellowish and are caseous, caseocalcareous or calcified and often encapsulated. Some tubercles are small enough to be missed by the naked eye unless the tissue is sectioned. In cattle, tubercles are found in the lymph nodes, particularly those of the head and thorax. They are also common in the lung, spleen, liver and the surfaces of body cavities. However, diagnosis while performing autopsies or inspection of carcasses in slaughterhouses presents considerable difficulty, since many pathogens, such as *Actinomyces bovis*, have granulomatous inflammation and morphological characteristics similar to *M. bovis*.
- **Histopathological diagnosis:** A presumptive diagnosis can be made by histopathology and/or microscopic demonstration of acid-fast bacilli. Direct detection of the bacterium in sputum samples or biopsies (mostly in humans) or at postmortem of tuberculous organ lesions can be carried out by Ziehl–Neelsen staining followed by light microscopy or auramine O staining and fluorescence microscopy.
- **Immunological diagnosis.**
  - *Delayed-type hypersensitivity (DTH) reaction:* The DTH reaction is represented by the tuberculin skin test (TST). The test in bovines is done with purified protein derivative (PPD) obtained from the *M. bovis* AN5 strain. Advantages of the use of PPD include low cost, ease of availability, long history of use and lack of alternative on-field methods to detect bovine TB. However, the limitations include difficulties in administration and interpretation of results, need for a second-step visit, low level of standardisation and imperfect test specificity. The TST and the interferon-γ test are based on detection of the early cell-mediated immune response in tuberculosis. However, during the late stages of the disease, the cell-mediated immune response can decline, so these tests can therefore show false-negative results.
  - *Interferon* (IFN)-γ *assays:* The IFNγ assay is used to verify the existence of cell-mediated immune response developed by the body of the animal in response to mycobacterial infection. The IFN-γ which is produced by T-lymphocytes of the infected animal is detected using monoclonal anti-IFN-γ antibodies.
  - *Enzyme-linked immunosorbent assays (ELISA):* The indirect ELISA technique measures the binding of specific antibodies to an antigen. An advantage of the ELISA is its simplicity; however, sensitivity is limited because of the late and irregular development of humoral immune response in many cattle during the disease.
- **Bacterial isolation:** The isolation of *M. bovis* is considered the gold standard for bovine tuberculosis diagnosis. However, isolation and biochemical identification of the pathogen may require more than 12 weeks, and also the procedure has low sensitivity.
- **Molecular diagnosis:** Nucleic acid-based technology, notably polymerase chain reaction and related methods, are rapid, sensitive and specific diagnostic tools. Restriction fragment length polymorphism analysis (DNA fingerprinting) could be useful in epidemiological studies that trace the spread of disease between cattle, other animals and humans or in the rapid differentiation of *M. bovis* within *M. tuberculosis* complex. The use of these modern molecular techniques is limited in most developing countries due to lack of diagnostic capacities.

Diagnosis in Humans

Zoonotic tuberculosis in humans remains highly underdiagnosed because routine diagnostic protocols were developed for patients with pulmonary tuberculosis caused by *M. tuberculosis*. The laboratory procedures frequently used for diagnosing tuberculosis, such as sputum smear microscopy or rapid molecular assays, cannot differentiate *M. tuberculosis* from *M. bovis*. Moreover, *M. bovis* is difficult to culture and type, and there are limited laboratory facilities in countries where tuberculosis is endemic. The most useable glycerol containing Löwenstein–Jensen medium for *M. tuberculosis* culture inhibits the growth of *M. bovis*, thereby increasing the number of undetected cases. Novel molecular diagnostic tools (e.g. spoligotyping) and whole-genome sequencing have been developed for the detection of *M. bovis*. However, these modern techniques require enhanced laboratory infrastructure and personnel training which are not currently available in many developing countries [2].

Vaccination and Treatment

Vaccination

Bacillus Calmette–Guérin (BCG) vaccine is the only registered tuberculosis vaccine for humans and was developed by Calmette and Guérin from a strain of *M. bovis* which was originally isolated by Nocard from a case of tuberculous mastitis. The strain was distributed to many countries during the 1920s and the continuing passage of the strain in differing conditions produced a considerable number of daughter strains, with varying antigenic profiles [7]. In many countries, it is part of the national childhood immunisation programme. BCG vaccine has a documented protective effect against meningitis and disseminated TB in children. It does not prevent primary infection and, more importantly, does not prevent reactivation of latent pulmonary infection, the principal source of bacillary spread in the community.

In cattle, many field trials of BCG vaccination were conducted in the first half of the twentieth century and the major caveats that restricted the use of vaccines in cattle were that protection was inadequate and vaccination could sensitise animals to respond during traditional diagnostic testing of tuberculosis [6]. Therefore, the development of a highly effective vaccine should be the priority in animal health research.

Treatment

In animals, the treatment of bovine tuberculosis is not recommended due to its infectious nature. If an animal is found to be infected, it should be separated and culled from the herd.

In humans, zoonotic TB also poses challenges for effective patient treatment and recovery. *M. bovis* is naturally resistant to pyrazinamide, one of the four essential medications used in the current first-line anti-TB treatment regimen. As healthcare providers often initiate treatment without drug susceptibility testing results, patients with zoonotic TB may receive inadequate treatment. This may lead to poor treatment outcomes and the development of further resistance to other anti-TB drugs. Resistance to additional drugs (including rifampicin and isoniazid) has also been detected in some *M. bovis* isolates, resulting in multidrug-resistant tuberculosis (MDR-TB).

Prevention and Control

Bovine tuberculosis results in major economic losses and trade barriers, as well as posing a risk to food safety and human health. In industrialised countries, animal TB control and elimination programmes (test and slaughter policies) have drastically reduced the incidence of disease caused by *M. bovis*. However, in developing countries, animal TB is widely distributed and control measures are not systematically applied. Raw dairy products are still consumed in many communities in endemic countries. There are very limited data on the zoonotic aspects of *M. bovis* in developing countries due to a lack of surveillance and awareness among the public.

Ten Priority Areas for Tackling Zoonotic TB

The WHO has identified 10 priority areas for tackling zoonotic TB in people and bovine TB in animals. These fall under three core themes [1].

1) Improving the scientific evidence base.
   - *Collect and report complete and accurate data from human and animal populations:* Systematically survey, collect, analyse and report better quality data on the incidence of zoonotic TB in people, and improve surveillance and reporting of the disease in livestock and wildlife.
   - *Improve diagnosis in people:* Expand availability of appropriate diagnostic tools and capacity for testing to identify and characterise zoonotic TB in people.
   - *Address research gaps:* Identify and address research gaps in zoonotic bovine TB, including epidemiology, diagnostic tools, vaccines, effective patient treatment regimens, health systems and interventions co-ordinated with veterinary services.
2) Reducing transmission at the animal–human interface.
   - *Ensure safer food:* Develop strategies to improve food safety.
   - *Improve animal health:* Develop the capacity of the animal health sector to reduce the prevalence of TB in livestock.
   - *Reduce the risk to people:* Identify key populations and risk pathways for transmission of zoonotic TB.
3) Strengthening intersectoral and collaborative approaches.
   - *Increase awareness, engagement and collaboration:* Increase awareness of zoonotic TB, engage key public and private stakeholders, and establish effective intersectoral collaboration.
   - *Develop policies and guidelines*: Develop and implement policies and guidelines for the prevention, surveillance, diagnosis and treatment of zoonotic TB, in line with relevant intergovernmental standards.
   - *Implement joint interventions:* Identify opportunities for community-tailored interventions that jointly address human and animal health.
   - *Advocate for investment:* Develop an investment case to advocate for political commitment and funding to address zoonotic TB across the sectors at global, national and regional levels.

References

1 World Health Organization (2017). Roadmap for zoonotic tuberculosis. https://apps.who.int/iris/bitstream/handle/10665/259229/9789241513043-eng.pdf

2 Abakar, M.F., Azami, H.Y., Bless, P.J. et al. (2017). Transmission dynamics and elimination potential of zoonotic tuberculosis in morocco. *PLoS Neglected Tropical Diseases 11* (2): e0005214.

3 Ashford, D.A., Whitney, E., Raghunathan, P., and Cosivi, O. (2001). Epidemiology of selected mycobacteria that infect humans and other animals. *Revue Scientifique et Technique 20* (1): 325–337.

4 Cosivi, O., Grange, J.M., Daborn, C.J. et al. (1998). Zoonotic tuberculosis due to *Mycobacterium bovis* in developing countries. *Emerging Infectious Diseases 4* (1): 59.

5 Daborn, C.J., Grange, J.M., and Kazwala, R.R. (1996). The bovine tuberculosis cycle – an African perspective. *Journal of Applied Bacteriology 81*: 27S–32S.

6 Neill, S.D., Bryson, D.G., and Pollock, J.M. (2001). Pathogenesis of tuberculosis in cattle. *Tuberculosis 81* (1–2): 79–86.

7 Buddle, B.M., Vordermeier, H.M., Chambers, M.A., and de Klerk-Lorist, L.M. (2018). Efficacy and safety of BCG vaccine for control of tuberculosis in domestic livestock and wildlife. *Frontiers in Veterinary Science 5*: 259.

12

Other Bacterial Zoonoses (including food-borne pathogens) of Public Health Importance

Melioidosis

Melioidosis is an infectious disease caused by the environmental Gram-negative bacterium *Burkholderia pseudomallei* which is mainly found in contaminated water and soil. It is predominantly a disease of tropical climates, mainly prevalent in Southeast Asia and Northern Australia; however, it is also emerging in other geographical regions of the world [1]. In 1912, pathologist Alfred Whitmore first described melioidosis in Rangoon (present-day Myanmar), so the disease is also known as Whitmore disease. Melioidosis (also known as the 'Vietnamese time bomb') received wide attention after the Vietnam War. During the war, when the USA helicopters landed troops throughout Vietnam, their blades kicked up dirt, exposing soldiers and pilots to hidden pathogens in the soil. Later on, occasional melioidosis cases were reported due to the lengthy disease latent period in war veterans.

Melioidosis spreads to humans and animals through direct contact with contaminated sources. The disease is grossly underdiagnosed worldwide, mainly due to the lack of diagnostic laboratories serving the low-income rural populations who are at the greatest risk of infection. In addition, there is a lack of awareness about the disease amongst physicians and laboratory staff in many endemic regions. Melioidosis tends to cause a wide range of symptoms similar to other conditions, leading to its nickname 'the Great Mimicker'. This makes differential diagnosis difficult and the disease may be mistaken for other diseases such as tuberculosis or common forms of pneumonia.

The organism is a facultative intracellular Gram-negative rod-shaped bacterium with bipolar staining that resembles a safety pin. *B. pseudomallei* produces a glycocalyx polysaccharide capsule that is probably an important virulence determinant for the disease [1]. *B. pseudomallei* is classified as a hazard group 3 pathogen [2]. Although healthy people may get melioidosis, the major risk factors are diabetes, liver disease, renal disease, thalassaemia, cancer or other immune-suppressing condition. Besides humans, goats, sheep and pigs are the most commonly infected animals. Additionally, cattle, horses, dogs, cats, rodents and other animals can become infected.

Naturally acquired infections in humans and animals result from exposure through broken skin, inhalation or ingestion of *B. pseudomallei*. Some environmental conditions, such as tropical storms, and specific occupations (e.g. rice farming) are known to increase the risk of exposure to the pathogen. Infected animals can shed the organism through wound exudates and other sources including nasal secretions, milk, faeces and urine. Human-to-human transfer is rarely reported.

Textbook of Zoonoses, First Edition. Jasbir Singh Bedi, Deepthi Vijay, and Pankaj Dhaka.

Burkholderia pseudomallei infection can be acute, chronic or latent. Usually, among the majority of immunocompetent individuals, the infection results in subclinical disease. The incubation period of acute infection is 9 days (range: 1–21 days) [1]. In humans, the majority of patients present with sepsis with or without pneumonia, or localised abscesses, but specific clinical presentations and their severity vary depending on the route of bacterial entry (skin penetration, inhalation, ingestion), host immune function and bacterial strain and load. The severe outcome includes pneumonia, meningoencephalitis, sepsis or chronic suppurative infection.

The disease in animals can be variable depending on the location of the infection. Many animals remain asymptomatic while others may have fever, loss of appetite or swollen glands. In severe cases, pneumonia, abscesses, lameness or nervous system signs can occur. Mastitis in goats is a common manifestation and the respiratory system is involved preferentially in sheep [3].

On the diagnostic front, organism culture remains the mainstay of melioidosis diagnosis. *B. pseudomallei* can grow on most routine laboratory media, but might not be recognised and could be dismissed as a contaminant. Therefore, Ashdown's media is preferred due to the growth of consistently distinctive colony morphology and odour. *B. pseudomallei* produce characteristic purple, dry and wrinkled colonies on this medium. Blood, throat swabs, rectal swabs, urine, sputum and pus are the samples of choice for culture. Most of the available serological tests are less sensitive and specific but novel enzyme-linked immunosorbent assay (ELISA) assays, immunochromatographic tests (ICTs) and antigen detection tests can be used as serological diagnoses in the absence of other suitable alternatives.

The laboratory diagnosis of melioidosis has advanced through development of sensitive tests such as polymerase chain reaction (PCR)-based diagnostics. Matrix-assisted laser desorption ionisation time-of-flight mass spectrometry (MALDI-TOF MS) has also emerged as an important technique for the rapid and accurate identification of the pathogen [4].

Early diagnosis and specific antimicrobial therapy are crucial for melioidosis treatment. Treatment generally starts with intravenous antimicrobial therapy for 10–14 days, followed by 3–6 months of oral antimicrobial therapy. However, in many cases, treatment can be difficult, as *B. pseudomallei* is often resistant to multiple antibiotics. Thus, a prolonged course of antibiotics is required to prevent disease relapse [2]. In untreated cases, the mortality is ≥40% [5].

In regions where the disease is widespread, contact with contaminated soil or water is considered an important risk factor for melioidosis. There is no vaccine currently available for human use. High-risk groups and persons with open skin wounds should avoid direct contact with soil and standing water and should wear protective clothing (such as boots and gloves). In endemic regions, always drink bottled or boiled water and avoid outdoor exposure to rain or dust clouds. Healthcare workers can use standard precautions when treating patients with melioidosis to prevent transmission. In animals, preventive measures are more practical and economical in intensive farming environments and involve raising the animals without soil bedding, especially avoiding exposure of animals to muddy or water-flooded regions and providing clean drinking water.

Tetanus

The disease tetanus is characterised by spastic paralysis and has a worldwide distribution in humans and animals. Tetanus is an example of a saprozoonosis (saprozoonoses are zoonoses that are transferred through a non-animal reservoir, such as a plant, or through the abiotic environment, such as water or soil) [6]. It is also considered an occupational hazard among farmers, veterinarians and zoo staff coming in contact with contaminated soil or animal faeces.

The aetiological agent for tetanus is *Clostridium tetani*. The organism is a Gram-positive, obligate anaerobe, sporulating saprophyte bacterium. *C. tetani* is commonly found in soil samples from all parts of the world. It can be detected in the intestine of animals but does not represent a significant part of the normal digestive flora [6].

Clostridium tetani produces one of the most poisonous bacterial toxins, i.e. neurotoxin – tetanus toxin. Infection and clinical signs often result from wound contamination with *C. tetani* spores which are present in the environment irrespective of geographical location. Different surfaces and objects contaminated with soil particles, dust or faeces may contain *C. tetani*. Tetanus spores are introduced into the body through wounds contaminated with soil, street dust or faeces, or injected contaminated drugs. The spores are round and terminal and provide a characteristic shape usually called a 'drumstick'. The spores generally survive moderate heating (75–80 °C for 10 minutes) but usually are destroyed within 1 hour at 100 °C [6].

Given that *C. tetani* is an obligate anaerobe, the deep anaerobic tissue wound provides an ideal environment for replication and growth of *C. tetani*. Following extensive bacterial replication at the wound site, expression of the genes encoding the toxins (tetanospasmin and tetanolysin) occurs. Tetanospasmin is taken up at the nerve terminals of the peripheral nervous system and can interfere with vesicular release of acetylcholine at the neuromuscular junction. Thus, an initial presenting symptom of tetanus is flaccid paralysis which can resemble the effects of *C. botulinum*. However, the toxin is transported in a retrograde fashion towards the central nervous system (CNS) and eventually reaches the spinal cord or brainstem. It is here that the tetanus toxin produces its characteristic satellite of symptoms. The toxin causes inhibition of the release of γ-aminobutyric acid (GABA) and glycine inside inhibitory nerve terminals that control the activity of the lower motor neurons. This results in a hyperactivity effect leading to involuntary contraction of the skeletal muscles. The signs of spastic paralysis are characteristic, and the diagnosis is often based on clinical observations.

The incubation period of tetanus varies from 8 days to several months based on the location of the injury site and its distance from the CNS. The severity of symptoms is incubation period dependent: the shorter the incubation period, the more severe the symptoms, and vice versa [7].

Another important manifestation is the neonatal form of tetanus. Newborns can become infected through contaminated instruments used to cut the umbilical cord or by improper handling of the umbilical stump. Neonatal tetanus is more likely to occur in low- and middle-income countries where unhygienic deliveries at home are common, and coverage of antenatal care services and maternal tetanus toxoid immunisation are usually inadequate [7].

All animal species are susceptible to tetanus but there is considerable variability in susceptibility between species. The most susceptible species are horse, guinea pig, monkey, sheep, mouse, and goat, whereas carnivores such as cats and dogs are less vulnerable, and birds are considered as resistant. Unlike sheep and goats, cattle are quite resistant to tetanus.

Among non-immunised horses, the acute form can be manifested with spastic paralysis which can rapidly spread from the head (muscles of mastication, ears, third eyelid) to the respiratory muscles and then to the limbs. The death of the animal can occur within 1–2 days due to respiratory failure. In the subacute form, the clinical signs develop in 1–3 weeks. Muscle stiffness involving the neck and back muscles resulting in a 'rocking horse stance' or stiffness of the masseter muscles resulting in 'lockjaw' appearance are often considered as the initial presenting signs. Affected horses are also often recognised due to characteristic facial changes including erect ears, dilated nares and prolapse of the third eyelid.

In cattle, the signs are comparable to those observed in horses, but the muscular hyperactivity in response to stimuli is less pronounced.

In humans, the incubation period ranges from 3 to 21 days (average 10 days) depending on the site of injury. Characteristic symptoms include painful muscular contractions, primarily of the masseter and neck muscles and secondarily of trunk muscles. Trismus or lockjaw is a common sign of tetanus in humans. In older children and adults, abdominal rigidity with generalised spasm (frequently induced by sensory stimuli) can be an important indication of the disease. The disease complications include laryngospasms, fractures, hypertension, pulmonary embolism, aspiration pneumonia and death.

Immunisation is the only effective prevention for tetanus. Tetanus toxoid is an effective, safe and affordable vaccine that can be given to all ages, including pregnant women and immunocompromised individuals. There are national and international guidelines/programmes for tetanus prevention through childhood immunisation, prophylaxis against neonatal tetanus and vaccination against adult tetanus. It is important to note that the protection from vaccines, or a prior infection, does not last a lifetime. This means that if an individual has had tetanus or received the vaccine, they still need to be vaccinated regularly to maintain an adequate level of protection against this serious disease. In addition, good wound care is important to prevent the entry of the pathogen. Never delay first aid of even minor, non-infected wounds like blisters, scrapes or any break in the skin. It is advisable to wash hands often with soap and water or use an alcohol-based handrub if washing is not possible. Always consult your doctor if you have concerns and need further advice [6].

There is no specific treatment available for clinical cases of tetanus. The toxin that has been taken into neuronal cells cannot be accessed by antitoxin antibodies. The focus of acute tetanus management should centre around toxin mitigation and aggressive symptom management, including airway protection. Patients who have tetanus due to open wounds should undergo immediate debridement to eradicate spores and to avoid further spread of the toxin from tissue to the bloodstream.

Regarding mitigation of the toxin, tetanus toxin binds irreversibly to tissue and so the focus of neutralisation is the unbound toxin. Human tetanus immune globulin should be given as soon as tetanus is suspected. Antimicrobial therapy is typically metronidazole as the preferred treatment for tetanus, with penicillin G as an option for second-line therapy with treatment duration of 1 week to 10 days. It is important to note that antimicrobial therapy plays a relatively minor role in the management of tetanus as wound debridement and toxin mitigation are of primary importance. Non-specific symptomatic treatments include sedation and muscle relaxation, and supportive nursing care (feeding, maintaining hydration, etc.) [8].

Dog Bite-Transmitted Bacterial Pathogens (*Capnocytophaga canimorsus* and *Pasteurellas spp.*)

Bites from pet dogs or cats may result in infections caused by a range of bacteria residing on the oral mucosa of the animal and the skin of the bite victim. The most common bacteria transmitted by dog bites are *Pasteurella* spp. (*P. multocida* and *P. canis*) and *Capnocytophaga canimorsus*. It is important to note that these pathogens do not make dogs or cats sick, so pets remain asymptomatic carriers of these bacteria. These are normally opportunistic pathogens of low virulence but they have been associated with high case fatality among the immunocompromised population. Brief descriptions of these pathogens are provided below [9].

- ***Capnocytophaga canimorsus:*** This bacterium is commonly found in the mouth of healthy dogs and cats, and can be transmitted to people through bites. Affected individuals may develop a localised bacterial infection or life-threatening systemic manifestations such as septicaemia

and meningitis. The bacteria can enter the bloodstream and cause infection in various parts of the body, including septicaemia, endocarditis, abscesses in various body tissues and inflammation of eyes, face, lymph nodes or meningitis. The disease mainly occurs in immunocompromised individuals. Important risk factors are pre-existing liver disease, alcoholism and immunological disorders like cancer, diabetes and human immunodeficiency virus (HIV) infection. *C. canimorsus* can cause serious illness in pregnant women and their unborn babies. Infection during the last few weeks of pregnancy can lead to chorioamnionitis (inflammation of the membranes that surround the baby in the womb). In newborns, the infection can cause low birth weight and serious outcomes can result in sepsis [10].
- ***Pasteurella* spp.:** *Pasteurella multocida* is a major and important pathogen of the group, but *P. canis* is also frequently isolated. Most human infections are associated with animal exposure, mainly from cats and dogs, and usually involve soft tissue sites after animal bites or scratches. Primary infection occurs in soft tissues while secondary infection may affect bones, joints, brain and respiratory tract [9].

Prevention measures involve education and awareness among pet owners on how to interact safely with pets. If you have been bitten by a dog or cat, wash the bite area immediately with soap and water, and call the doctor, even if you don't feel sick. This is because dog and cat bites can pose a risk for deadly pathogens like rabies [10]. Immunocompromised patients, regardless of wound size, should consult their physician for appropriate antimicrobial prophylaxis.

Rat Bite Fever Agents

Rats are responsible for 1% of animal bites in humans each year [11]. The main bacteria detected in rat bite wounds are staphylococci, *Leptospira* spp., *Pasteurella* spp., *Corynebacterium* spp., *Fusobacterium* spp. and the rat bite fever (RBF) agents (*Streptobacillus moniliformis* and *Spirillum minus*) [12]. RBF is a systemic illness caused by infection with *Streptobacillus moniliformis*, *Spirillum minus* or *Streptobacillus notomytis*. *S. moniliformis* is a more common cause of RBF occurring worldwide. In Japan, RBF is known as sodoku (*so*: rat, and *doku*: poison) and it is primarily caused by *Sp. minus* which occurs mainly in Asian countries although occasional cases of RBF are attributed to this organism in North America, Europe and Africa [13]. Infection with *S. notomytis* has rarely been reported [14].

Rats are considered to be the reservoir hosts for *S. moniliformis*, and they usually carry this organism asymptomatically as a part of the normal nasopharyngeal flora. It can be found in *Rattus rattus* (the black rat) and *R. norvegicus*, the ancestor of most laboratory and pet rats. Mice can be infected either subclinically or symptomatically with *S. moniliformis*. Gerbils and African squirrels are considered potential hosts, based on their association with human cases of RBF. Animals that eat rodents, including cats, dogs, ferrets, weasels and pigs, might be infected or colonised with the organisms, as they have been implicated in a few human cases [13].

Rats are also thought to be the reservoir hosts for *Sp. minus*, and carry it asymptomatically. In addition to rats, *Sp. minus* is reported to infect mice, and the illness has been reported in experimentally infected guinea pigs and rhesus macaques.

The organism *S. moniliformis* is a Gram-negative pleomorphic bacterium showing filaments in chains with numerous bulbous swellings. Two distinct clinical syndromes that have been identified in association with *S. moniliformis* infection are RBF and Haverhill fever.

- ***S. moniliformis* RBF** is is the common syndrome associated with rat bites and scratches. Clinical symptoms include an abrupt onset of high fever, followed by headache, chills, vomiting and rash. The petechial rash develops over the extremities, in particular the palms and soles, but sometimes it is present all over the body. In 20% of cases, the rash desquamates, and later a symmetric polyarthritis develops in about 50–70% of patients.

- **Haverhill fever (HF)** is a form of *S. moniliformis* infection that is believed to develop after the consumption of water, milk or food contaminated by rat excreta. Haverhill fever symptoms include fever, chills, pharyngitis and pronounced vomiting, which may be followed by skin rashes and polyarthralgia.

Spirillum minus is a spiral-shaped Gram-negative bacterium, actively motile via 2–6 spirals and bipolar bundles of flagella. *Sp. minus* RBF usually manifest at a later stage than RBF by *S. moniliformis*. The infection has an incubation period of 2–3 weeks (with a maximum of 4 months). The clinical course is similar to streptobacillary RBF. However, an indurated, painful and often ulcerated lesion occurs at the site of the bite in this form of the disease. This skin lesion may appear as the fever develops. The regional lymph nodes are often swollen and tender. Febrile relapses separated by afebrile periods are often seen in spirillary RBF, and these relapses can recur several times over 1–3 months. Although the rash is less common compared to the streptobacillary form, some patients develop a distinctive rash consisting of large violaceous or reddish macules. Arthritis and myalgia occur infrequently. Asymmetrical polyarthritis is less frequently observed compared to *S. moniliformis* RBF. There will be regional lymphangitis and lymphadenopathy. Diarrhoea, vomiting, arthralgias, neuralgias and CNS symptoms may occur. Endo- and myocarditis, hepatitis and meningitis are the possible complications.

Person-to-person transmission has not been reported in RBF. Historically, over 50% of reported cases occurred in children living in poverty [15]. However, the disease is expanding its horizon, and now also includes pet store workers and laboratory technicians as rats have become popular pets and research subjects.

Many cases go undiagnosed since these bacteria are difficult to identify and are likely to respond to empiric antibiotic therapy. Penicillin is the treatment of choice for both forms of RBF, but streptomycin, tetracycline, doxycycline, cephalosporin and other antibiotics have also been used in the treatment. Although tedious, *S. moniliformis* and *S. notomytis* can be grown in culture. By contrast, *Sp. minus* cannot be cultured in artificial media. *S. moniliformis* is fastidious and requires media enriched with 10–20% blood, serum or ascitic fluid for growth. In liquid media with serum, bacterial growth shows a typical 'puff-ball' or 'bread crumb-like' appearance. They can develop into 'L-forms' which have a 'fried egg' appearance and it is difficult to distinguish them from *Mycoplasma* colonies. For rapid diagnosis of infection by *S. moniliformis*, enzyme-linked immunosorbent assays, indirect immunofluorescence, immunoblotting (Western blotting) and PCR tests can be used.

Spirillary RBF is usually diagnosed by identifying spirilla consistent with *Sp. minus* in blood, exudates or tissues, including lymph node aspirates, the bite wound or erythematous plaques by dark-field microscopy. Because *Sp. minus* cannot be cultured, no serological or molecular (PCR) tests are available for diagnosis.

The risk of infection can be reduced by avoiding exposure to rats, particularly wild rats. Wild rat populations around homes should be controlled. Food and water storage should be designed to prevent contamination by rodents, and potentially contaminated water and food sources should be avoided. Pasteurisation of milk and sterilisation of drinking water decrease the risk of Haverhill fever. Specific pathogen-free (SPF) rodents, rather than conventional animals, should be used in laboratories or when breeding pets. The laboratory animals should be housed in areas free of wild rodents. Bites from rodents should be avoided as much as possible by adopting proper handling techniques during laboratory experimentation. Protective clothing, including gloves, can also be helpful. Hand-to-mouth contact should be avoided when handling a rodent or cleaning its cage, and hands should be washed after contact. Bite wounds or scratches should be cleaned promptly and thoroughly. In case of emergency, contact your physician for the proper treatment.

Bacterial Food-borne Pathogens

Introduction

Unsafe food due to microbial contamination poses global health threats. There are more than 250 food-borne diseases (FBD) that can infect humans, and particularly vulnerable populations of infants, young children, pregnant women, the elderly and those with an underlying illness (immunocompromised individuals). Compromised food safety creates a vicious cycle of diarrhoea and malnutrition, thereby threatening the nutritional status of the most vulnerable part of the society especially in low- and middle-income countries where the burden of FBD is highest. Therefore, food safety plays a crucial role in achieving relevant Sustainable Development Goals (SDGs). Three important health-related goals are SDG 3 'Good health and wellbeing', SDG 2 'Zero Hunger' and SDG 6 'Clean water and sanitation'. These SDGs are directly or indirectly dependent on food safety and food security.

Food-borne diseases (also referred to as food-borne illness or food poisoning) are illnesses caused by contaminated, or naturally harmful, food or drink. These diseases are the result of ingestion of food safety hazards that can harm consumers' health. The hazards are often classified as: biological (e.g. bacteria, virus, parasites, etc.), chemical (e.g. heavy metals, pesticides, etc.), and physical (e.g. fragments of metal or glass). Many FBDs are zoonotic. Many of these zoonotic FBDs are emerging diseases in nature with the potential to cause huge socio-economic and public health impacts. Lack of evidence on the burden of FBD, due to their self-limiting nature and the difficulty of establishing causal relationships between food contamination and resulting illness or death, often results in under-reporting and therefore negligence in the development of public health regulatory frameworks and establishment of food security policies.

The important food-borne bacterial pathogens along with their disease characteristics are listed in Table 12.1 and the details of these pathogens are discussed below.

Bacillus cereus

Aetiology

Bacillus cereus (also known as *Bacillus cereus sensu lato*) is a Gram-positive, spore-forming, facultative anaerobic rod-shaped bacterium which is ubiquitously found in the environment. *B. cereus* is well associated with food poisoning-related outbreaks, and also plays an important role as a food spoilage organism due to its proteolytic and lipolytic properties (e.g. sweet coagulation or ropiness of milk and milk products) [16].

Organism Characteristics

Bacillus cereus grows at temperatures between 4 and 48 °C (with an optimal growth temperature of 28–35 °C) and a pH range of 4.9–9.3 [17]. *B. cereus* strains can vary in their growth and survival characteristics and are divided into psychrotrophic and mesophilic groups. The psychrotrophic strains grow well at temperatures below 10 °C (but grow poorly at 37 °C) and are generally found in chilled foods and sometimes in fresh foods whereas the mesophilic strains grow well at 37 °C (but can survive at temperatures below 10 °C) [18].

Table 12.1 Food-borne bacterial pathogens along with their disease characteristics.

Name	Sources	Onset of disease	Symptoms
Bacillus cereus	Improperly refrigerated starchy foodstuffs such as cooked rice and other cereals, pasta, potatoes, cooked vegetables and meat	*Diarrhoeal toxin:* 6–15 h *Emetic toxin:* 30 min to 6 h	*Diarrhoeal toxin:* Watery diarrhea and abdominal cramps *Emetic toxin:* Nausea and vomiting
Campylobacter jejuni	Undercooked meat and meat products, unpasteurised dairy products, contaminated water, and direct contact with farm animals/birds	24–72 h	Fever, vomiting and headaches Sometimes followed by severe abdominal cramps with watery or bloody diarrhoea
Clostridium perfringens	Undercooked contaminated meat and meat products (poultry, beef, gravies, etc.)	8–14 h	Abdominal cramps, watery diarrhoea, nausea (generally without fever and vomiting)
Clostridium botulinum	Improperly canned food, vacuum-packed and refrigerated food, low acid preserved vegetables, meat products and sausage Contaminated honey is an important source of infant botulism	Children and adults: 12–72 h Infants: 3–30 d	*Children and adults*: Nausea, vertigo, double vision or blurred vision, drooping eyelids, slurred speech, difficulty in swallowing, dry mouth, muscle weakness *Infants:* Lethargy, poor feeding, constipation and poor muscle tone (appear 'floppy')
Diarrhoeagenic *E. coli*	Faecal contaminated food, especially undercooked ground beef, unpasteurised (raw) milk and milk products, raw fruits and vegetables, and contaminated water	Depend on pathotype (range: 8 h to 10 d)	Most pathotypes are associated with severe diarrhoea, stomach pain and vomiting. Enterohaemorrhagic *E. coli* may cause haemolytic uraemic syndrome (HUS) and/or haemorrhagic colitis (HC)
Listeria monocytogenes	Raw milk and dairy products. Soft cheese made with unpasteurised milk. Contaminated ready-to-eat food products, and raw fruits and vegetables (such as sprouts), etc.	Invasive listeriosis: 8 d (range: 1–67 d)	The gastrointestinal form is mild with fever and diarrhoea. Symptoms of invasive listeriosis include stiff neck, delirium and convulsions along with fever and myalgia. In severe form, it causes meningitis and encephalitis. Pregnant women may experience foetal death, preterm labour or infection of the newborn.

(*Continued*)

Table 12.1 (Continued)

Name	Sources	Onset of disease	Symptoms
Salmonella spp.	Contaminated eggs, meat, vegetables, fruits and sprouts. Animals and their environments, particularly reptiles (snakes, turtles, lizards), amphibians (frogs), birds (baby chicks) and pet animals (cats and dogs)	6–72 h	Stomach cramps and diarrhoea, but other possible symptoms include vomiting, nausea, fever, muscular pain and loss of appetite. Bacteraemia may develop in 5–10% of patients that may lead to focal infections, such as meningitis, endocarditis, arthritis and osteitis
Staphylococcus aureus	Humans (skin, hand, nose) are an important source of food contamination. Food that is prepared by human contacts like sliced meats, puddings, pastries, sandwiches and milk products are especially risky if hygiene is not maintained	30 min to 6 h	Nausea, vomiting, chills, headache and abdominal cramping with or without diarrhoea (usually without fever)
Vibrio cholerae	Humans are the natural host for *V. cholerae*. Transmission is mainly through the faecal–oral route. Occasional outbreaks have been reported from shellfish consumption	1–2 d	Acute gastroenteritis leads to characteristic 'rice-water' stools. Large volumes of watery stool can cause rapid dehydration that can progress to hypovolaemic shock and metabolic acidosis
Vibrio parahaemolyticus	Raw or undercooked shellfish, particularly oysters	2–10 d	Acute gastroenteritis characterised by diarrhoea, headache, vomiting, nausea and abdominal cramps
Vibrio vulnificus	Environmental sources (sea water and sediment) and seafood	Within 24 h of exposure	Range from mild gastroenteritis and abdominal cramps to the lethal septicemic form
Yersinia enterocolitica	Uncooked pork and other meats, unpasteurised milk and contaminated water	4–6 d	Fever, abdominal pain, vomiting, watery or bloody diarrhoea

The organism can persist and survive in harsh environmental conditions by the production of endospores and the formation of biofilms. The bacterial spores have no metabolic activity and are resistant to heating, freezing, drying, γ-ray and ultraviolet radiation. Moreover, the ability of the bacterium to form biofilms complicates cleaning and disinfection measures on surfaces of food establishments [19].

Epidemiology and Transmission Routes

Food-borne outbreaks due to *B. cereus* have been documented worldwide. However, like other common food-borne pathogens, due to the self-limiting nature of the infection coupled with the lack of laboratory testing facilities, globally *B. cereus* infection is highly under-reported [19].

Symptoms

Bacillus cereus can cause two different types of gastrointestinal diseases: emetic and diarrhoeal syndromes [20].

- **Emetic syndrome:** Emetic *B. cereus* strains are mainly associated with starchy foodstuffs such as rice, pasta and pastries. The emetic form resembles *Staphylococcus aureus* intoxication and is caused by the emetic toxin, cereulide. Cereulide is a small, heat-resistant, ring-shaped dodecadepsipeptide that remains stable even after heating at 121 °C for 30 minutes, cooling at 4 °C for 60 days, and at a pH range of 2–11 [17]. The emetic syndrome is characterized by nausea and vomiting within 30 minutes to 6 hours of consumption of contaminated food. Generally, the symptoms are self-limiting and of short duration (lasting not more than 1 day), but occasionally severe intoxication cases may require hospitalisation, where acute liver failure and encephalopathy may occur [21].
- **Diarrhoeal syndrome:** Enteropathogenic strains of *B. cereus* are found in all kinds of foods including milk products, vegetables, meat products, puddings, spices, poultry and sprouts. The symptoms of the diarrheal form of *B. cereus* food poisoning usually start within about 6–15 hours and are characterised by abdominal pain and watery diarrhoea which resemble the symptoms of *Clostridium perfringens* infection. In contrast to the emetic toxin, diarrhoea-associated enterotoxins are not produced in the food matrix itself, but in the intestine due to ingestion of contaminated food containing toxin-producing *B. cereus* strains. The diarrhoeal symptoms are mainly due to enterotoxins (heat sensitive), which form pores in the membranes of epithelial cells in the small intestine. Two tripartite protein toxin complexes, the non-hemolytic enterotoxin complex (Nhe) and the hemolytic enterotoxin complex (Hbl), and the single protein cytotoxin K (CytK) have been linked to the diarrhoeal syndrome.

Isolation and Identification

The conventional method of detecting *B. cereus* in food products includes plating on 'mannitol–egg yolk–polymyxin agar' as a standard medium. Molecular techniques such as PCR have long been adopted for the rapid detection of *B. cereus*. Immunological methods using double-antibody sandwich enzyme-linked immunosorbent assay (ELISA) or endolysin cell wall binding domain from bacteriophage have also been reported.

Prevention and Control

The vegetative form of *B. cereus* can be eliminated by heat treatment. However, the spores can survive at high temperatures, such as pasteurisation treatment. It has been recommended that foods which are sensitive for *B. cereus* contamination (e.g. meat, poultry, starchy foods like rice and potatoes, cooked vegetables, etc.) should not be held in the danger temperature zone of 4.4–60 °C, in which pathogenic bacteria can grow rapidly in food products [17].

During long holding of foods at ambient temperature, the spores can turn into vegetative *B. cereus* bacteria, and therefore the more bacteria, the more toxin is produced, and this increases the risk of food poisoning. The reheating of food may kill the vegetative forms of the bacteria, but might not disable the toxin that causes the emetic type of illness [19]. Therefore, it is recommended that food should be properly stored at refrigeration temperature. However, many psychrotrophic strains of *B. cereus* can survive and grow at refrigeration temperature. Therefore, other food safety measures like keeping raw and cooked foods separate and maintaining good hygiene practices are important to prevent *B. cereus*-related food poisoning outbreaks.

Campylobacteriosis

Campylobacter spp. is a commonly reported zoonotic food-borne pathogen associated with food poisoning outbreaks in many countries. The colonisation capacity of *Campylobacter* spp. in livestock and avian species is considered an important route of transmission. In humans, campylobacteriosis is associated with gastroenteritis and the possibility of other serious chronic manifestations, such as Guillain–Barré syndrome (GBS) and Miller Fisher syndrome (MFS).

Aetiology

Campylobacter (Greek for 'curved rod') is a Gram-negative bacterium, with slender, spiral or curved shape and characterised by its ability to grow under microaerophilic conditions. The organism exists as commensals in the gastrointestinal tract of mammals and birds. Among the 29 species of *Campylobacter*, *C. jejuni* and *C. coli* are associated with the majority of human campylobacteriosis cases [22].

Pathogen Characteristics

Campylobacter spp. grow optimally at pH 6.5–7.5 and do not survive below pH 4.9 and above pH 9.0. Both *C. jejuni* and *C. coli* prefer to grow at 42 °C and therefore are generally called thermophilic *Campylobacter* species. The thermophilic *Campylobacter* species are unable to grow below 30 °C due to the absence of genes for cold shock proteins [23].

Exposure of the organism to the environment and other food processing and storage conditions can pose stresses, which lead to a change in their shape from spiral to coccoid forms. This survival strategy is known as 'viable but non-culturable' (VBNC) state. The VBNC state is characterised by decreased metabolic activity, increased production of degradative and substrate-capture enzymes and cell shrinkage, which is found to be associated with enhanced virulence [24]. This characteristic of the organism poses difficulties for the accurate detection and enumeration of *Campylobacter* species in food or environmental samples.

Epidemiology and Transmission Routes

The global distribution of *Campylobacter* spp. is attributed to its ability to colonise and form a part of the commensal flora of a wide range of species including poultry, pigs and cattle. Globally, *C. jejuni* is more prevalent in poultry, whereas *C. coli* is more common in pigs. The majority of gastrointestinal cases (>90% of cases) are caused by *C. jejuni* and to a lesser extent by *C. coli*. Poultry is the natural host for *C. jejuni*, where the intestinal microaerophilic conditions and optimal temperature of around 40–42 °C allow the continuous replication of the organism without any clinical signs [22]. The colonisation of *C. jejuni* in poultry is mainly associated with horizontal transmission at the farm level.

Transmission to humans is commonly through faecal contamination of food due to *Campylobacter*-shedding animals or birds during slaughtering/food processing/post-processing. It can also be transmitted from human to human by cross-contamination through the faecal–oral route.

Important risk factors for infection include consumption of undercooked meat and meat products, unpasteurised milk and dairy products, contaminated drinking water and/or direct contact with farm animals and birds. In addition, rats, mice, wild birds, insects and houseflies can act as vectors or vehicles for the pathogen, and thereby contaminate food, farm animals/birds, utensils, equipment and other items.

Symptoms

The ingestion of only a few hundred cells (500–800 colony forming units [CFU]) may be sufficient to initiate the disease. An incubation period of 24–72 hours is observed before the onset of illness. After ingestion of the pathogen by humans, *C. jejuni* colonises the lower gastrointestinal tract (i.e. ileum, jejunum and colon) and often will not exhibit any symptoms. The severity of infection depends on factors like the immune status of the host, ingested bacterial load and virulence of the *Campylobacter* strain, etc. In most symptomatic cases, campylobacteriosis manifests as mild self-limiting gastroenteritis characterised by fever, vomiting and headaches sometimes followed by severe abdominal pain with watery or bloody diarrhoea. However, *Campylobacter* enteritis has recently been identified as an important risk factor for the development of inflammatory bowel syndrome [25].

In some individuals, the infection can result in serious illness, including immunoreactive complications such as GBS and MFS, a chronic and potentially fatal form of paralysis. GBS is a rare autoimmune disease characterised by the demyelination of motor and sensory nerves or deterioration of axonal nerves of the peripheral nervous system. It is reported that 'GBS has become the most frequent cause of acute flaccid paralysis since the near elimination of poliomyelitis in the world'. The axonal degeneration in patients with GBS has been reported to be associated with the molecular mimicry between GM1 and GD1a gangliosides of human neurons and the lipo-oligosaccharides of *C. jejuni* [26].

Isolation and Identification

For isolation and identification of the organism, fecal specimens can be collected from suspected cases and should be transported in Cary–Blair transport medium. *Campylobacter* can pass 0.45 μm cellulose acetate membrane filters while most of the other faecal flora do not, so this characteristic can be used in the filtration of the organism from the sample. Selective broths, including Bolton broth (BB), *Campylobacter* enrichment broth (CEB) and Preston broth (PB), can be used for the enrichment of samples. The commonly used selective media are Skirrow's medium, Butzler's medium, Campy-BAP medium and charcoal cefoperazone deoxycholate (CCDA) medium. All these basal media should be enriched with sheep or horse blood and supplemented with antibiotics to inhibit the normal enteric flora.

Campylobacter spp. are considered as microaerophilic as they require an atmosphere with an oxygen concentration of 5–10% for optimal growth. After incubation of cultures under suitable conditions (temperature 42°C, time 24–48 hours), colonies that are mucoid or wet appearing should be suspected and confirmed further by biochemical (oxidase and catalase positive) and other molecular methods.

For epidemiological studies and outbreak investigations, many molecular typing tools are available, such as PCR, random amplification of polymorphic DNA (RAPD), multilocus sequence typing (MLST) and pulsed-field gel electrophoresis (PFGE).

Prevention and Control

Campylobacter spp. are generally regarded as sensitive to environmental conditions, drying, freezing, oxygen exposure, etc. However, the organisms can be resilient due to their ability to attain the VBNC state and the formation of biofilms. Moreover, the genome of *Campylobacter* poses high plasticity which enables them to secrete extracellular proteins associated with stress tolerance [27].

Poultry meat remains the main source of human campylobacteriosis, so the control of cross-contamination in the poultry meat production chain should be the main focus to reduce human illness. It is important to minimise contamination of poultry farms from wild and domestic animals. Installing hygienic barriers and implementation of strict farm biosecurity protocols, including strict hygienic routines such as washing and sanitising of hands, controlling the entry of farm visitors, changing boots, etc., can be effective in reducing the entry of pathogens in farms. There must be adequate precautionary measures during the evisceration stage of slaughter, as the rupture or leakage of intestinal contents can increase the chances of contamination of carcasses and the processing environment. In addition, other upcoming control measures like the use of probiotics, bacteriocins, bacteriophages and feed and water additives, and the development of suitable vaccine candidates, can reduce the colonisation of the organism in poultry flocks [23].

Since *Campylobacter* spp. is heat sensitive, in domestic and catering settings, cooking temperatures and times are sufficient to eliminate the organism, as long as this critical control point (CCP) is not compromised by later cross-contamination (e.g. from working surfaces and contaminated utensils). The washing of food-processing surfaces with hot water and hypochlorite can significantly reduce the contamination load. At the consumer level, preventive measures for cross-contamination are important for ready-to-eat (RTE) products and other foods which do not require heat treatment before consumption.

Clostridium perfringens

Clostridium perfringens is a common pathogen associated with enteric diseases in animals and humans which include histotoxic and enteric infections, food poisoning (toxico-infection) and enterocolitis.

Aetiology

Clostridium perfringens is a Gram-positive, anaerobic, spore-forming, rod-shaped bacterium. The organism is considered a saprophyte which is widespread in soil, feed, litter and sewage, and also inhabits the intestinal tract of mammals and birds. The organism can form spores that are resistant to many environmental stressors including heat, desiccation, acids and many of the commonly used disinfectants.

Pathogen Characteristics

Clostridium perfringens possesses an arsenal of toxins, and toxin production varies significantly among the strains of the organism. *C. perfringens* has been classified into seven toxinotypes (A, B, C, D, E, F, G), based on the presence of genes encoding for α (CPA), β (CPB), ε (ETX), and ι (ITX) toxins, and the recently included enterotoxin CPE and necrotic enteritis B-like toxin (NetB) [28]. The food poisoning-associated enterotoxin CPE was genotyped in type F strains (previously named CPE-positive type A). It is important to note that no single strain of *C. perfringens* is known to produce all these toxins [29]. *C. perfringens* has a very short generation time (8–12 minutes) when cultured at optimal conditions, which could represent an effective mechanism for outgrowing other resident bacteria, thus leading to efficient gut colonisation of the organism.

Epidemiology and Transmission Routes

The ability to sporulate and wide temperature range adaptation of *C. perfringens* allow the bacteria to survive in extreme or nutrient-depleted conditions. This results in the transmission of this organism from diverse environments to the hosts. After cooking of food, slow cooling at room temperature allows the spores to germinate (since heating removes oxygen and creates a favourable anaerobic environment). Therefore, food items that require high-temperature treatment and then are cooled down too slowly, and then frozen and reheated insufficiently are considered at high risk for *C. perfringens* food poisoning. Toxinotype A is considered to be responsible for most of the food poisoning and non-food-borne diarrhoeal disease outbreaks. The most common foods which act as vehicle for transmission are undercooked contaminated meat and meat products.

Symptoms

Clostridium perfringens has been associated with various systemic and enteric diseases in humans as well as animals, which include gas gangrene in contaminated wounds (also known as clostridial myonecrosis), gastroenteritis (including food-borne and non-food-borne diarrhoea) and enterocolitis, and more recently it has been linked to necrotising enterocolitis (NEC) in preterm infants [29]. The gas gangrene (clostridial myonecrosis) is accompanied by profuse gas production and readily permeable toxic substances, which when produced in excess are associated with other intestinal inflammatory diseases (e.g. ulcerative colitis).

Some of the important clinical manifestations of *C. perfringens* infection are as follows.

- **Food poisoning (acute watery diarrhoea):** Globally, food poisoning due to *C. perfringens* type A is ranked among the most prevalent causes of bacterial food poisoning. The hallmark symptoms include rapid onset within 8–14 hours after ingestion of contaminated food, intestinal cramps and watery diarrhoea (without fever or vomiting). Currently, food poisoning *C. perfringens* cases are thought to be caused by CPE (encoded by the *cpe* gene). This secretes pore-forming toxin which is also associated with disruption of intestinal tight junction barriers and initiates disease development.
- **Non-food-borne diarrhoea:** *C. perfringens* has also been associated with non-food-borne diarrhoea which is considered a disease entity distinct from food poisoning, and characterised by severe symptoms and longer course. This includes antibiotic-associated diarrhoea (AAD) and sporadic diarrhoea (SD) [30]. AAD typically occurs after the administration of broad-spectrum antibiotics and mainly affects the older age group and immunocompromised individuals. The clinical symptoms are abdominal pain, prolonged diarrhoea (more than 3 days to several weeks) and dysentery. Other pathogenic bacteria including *C. difficile* (the most common pathogen associated with AAD) and *S. aureus* have also been implicated in AAD.
- **Preterm infant NEC:** Since the 1970s, preterm infant NEC has been clinically linked with *C. perfringens* type A. The organisms were isolated from necrotic tissues in many NEC cases and were also termed as 'gas gangrene of the bowel' owing to its reflection of the highly similar disease histology with the infamous tissue myonecrosis [31]. Both *Klebsiella* spp. and *C. perfringens* have been linked to clinical NEC in recent years. Being universal in habitable niches, the spore former *C. perfringens* may readily pass to in-hospital neonates through environmental contamination or oral transmission. The underlying mechanisms for *C. perfringens*-associated NEC include the following.
  - Reduced bowel peristalsis in preterm infants can increase pathogen retention time.
  - Administration of broad-spectrum antibiotics can lead to a reduction in microbiota diversity which can support rapid overgrowth of resistant spores.
  - Weak gut barrier integrity (non-existent mucus layer), lack of protective bacteria (including *Bifidobacterium* spp.) and immature/underdeveloped immune system in preterm infants can favour the invasion of *C. perfringens*.

- **Darmbrand (which means 'burning bowels' in German):** This term was used to describe a type of necrotic inflammatory gut disease (also known as enteritis necroticans) associated with *C. perfringens*. An epidemic of Darmbrand occurred after the Second World War (1944–1949) in northwest Germany.
- **Pigbel (also known as enteritis necroticans):** This is a form of inflammatory gut disease. The first documented outbreak was in 1966 which was associated with pork-feasting activities among Papua New Guinea Highlanders. The classic description of the symptoms is 'spontaneous gangrene of small intestine, without obvious vascular or mechanical cause'. The clinical form resembles Darmbrand and occurs mainly in children.

Isolation and Identification

The commonly used enrichment medium for isolation of *C. perfringens* is thioglycollate and Robertson's cooked meat medium (RCM). The selective agars for isolation of *C. perfringens* are sulfite polymyxin sulfadiazine agar (SPS) and tryptose sulfite cycloserine agar (TSC). The characteristic black colony of *C. perfringens* will appear after incubation at 37 °C for 24–48 hours under anaerobic conditions.

Clostridium perfringens causes β-hemolysis on sheep blood agar and exhibits Nagler's reaction (lecithinase test) on egg yolk agar plates, due to the hydrolysis of lecithin by lecithinase enzyme (phospholipase-C) produced by *C. perfringens* type A. In the reverse CAMP test, *Streptococcus agalactiae* is streaked on blood agar and *C. perfringens* is streaked perpendicular to *S. agalactiae*. After 24–48 hours of anaerobic incubation, a 'bow-tie' zone will be formed by *C. perfringens* due to synergistic haemolysis.

In suspected *C. perfringens* infections, analysis of stool samples should be performed as stool culture and ELISA testing for CPA toxin. Molecular detection of faecal CPE or PCR confirmation of *cpe* gene is the widely used clinical diagnostic method for identification of *C. perfringens* AAD. The isolates can be further confirmed and characterised by using animal inoculation test, *in vitro* testing, and novel microbial source tracking (MST) tools (e.g. real-time PCR, loop-mediated isothermal amplification [LAMP], MLST, PFGE, etc.).

Prevention and Control

Prevention and control measures include proper biosecurity of animal farms and the application of hygienic measures across the food production chain. In food-processing units, care must be taken to avoid the cross-contamination of food products. At the consumer level, proper cooking of foods should be followed and food should be served hot, and leftover food should be refrigerated at 40 °F or below as soon as possible (preferably within 2 hours of preparation), and the food must be reheated at least to 165 °F (74 °C) before serving.

Clostridium botulinum

Clostridium botulinum is associated with the production of botulinum toxin that causes botulism in humans and animals. The term 'botulism' is derived from the Latin word *botulus* which means 'sausage'. In the eighteenth century, the disease was frequently linked with the consumption of blood sausage in central Europe.

Aetiology

Clostridium botulinum is a Gram-positive, anaerobic, rod-shaped spore-forming bacterium that produces a toxin with characteristic neurotoxicity. The spores of *C. botulinum* are heat resistant and widely distributed in environmental sources. In the absence of oxygen, the spores germinate, grow and excrete toxins in contaminated foods.

Pathogen Characteristics

Clostridium botulinum produces three types of toxins: botulinum neurotoxin (BoNT), C2 toxin and C3 toxin. BoNT affects neurons, while C2 and C3 toxins induce epithelial cell damage and facilitate the spread of BoNT to deeper tissues [32].

The botulinum toxins are classified into eight distinct types (A, B, C, D, E, F, G, H) and subtypes of A (A1, A2, A3, A4, A5), which are antigenically distinct [32]. Types A, B, E, H and, in rare cases, F cause human botulism while types C, D and E cause illness in other mammals, birds and fish [33]. The toxin is produced when the clostridial cells are lysogenised by the bacteriophage or due to autolysis of cells during the late phase of the growth cycle [32].

Epidemiology and Transmission Routes

Clostridium botulinum toxin type A can result in food-borne, wound and infant botulism. Toxin types B and E can be associated with such botulism cases, but to a lesser extent. Botulinum toxin A is considered one of the most lethal biological substances. The human lethal dose for toxin A is estimated to be approximately 1 ng/kg by parenteral or oral routes [34]. Food-borne botulism is considered as an intoxication (as the preformed toxin is responsible for the disease, even without the bacterium).

Globally, food-borne botulism outbreaks occur when *C. botulinum* grows and produces toxins in food before consumption. The botulinum toxin has been detected in a variety of foods, including low-acid preserved vegetables (such as green beans, spinach), fish, meat products and sausage. Outbreaks are mainly associated with inadequately processed, home-canned or home-bottled foods. Conditions like low-oxygen or anaerobic environment and low-acid foods without adequate preservatives (e.g. sugar and salt) with high water content are favourable for spore germination. The consumption of foods contaminated with spores is generally not associated with the disease in healthy adults. Spore germination may take place in the colon, but the organisms are unable to survive because of the competent resident microflora. Food contamination after proper heating (around 85 °C) and later cooling at room temperature at a slow rate promotes the germination of spores. The heating of foods removes the oxygen and creates an anaerobic environment which allows germination and growth of the organism and subsequent botulinum toxin production in contaminated foods.

Symptoms

The clinical symptoms associated with various types of botulism are described below.

- **Food-borne botulism:** The incubation period of botulism depends on the rate and the amount of the toxin consumed, which can occur as early as 2 hours or as long as 8 days (typically within 12–72 hours) [32]. After consumption, the toxin is absorbed and reaches the blood circulation where it blocks the release of the neurotransmitter acetylcholine. This causes flaccid paralysis by preventing nerve impulse propagation in peripheral neurons and thereby affecting the parasympathetic and sympathetic nervous systems and neuromuscular junctions. Symptoms include nausea, vomiting, headache, double vision, slurred speech, muscle spasm (dystonia) and muscle weakness. The toxin first affects the upper limbs then the lower limbs and later causes breathing difficulty due to pharyngeal and diaphragm muscle weakness. Heart function also weakens and death follows. Autonomic symptoms include dry mouth, postural hypotension, urinary retention and pupillary abnormalities.

- **Infant botulism:** There are several possible sources of infection for infant botulism, but spore-contaminated honey has been associated with a large number of cases. Infants under 6 months of age remain the most susceptible group. As infants do not have developed colonic microflora populations, there are no antagonistic effects from resident flora or bile salts. The spores germinate in the intestinal tract of the infant and the vegetative cells colonise the gut. Progression of the disease is very slow because of poor absorption of toxins through the colonic cell layers. In adults and children older than about 6 months, this would not happen because of the natural defences in the intestines that develop over time, which prevent germination and growth of the bacterium. The symptoms of infant botulinum are similar to adult botulism; however, nausea and vomiting are absent. Early signs are weak cry, muscle weakness, difficulty in feeding, i.e. poor suckling ability, hypotonia ('floppy baby syndrome') and a decrease in spontaneous movement. Symptoms such as constipation, tachycardia and dry mouth are due to the blockade of parasympathetic nerve impulses. Most cases recover with adequate supportive therapy and interventions; however, death may occur in severe cases.
- **Wound botulism:** This can occur in patients with traumatic and surgical wounds and in users of contaminated intravenous drugs. The condition is also common in soldiers on the battlefield. The spores lodge in the deep wound or at the injection sites of drug users, where the anaerobic environment created by tissue destruction helps in the germination and growth of *C. botulinum*. The incubation period for wound botulism is 4–14 days. Botulinum toxin is produced and absorbed through the mucous membranes, broken skin or wounds, leading to botulism.
- **Inhalation botulism:** Inhalation botulism is rare and does not occur naturally. It is mainly associated with accidental or intentional events (such as bioterrorism) which result in the release of the toxins as aerosols. Inhalation botulism exhibits a similar clinical footprint to food-borne botulism.
- **Other types of intoxication:** Water-borne botulism has been reported from ingestion of the preformed toxin. However, common water treatment processes (such as boiling, disinfection with 0.1% hypochlorite bleach solution) destroy the toxin so the risk is considered low. Sometimes botulism of undetermined origin involves adult cases where no food or wound source could be identified. These cases are comparable to infant botulism and may occur due to alteration of gut flora as a result of surgical procedures or antibiotic therapy. Also, adverse effects of the pure botulism toxin (Botox®) have been reported as a result of its medical or cosmetic use in patients.

Isolation and Identification

Apart from the clinical manifestation(s) and patient history, diagnosis can be supplemented by positive laboratory findings. Blood, stool or food samples can be tested for the presence of *C. botulinum* or its toxin. Food samples should be enriched in RCM or trypticase-peptone-glucose-yeast extract (TPGY) at 28 or 35 °C for around 5 days under strict anaerobic conditions. Gram staining or observations under bright-field microscopy should reveal the presence of typical cells with a 'tennis racket' appearance when forming spores. For isolation, mix the enriched culture with alcohol or provide heat treatment of 80 °C for 10–15 min, then streak it onto egg yolk agar or liver-veal-egg yolk agar and incubate at 35 °C for 48 hours under anaerobic conditions. The typical *C. botulinum* colonies appear as raised or flat, smooth or rough with spreading and irregular edges. On egg yolk agar, colonies show a lustrous zone (referred to also as a pearly zone), when observed under oblique light. Immunoassays like ELISA are widely used for the detection of toxins. The mouse bioassay can also be used but it is expensive and requires special facilities. On the molecular front, specific PCR assays can be used for toxinotyping and detection of virulence genes associated with *C. botulinum* types [35].

Prevention and Control

The typical outcome of botulism is descending flaccid paralysis that, unless treated immediately, may lead to death due to failure of respiratory musculature. Prevention of food-borne botulism is based on hygienic food preparation practices. Though the spores of *C. botulinum* are heat resistant, the toxin produced by bacteria growing out of the spores under anaerobic conditions can be destroyed by boiling (e.g. internal temperature >85 °C for 5 minutes or longer is sufficient to destroy the toxin) [33]. Moreover, *C. botulinum* will not grow in acidic conditions (pH <4.6), and therefore the toxin will not be formed in acidic foods (note: a low pH will not degrade any preformed toxin in the food). Combinations of low storage temperature and salt contents and/or pH are also used to prevent the growth of the bacteria or formation of the toxin [33]. Precautions for the cross-contamination of high-risk foods (e.g. ready-to-eat (RTE) foods, canned foods, honey, etc.) should be taken throughout the food supply chain.

Diarrhoeagenic *Escherichia coli*

Escherichia coli (*E. coli*) is a Gram-negative, non-spore-forming, rod-shaped facultative anaerobic bacterium that belongs to the family Enterobacteriaceae. *E. coli* was first isolated from the stool of an infant by Theodor Escherich in the year 1885. The bacterium is widely distributed and is considered commensal, where it inhabits the colon of humans and warm-blooded animals. Most of these commensal *E. coli* strains are considered beneficial to their hosts and lack virulence factors. However, several highly adapted *E. coli* clones have acquired specific virulence features which lead to an increase in their ability to adapt to new niches and allows them to cause a broad range of diseases with intraintestinal and extraintestinal manifestations [36, 37]. The three clinical syndromes that can result from infection with these pathotypes are (i) diarrhoeal disease by diarrhoeagenic *E. coli* pathotypes, (ii) urinary tract infections (UTIs) by uropathogenic *E. coli* (UPEC) and (iii) sepsis/meningitis by neonatal meningitis *E. coli* (NMEC) [38].

Diarrhoeagenic *E. coli* Pathotypes

The group of *E. coli* pathotypes responsible for diarrhoea in humans and animals is commonly known as diarrhoeagenic *E. coli* pathotypes (DEC). Diarrhoeagenic *E. coli* remains one of the most important causes of diarrhoea-related mortality of children under 5 years of age [39]. The DEC pathotypes differ regarding their preferential host colonisation sites, virulence mechanisms and the resulting clinical symptoms and consequences, and are classified as follows.

- **Enteropathogenic *Escherichia coli* (EPEC):** EPEC belongs to a group of bacteria collectively known as attaching and effacing (A/E) pathogens. They are characterised by the presence of the locus for enterocyte effacement (LEE) pathogenicity island, which carries multiple virulence factors, including the *eae* gene that encodes for intimin and the *tir* gene (intimin receptor) that allows intimate adherence of EPEC to the intestinal epithelial cells. EPEC causes a profuse watery diarrhoeal disease and is considered as one of the leading causes of diarrhoea, especially among infants up to 2 years of age via faeco-oral transmission in unhygienic conditions [38]. EPEC has been isolated from human as well as animal species and many are clonally related with the sharing of various virulence properties [40].
- **Enterohaemorrhagic *Escherichia coli* (EHEC):** The EHEC pathotype constitutes a subset of Shiga toxin (Stx)-producing *E. coli* (STEC) which are associated with serious illnesses in humans. EHEC are characterised by the production of Stx, including Stx1 and/or Stx2, and the presence of LEE ('locus for enterocyte effacement'), a pathogenicity island that encodes for intimin which enables bacterial attachment to epithelial cells. Ruminants are considered as the primary

reservoir for EHEC, but the pathotype has been reported from a variety of animals, including dogs, cats, chickens and pigs. EHEC is considered as an emerging pathotype responsible for causing haemorrhagic colitis (HC) and haemolytic uraemic syndrome (HUS) in humans where the infective dose of STEC is very low (i.e. $10–10^2$). The most reported serotype of EHEC is O157:H7, which was first linked to HC and HUS cases in the early 1980s. Since then this serotype has been responsible for numerous lethal outbreaks and sporadic cases of severe diseases globally and is therefore considered to be the prototype of this pathogenic group of bacteria. The acute symptoms include HC, characterised by severe abdominal cramps and bloody diarrhoea, which may progress to life-threatening complications such as HUS or thrombotic thrombocytopenia purpura (TTP) conditions. Young children and the elderly are more susceptible and at high risk of the illness progressing to severe complications. Apart from EHEC O157:H7, other non-O157 EHEC serotypes are also emerging as a cause of food-borne illnesses; in the USA, a group often referred to as the 'big 6' (O111, O26, O121, O103, O145, O45) accounts for the majority of the non-O157:H7 serotypes isolated from clinical infections [41]. Moreover, in recent years, the emergence of particular hybrid clones such as O104:H4 enteroaggregative *E. coli* carrying *stx2* genes, which was responsible for the severe outbreak of HUS in Germany during 2011, and the spread of a new O26:H11 clone in Europe suggest that the mobility of these virulence genes is an important feature in their pathogenic potential [37]. The presence of EHEC/STEC in the environment is another issue of concern, since they can survive in the soil, manure, pastures and water, which thus represent important vehicles of transmission.

- **Enterotoxigenic *Escherichia coli* (ETEC):** The ETEC pathotype is considered a major cause of travellers' diarrhoea and is endemic in many regions of the world where hygiene is compromised. The pathogenicity of this strain is associated with the heat-labile (LT) and/or heat-stable (STa and STb) toxins as well as several colonisation factor antigens [36, 37]. Globally, ETEC is involved in the diarrhoeal infections of human infants and animals such as neonatal calves, pigs and lambs. It generally causes watery diarrhoea that can be mild or in some instances severe, resembling cholera-like illness with up to five or more daily passages of rice water-like stools. Rapid dehydration due to the continuous episodes of diarrhoea can be life-threatening.
- **Enteroaggregative *Escherichia coli* (EAEC):** The EAEC pathotype emerged as an important cause of acute and persistent diarrhoea which results in the stunting of malnourished children in developing countries. Its persistent nature seems to be more aggravated with its biofilm-producing tendency and it is difficult to treat with commonly used antibiotic therapies [42].
- **Enteroinvasive *Escherichia coli* (EIEC):** This pathotype is closely related to *Shigella* spp. EIEC dysentery resembles the mild form of bacillary dysentery produced by *Shigella dysenteriae*. Infection can occur through contaminated food or water, or mechanical vectors such as flies. The illness generally is self-limiting with no known complications [38, 43].
- **Diffusely adherent *Escherichia coli* (DAEC):** DAEC is defined by the presence of the characteristic diffuse pattern of adherence to HEp-2 cell monolayer. DAEC has been implicated as a cause of diarrhoea in several studies, particularly in children less than 12 months of age [43].

Isolation and Identification

The definitive diagnosis of diarrhoeagenic *E. coli* (DEC) requires isolation of the organism from suspected specimens such as food sample, stool, rectal swab, vomit, etc. The isolation of *E. coli* also permits additional characterisation of the bacteria by a variety of methods, including O:H serotyping, virulotyping of pathotypes, phage typing, restriction fragment length polymorphism (RLFP), pulsed-field gel electrophoresis (PFGE) and amplification-based DNA typing.

Escherichia coli from food and faecal samples are most often recovered on MacConkey or eosin methylene blue (EMB) agar. However, unlike generic *E. coli*, EHEC O157:H7 does not ferment the sugar sorbitol, so an effective method of its isolation is to plate the suspected samples onto sorbitol MacConkey medium to screen for sorbitol non-fermenting isolates. These are then typed serologically using antibodies to the O157 and H7 antigens.

Currently, there are novel rapid molecular and immunological methods available to diagnose DEC, such as ELISA, latex agglutination, *in vitro* immunochemical assays, gene probes and PCR. The PCR has been successfully used to detect virulence genes among the recovered DEC pathotypes, where the virulence marker genes are targeted in detecting the respective pathotypes [38, 43].

Prevention and Control

Diarrhoeagenic *E. coli* infections are still common in many developing countries due to poor living conditions, including inadequate water supplies, poor environmental hygiene and sanitation, and insufficient hygiene education and related awareness. The most common transmission route is faeco-oral, where outbreaks have been linked with faecal/sewage contamination of food or water supplies. Raw milk and undercooked ground beef and beef products remain important vehicles during the investigation of past O157:H7 outbreaks [38, 41]. Due to inadequate hygiene, direct contact with animals at farms or zoos has been found to transmit the pathogen to humans. Therefore, adequate personal and food hygiene is important to prevent DEC infections. Faecal contamination of the farm environment by wild animals should be avoided to prevent the entry of DEC pathotypes into the agricultural environment and hence, into a wide variety of raw foods. Finally, consumer awareness of food and personal hygiene is one of the most important interventions to prevent DEC outbreaks.

Listeria monocytogenes

Listeriosis is an important food-borne bacterial zoonosis with most of the cases predominantly associated with the species *Listeria monocytogenes*. The organism is commonly found as a saprophyte in the environment, in foods and also inhabits the intestine of animals and birds. *L. monocytogenes* mainly causes gastroenteritis and invasive listeriosis. The invasive form of the disease causes meningitis, encephalitis, miscarriage and stillbirth, where it typically affects the elderly, pregnant women, neonates and immunosuppressed individuals.

Aetiology

Listeria monocytogenes is a Gram-positive, non-sporulating, rod-shaped aerobic or facultative anaerobic micro-organism. It is an intracellular bacterium that is capable of growing at a temperature ranging between −0.5 and 50 °C (although 30–37 °C is the optimal growth temperature). Based on somatic (O) and flagellar (H) antigens, *L. monocytogenes* is classified into 13 serotypes, and three of them (1/2a, 1/2b, and 4b) are associated with most food-borne cases of human listeriosis [44].

Organism Characteristics

The versatile combination of virulence properties and the potential for biofilm formation means the bacteria are able to withstand an array of external stresses such as dry environments, high salt concentrations (10%, wt/vol), low temperatures (down to −0.5 °C) and a wide pH range (4.7–9.2) [45]. The infective dose is suspected to be high and the contamination levels in foods responsible for listeriosis cases are estimated to be more than 10^4 CFU/g [46]. On ingestion, *L. monocytogenes* can survive in phagocytes by escaping its internalisation vacuole through the action of pore-forming toxin listeriolysin O [47]. In the cytosol, the organism can polymerise actin via its surface protein ActA, and this propels the bacteria intracellularly and from one cell to its neighbours, which allows the propagation of the infection into foci without contact with the extracellular milieu.

Epidemiology and Transmission Routes

Listeria monocytogenes is ubiquitously present in nature where the soil, decaying vegetation, silage, sewage and animal intestine are considered as natural habitats of the organism. *L. monocytogenes* can colonise plants, which later can be ingested by herbivorous animals, and mostly the animals asymptomatically shed the organism in the environment through faeces [48].

In animals, the disease causes considerable mortality and production losses. The disease in animals arises mainly from the ingestion of contaminated food and water and is particularly common in ruminants fed on contaminated silage. Listeriosis in animals is also known as 'silage disease', due to its association with the feeding of poorly processed silage, and 'circling sickness' as it affects the central nervous system (CNS), which leads to unilateral circling movements of the infected animal. Listeriosis is considered a well-recognised cause of abortion, endometritis, repeat breeding, encephalitis, septicaemia and mastitis in animals.

In humans, the food-borne origin of the pathogen was formally proven in the mid-1980s during epidemiological investigations of an outbreak in Canada, which was linked to the ingestion of contaminated cole slaw [49]. The consumption of contaminated food is believed to be the principal route of infection in most human cases. Various concomitant factors which have contributed to the emergence of *L. monocytogenes* as a major food-borne pathogen are: (i) globalised industrialisation of the food chain which can result in wider distribution of contaminated food, (ii) generalisation of food refrigeration facilities which provide the opportunity for selective growth of *L. monocytogenes*, and (iii) increase in the prevalence of at-risk segments of the population, such as patients under immunosuppressive therapies, chronic immunosuppressive conditions, HIV positive patients, elder population, etc. [50].

Symptoms

The infection in humans causes a wide spectrum of illnesses, ranging from febrile gastroenteritis to invasive disease, including bacteraemia, sepsis, abortions and meningoencephalitis, especially in high-risk patients such as the elderly, immunosuppressed patients, pregnant women and unborn or newly delivered babies. In pregnant women, *L. monocytogenes* invades the foetus through the placenta and results in the development of chorioamnionitis. It may either lead to abortion from 5 months of gestation onward or the birth of a stillborn foetus or baby with a clinical syndrome known as granulomatosis infantiseptica, which is differentiated by the presence of pyogranulomatous microabscesses all over the body with a high mortality rate of 50% [51].

The infection can be treated successfully with antibiotics but despite this, high rates of hospitalisation and mortality (i.e. 20–30%) affect at-risk group including nursing infants, immunocompromised and elderly individuals [52].

Isolation and Identification

The standard microbiological culture method for detection of the presence or absence of *L. monocytogenes* in food or other clinical samples remains the gold standard. Clinical/food samples are first enriched in *Listeria* enrichment broth followed by plating onto *Listeria* selective agar(s) (e.g. ALOA agar, chromogenic agar, *L. monocytogenes* blood agar, lithium chloridephenylethanol-moxalactam [LPM] agar, Oxford agar, or PALCAM agar). The incubation of the samples is done under aerobic conditions at 30–35 °C for 24–48 hours.

Serological and molecular methods are rapid and reliable tools for the detection of *Listeria* in food and clinical samples. These include immunological methods, amplification methods, biosensor-based methods, microarray-based methods, matrix-assisted laser desorption ionisation time-of-flight mass spectrometry (MALDI-TOF MS) methods, and fluorescent *in situ* hybridisation (FISH) methods. Further, molecular typing techniques allow rapid and sensitive differentiation between *L. monocytogenes* strains, which include RAPD, PFGE, MLST, multilocus enzyme electrophoresis (MEE), etc.

Prevention and Control

Listeria monocytogenes is a ubiquitous organism with special growth abilities, attachment potential and biofilm formation on inert surfaces, which assist it to colonise and persist in the food-processing environment. Therefore, its microbiological and epidemiological surveillance, control and elimination constitute a major challenge for the food industry and public health.

RTE foods of animal or plant origin (e.g. meat, dairy products, fruits and vegetables) are considered as the primary source of the pathogen as the organism is highly tolerant to the detrimental effects of processing, such as freezing, drying and heating. *L. monocytogenes* is also able to colonise the inert surfaces of food-processing plants to form biofilms. Post-processing contamination of these products also remains a major concern since most of these products are consumed without further cooking. Hence, the primary intervention to prevent disease is to eliminate or reduce this bacterium from the food-processing chain.

The occurrence of *L. monocytogenes* in processed food is inevitable, but contamination can be reduced by providing attention to hygiene and processing practices. Standard operating protocols should be undertaken to target the pathogen in the environment, farm or food-processing plants. Cleanliness should be maintained in the farm environment. Livestock houses should be cleaned and disinfected regularly. The feed may also be an important source of *L. monocytogenes* contamination in animals; therefore, animal feed should be stored in hygienic conditions as per the standard protocol to check microbial growth. Entry of wild and stray animals to the farm and feed storage area should be restricted. Plans for the proper monitoring of personal hygiene of workers should be implemented by food-processing units. Proper sanitary conditions can reduce the colonisation, transmission and cross-contamination of the pathogen among various food products and the environment.

At the consumer level, ways to prevent the disease include the following.

- Keep uncooked meats separate from vegetables and cooked foods and RTE foods.
- Raw food from animal sources (e.g. mutton, beef, pork, poultry meat) must be cooked properly and wash raw vegetables thoroughly before eating.
- Avoid the consumption of raw (unpasteurised) milk or milk products.
- Wash hands, knives and cutting boards after handling uncooked foods.
- When using a microwave oven to cook or reheat food, observe the standing times recommended by the oven manufacturer to ensure that food attains an even temperature before it is eaten.

Salmonellosis

Salmonellosis is caused by the bacteria *Salmonella*, and the clinical form of the disease ranges from common gastroenteritis (diarrhoea, abdominal cramps, fever) to enteric fever (including typhoid fever). More than 2500 different serotypes or serovars of *Salmonella* have been identified which can affect a broad range of hosts, including humans. Due to the ubiquitous and hardy nature of the organism, *Salmonella* can survive several weeks in various foods and environments, thereby posing a significant threat to the food industry.

Aetiology

Salmonella is a Gram-negative, facultatively anaerobic, non-sporulating, rod-shaped bacterium belonging to the family Enterobacteriaceae. There are more than 2500 serotypes identified according to differences in the structure of the lipopolysaccharide O-antigen (somatic) and H-antigen (ciliary) [53].

The nomenclature of the *Salmonella* genus is complex. Based on genetic relatedness and biochemical characteristics, the genus is divided into two species: *S. bongori* and *S. enterica* [54]. Based on their usual habitat, biochemical and genetic criteria, the genus is divided into seven subspecies: I, II, IIIa, IIIb, IV, V and VI [54]. *S. bongori* species has serotypes belonging to subspecies V whereas *S. enterica* has subspecies I, II, IIIa, IIIb, IV and VI. They are *S. enterica* subsp. *enterica*, *S. enterica* subsp. *salamae*, *S. enterica* subsp. *arizonae*, *S. enterica* subsp. *diarizonae*, *S. enterica* subsp. *hountanae* and *S. enterica* subsp. *indica*, respectively.

Organism Characteristics

The genus *Salmonella* contains intracellular facultative pathogens. They can grow at temperatures ranging between 8 and 45 °C (optimum temperature 37 °C), at pH range 4.0–9.5 (optimum pH 6.5–7.0) and in conditions of low water activity (a_W) of 0.94.

Salmonella enterica subsp. *enterica* (subspecies I) harbours most of the serotypes and they are responsible for around 99% of salmonellosis cases in humans, warm-blooded animals and birds [55]. The ability to adapt to the specific host and the resultant pathogenicity depend on the serotype; for example, *S. typhi* and *S. paratyphi* A, B and C are pathogenic for humans but their presence in animals is asymptomatic. Serotype *S. cholerasuis* mostly affects pigs, but also causes salmonellosis in humans, and the common serotypes *S. enteritidis* and *S. typhimurium* cause gastrointestinal tract infections in humans, as well as various symptoms in infected animals.

Epidemiology and Transmission Routes

Salmonella spp. have various attributes for wider distribution, which include broad host range, efficient faecal shedding from carrier animals, long survival in the environment, and effective transmission through vectors (e.g. feed, fomites, vehicles, etc.). In addition, most of the host species remain asymptomatic and become long-term carriers, which can continuously or intermittently shed the organism in faeces. Shedding of the organism can be exacerbated by stressors, such as improper animal transportation, concurrent diseases, antibiotic therapy, etc.

In humans, infection with *Salmonella* spp. might be the result of direct contact with infected animals/birds or indirect contact through food or environment. Animal foods (e.g. meat, eggs, raw milk) and vegetables contaminated with animal faecal microbiota can be important sources of pathogenic *Salmonella*.

The intestines of poultry and other animals are asymptomatically colonised by *Salmonella* spp. During unhygienic food production, the meat of these animals can be contaminated with *Salmonella* spp. on contact with gastrointestinal contents during slaughter. In addition, the vertical route of transmission of *Salmonella* spp. is also possible, which includes the transovarial transmission of the organism to the offspring/eggs. Due to the bacterial colonisation of the hen's genital system, the eggs may be infected at the stage of formation. Moreover, eggs may also be infected through the environment, as the bacteria may not only be present on the surface of an eggshell but also penetrate the inside of the eggs.

Symptoms

The pathogenic strains of *Salmonella* spp. are associated with two types of clinical manifestations in humans: (i) non-typhoidal *Salmonella* and (ii) typhoidal *Salmonella* (*S. enterica* serovars *typhi*, *paratyphi* A, *paratyphi* B and *paratyphi* C).

Non-typhoidal Salmonellosis

Salmonellosis can be caused by many of the non-typhoidal serotypes of the *Salmonella* genus (excluding *S. typhi* and *S. paratyphi* A, B and C), isolated both from humans and animals. The serotypes *S. typhimurium*, *S. enteritidis*, *S. newport* and *S. heidelberg* are often responsible for food poisoning cases in humans, and others like *S. cholerasuis* and *S. dublin* can also cause diarrhoeal diseases [56]. The infective dose for salmonellosis ranges between 10^6 and 10^8 cells [53]. The incubation period lasts for 6–72 hours, which depends on the infective dose and the host's immune status [56]. The common clinical signs of infection are stomach aches and diarrhoea, but other possible symptoms include vomiting, nausea, fever, muscular pain, cramps and loss of appetite. Even after the clinical phase, *Salmonella* spp. may still reside in the intestinal tract of an adult for 4 weeks and in children for up to 7 weeks. A small number of people demonstrate an asymptomatic carrier stage for a year after the disappearance of symptoms. Bacteraemia may develop in 5–10% of patients infected with *Salmonella* spp. that may lead to focal infections, such as meningitis, endocarditis, arthritis and osteitis [57].

Typhoidal and Paratyphoid Fever

The serotype *S. typhi* causing typhoid fever can be transmitted between humans (without the involvement of animals) through the ingestion of contaminated food or water as a result of poor hygiene. The symptoms of typhoid fever include headache, fever, stomach pain, diarrhoea or constipation, and loss of appetite. In severe cases without proper treatment, respiratory problems, neurological changes, perforation of the intestine, and hepatic and splenic injury may be observed.

Isolation and Identification

Isolation of *Salmonella* spp. from food and clinical samples (e.g. stool samples, body tissue or fluids) can be carried out by the enrichment of the samples in suitable media (e.g. tetrathionate broth, selenite broth, etc.), followed by plating on selective agar (e.g. brilliant green, bismuth sulfite, blood agar, *Salmonella-Shigella* agar or MacConkey agar). However, the standard protocol may vary for different serovars.

Among serological tests, the Widal test measures agglutinating antibodies against LPS (O) and flagellar (H) antigens of *S. typhi* in the sera of individuals with suspected enteric fever. Enzyme-linked immunosorbent assays (ELISAs) have been used to detect the antibody response to LPS, flagella, Vi capsular polysaccharide or outer membrane protein antigens. Molecular tools including PCR and real-time PCR can be used for detection of virulence genes and characterisation of isolates. Novel proteomic and immunoscreening approaches have been recently developed to detect antibodies and antigens that have a higher level of specificity than those used currently [58].

Prevention and Control

Prevention and control measures for salmonellosis depend on efforts to minimise the exposure of animals and humans to the pathogen. Prevention requires control measures at all stages of the food chain, from agricultural production to processing, manufacturing and preparation of foods at the consumer end. Contact between infants/young children and pet animals (such as cats, dogs and turtles) needs careful supervision. National and regional surveillance systems should be in place to monitor FBDs and also to detect and respond to salmonellosis and other enteric infections in early stages, thus preventing them from further spread. Other precautions include the following.

- Ensure food is properly cooked and still hot when served.
- Avoid raw milk and milk products.
- When the safety of drinking water is questionable, boil it or if this is not possible, disinfect it with a reliable disinfectant.
- Wash fruits and vegetables carefully, particularly if they are eaten raw.
- Wash hands thoroughly and frequently using soap, in particular after contact with pets or farm animals, or after having been to the toilet.
- Food handlers should observe hygienic rules of food preparation. Food handlers who suffer from fever, diarrhoea, vomiting or visible infected skin lesions should report to their employer immediately.

Staphylococcus aureus

Aetiology

The genus *Staphylococcus* (*staphyle* in Greek means 'bunch of grapes') comprises several species and subspecies. Among these, the bacterium *S. aureus* is globally considered as one of the most common food-borne pathogens and is predominantly associated with staphylococcal food poisoning [59]. The organism is a Gram-positive, non-motile, catalase-positive, facultative anaerobic coccus, which appears in pairs, short chains or bunched in grape-like clusters on microscopic examination. *S. aureus* is an opportunistic pathogen that can cause multiple infectious diseases of diverse severity in both humans and animals.

The pathogen came to public attention due to its high mortality associated with the emergence of resistant strains such as methicillin-resistant *Staphylococcus aureus* (MRSA), which was first reported in the 1960s and is now regarded as a common hospital-acquired nosocomial pathogen. In addition, the emergence of MRSA in livestock and the possibility of human cross-contamination are serious concerns due to its zoonotic potential [60].

Organism Characteristics

Staphylococcus aureus is one of the most resistant among non-spore forming human pathogens. The organism can grow in a wide range of temperatures (7–47.8 °C, with an optimum of 30–37 °C for growth), pH (4.2–9.3, with an optimum of 7.0–7.5) and sodium chloride concentrations (up to 15% NaCl). The organism is peculiar in its ability to grow at a level of water activity (a_W) as low as 0.83 (optimal growth occurs at a_W >0.99). These characteristics enable the bacteria to survive in a wide variety of foods, mainly those of animal origin [61]. The organism has a variety of virulence factors that, singly and in combination, can result in severe infection. The extracellular active substances which contribute to the pathogenicity include coagulase, haemolysins, nuclease, acid phosphatase, lipase, protease, fibrinolysin, enterotoxins and toxic shock syndrome toxins [62].

Several species of *S. aureus* (including both coagulase-positive and -negative strains) can produce heat-stable enterotoxins that cause gastroenteritis in humans. These toxins are resistant to proteolytic enzymes, such as trypsin and pepsin, which allow them to transit intact through the digestive tract [63]. Around 26 staphylococcal enterotoxins (SE) and enterotoxin-like types have been described and the classic types, which include SEA, SEB, SEC (with SEC1, SEC2, SEC3, SEC ovine and SEC bovine variants), SED and SEE, are mainly involved in food-borne outbreaks [63].

Epidemiology and Transmission Routes

Staphylococcus aureus is ubiquitous in the environment with a broad host range, including humans, food-producing animals and birds [59]. The organism is present in the nasal passage, throat and skin of 50% or more of healthy individuals [62]. Therefore, food contamination with *S. aureus* may occur directly from infected food-producing animals, may result from poor hygiene protocols during food processing, the retail and storage of food or due to cross-contamination at the consumer's end due to lack of hygiene. Several foods of animal origin, including milk and dairy products, meat, poultry and eggs, are common vehicles that are frequently associated with staphylococcal food poisoning outbreaks [63].

Symptoms

The bacteria can cause various disease conditions, ranging from skin infection to serious infections such as septicaemia, necrotising fasciitis, endocarditis, necrotising pneumonia and toxic shock syndrome [62]. Moreover, MRSA has been associated with severe nosocomial infections which can result in potentially life-threatening conditions [60].

Food poisoning outbreaks are mainly associated with the consumption of food contaminated with enterotoxigenic *S. aureus* or ingestion of the preformed enterotoxin (i.e. intoxication). The organism can be destroyed by common heat processing but the destruction of viable cells by heat does not destroy the biological activity of preformed staphylococcal enterotoxins. The intoxication dose of staphylococcal enterotoxins is less than 1.0 μg and usually, this toxin level is reached when *S. aureus* populations exceed 100 000 organisms/g in food. This level is indicative of unsanitary conditions in which the product can be rendered injurious to health [62]. Moreover, staphylococcal enterotoxins can act as superantigens which can stimulate large population of T-cells (approximately 20–30%) leading to the production of a cytokine bolus [64]. The enterotoxins stimulate the emetic center of the CNS and inhibit water and sodium absorption in the small intestine. They are responsible for symptoms of acute gastroenteritis.

The disease has a short incubation period and clinical signs appear within 2–4 hours after food consumption. It is characterised by nausea, vomiting, chills, headache and abdominal cramping with or without diarrhoea and usually without fever. Severe outcomes occasionally occur among susceptible individuals, such as children, immunocompromised and the elderly population [62, 63].

Isolation and Identification

The widely used criterion for the identification of pathogenic staphylococci is their ability to produce coagulase. Gold colony pigmentation, production of coagulase, fermentation of mannitol and trehalose, and production of heat-stable thermonuclease distinguish *S. aureus* from other staphylococcal species. The common media used for the isolation of staphylococci are mannitol salt agar and Baird–Parker agar. Molecular-based assays (e.g. real-time PCR and quantitative PCR) and immunological techniques (ELISA, agglutination test, gel diffusion tests, fluorescent immunoassays, etc.) are rapid tools for the identification of *S. aureus* contamination. Molecular subtyping tools used to assess genetic relatedness among the recovered isolates include PFGE and MLST [62].

Prevention and Control

The prevention of staphylococcal infection and/or intoxication requires strategies to interrupt various chains of transmission. In the past, many outbreaks were linked to foods that require a lot of handling when they are being processed or prepared and/or are not kept at proper refrigerator temperature (40 °F or below). If food is stored at room temperature for a prolonged time, the organism can produce its toxin while multiplying in the food. Therefore, avoiding the time and temperature abuse of food products at high risk of containing *S. aureus* is essential in preventing proliferation of the bacterium and subsequent production of enterotoxin. Some prevention strategies include the following.

- Cook the food thoroughly and prevent contamination and cross-contamination.
- Public awareness regarding hygienic handling of foods of animal origin, decontamination of equipment and surfaces, proper cooking and storage of food, etc.
- Preventive systems like Hazard Analysis and Critical Control Points (HACCP), Good Manufacturing Practices (GMP) and Good Hygienic Practices (GHP) should be implemented by food establishments.

Vibriosis

Vibrio species are natural inhabitants of the aquatic environment, mainly in brackish and salt water. *Vibrio* spp. include well-known as well as emerging pathogens, such as *V. cholerae*, *V. parahaemolyticus* and *V. vulnificus*. The pathogenic strains of *Vibrio* can cause serious food-borne illnesses in both humans and animals, and also pose a significant threat to the aquaculture industry.

Vibrio cholerae

Aetiology

Vibrio cholerae is a motile, comma-shaped Gram-negative bacteria with a single polar flagellum. The organism is a natural inhabitant of the aquatic environment, particularly brackish riverine, estuarine and coastal waters. *V. cholerae* is associated with the disease known as cholera, which is an acute intestinal infection that leads to rapid and severe dehydrating diarrhoea. More than 200 serogroups are reported within the species *V. cholerae*, and among these *V. cholerae* serogroup O1 is considered the most notorious strain causing epidemic or pandemic diarrhoeal disease [65]. Based on phenotypic and genotypic characteristics, *V. cholerae* O1 is subdivided into two biotypes, classical and El Tor.

Epidemiology and Transmission Routes

The disease cholera has had devastating effects on civilisations throughout history. To date, a total of seven pandemics have been recorded across the globe. The first pandemic started in 1817, and subsequent pandemics started during 1829, 1852, 1863, 1881, 1889 and 1961, and the last is still persisting. The current seventh pandemic of cholera began in 1961 and is attributed to *V. cholerae* O1 biotype El Tor lineage, which is different from the classical biotype *V. cholerae* O1 (which was associated with previous pandemics). Cholera is now considered endemic in many countries. Emerging infections due to the strain of non-O1 *V. cholerae*, designated as *V. cholerae* 0139, was first identified in Bangladesh in 1992 and later reported from various parts of Bangladesh, India and other countries. There is no difference in the illness caused by the two serogroups.

Cholera is endemic to regions with poor water, sanitation and hygiene infrastructures, such as sub-Saharan Africa and regions of the Middle East and Southeast Asian countries. Typical at-risk areas include periurban slums and camps for internally displaced persons or refugees, where minimum requirements of clean water and sanitation are not met.

Humans are the natural host for *V. cholerae* and transmission is mainly through the faecal–oral route. However, *V. cholerae* is also found as a free-living organism in brackish water and can survive in fresh or salt water, which explains the occasional outbreaks associated with shellfish.

Cholera spreads through the faecal–oral route, either directly from person to person or indirectly through contaminated fluids from environmental reservoirs, foods and vectors (e.g. flies), and fomites. The bacteria alternate between states of free-swimming cells and biofilm-like aggregates to efficiently colonise the small intestine. Bacteria in the biofilm state are more resistant to stressful conditions in the host, exhibit a lower infective dose, and may enhance the dissemination of the disease with more severity [66].

Symptoms

Cholera has a typical incubation period of 1–2 days (the median incubation period is reported to be 1.5 days) [67]. Acute gastroenteritis is the most common clinical manifestation of non-O1 *V. cholerae* infection for both sporadic and outbreaks cases. Infected persons excrete *V. cholerae* in their stool, where the duration may be as short as one day among asymptomatic infected contacts, whereas symptomatic patients may excrete the organism for up to 1–2 weeks and can potentially contaminate the environment. The classic diarrhoeal presentation consists of watery foul-smelling mucus described as 'rice water' stools. Many times, this potentially fatal diarrhoeal disease results in large volumes of watery stool, causing rapid dehydration that can progress to hypovolaemic shock and metabolic acidosis. If treatment does not start immediately, death rates as high as 70% have been reported [68].

Isolation and Identification

The confirmatory diagnosis of *V. cholerae* consists of isolation of the organism in stool cultures, PCR and other rapid tests. Isolation and identification of *V. cholerae* serogroup O1 or O139 by the culture of stool specimen remains the gold standard diagnosis. Cary–Blair medium is considered ideal for transport, and selective thiosulfate–citrate–bile salts–sucrose (TCBS) agar is ideal for isolation and identification. As an adequate diagnosis can be achieved clinically, treatment should never be delayed for the results of diagnostic testing.

Prevention and Control

The risk factors for cholera include lack of access to safe water, poor hygiene and sanitation, and unsafe food handling behaviours. A multifaceted approach is key for controlling cholera and reducing mortality. A combination of public health efforts including water sanitation and hygiene, social mobilisation, treatment facilities and oral cholera vaccines (OCV) can be applied in endemic regions. To prevent the bacteria from spreading, all faeces (human waste) from sick persons should be disposed of carefully to ensure that it does not contaminate surroundings. People caring for cholera patients must wash their hands thoroughly after touching inanimate object(s) that might be contaminated with patients' faeces.

Cholera is an easily treatable disease. The majority of cases can be treated successfully through prompt administration of oral rehydration solution (ORS). Currently, there are three World Health Organization (WHO) prequalified OCV: Dukoral®, Shanchol™ and Euvichol-Plus®.

Vibrio parahaemolyticus

Vibrio parahaemolyticus is the cause of food-borne diarrhoeal disease associated with seafood worldwide. The organism occurs naturally in marine environments and is frequently isolated from varieties of raw seafood. The consumption of raw or undercooked seafood contaminated with *V. parahaemolyticus* may lead to the development of acute gastroenteritis characterised by diarrhoea, headache, vomiting, nausea and abdominal cramps. The pathogen is a common cause of food-borne illnesses in many Asian countries, including China, Japan and Taiwan, and is recognised as the leading cause of human gastroenteritis associated with seafood consumption in the United States [69].

Organism Characteristics

Vibrio parahaemolyticus is a Gram-negative, halophilic non-spore-forming rod-shaped organism. It is a multiserotype bacterium, containing at least 12 different O antigens and more than 70 different K antigens in its capsule. Consequently, serotyping has been widely used to characterise *V. parahaemolyticus* and to study its pathogenesis. Among the serotypes, three serotypes (O3:K6, O4:K68 and O1:K untypeable) are extremely virulent and pathogenic to humans [70]. Since 1996, increased incidences of gastroenteritis caused by *V. parahaemolyticus* serotype O3:K6 have been reported in many countries [71].

Clinical strains of *V. parahaemolyticus* can be differentiated from environmental strains by their ability to produce thermostable direct haemolysin (TDH), an enzyme that can lyse red blood cells on Wagatsuma blood agar plates. The haemolytic activity of TDH, also named the Kanagawa phenomenon, is reported to be commonly associated with strains isolated from humans with gastroenteritis but were rarely observed in environmental isolates. Despite epidemiological investigations which revealed a strong association between the Kanagawa phenomenon (KP) and the pathogenicity of *V. parahaemolyticus*, KP-negative strains that did not produce TDH but a TDH-related haemolysin (TRH) have also been isolated from outbreak patients. Therefore, the pathogenicity of *V. parahaemolyticus* appears to be linked to the presence of *tdh* and *trh* genes. Thermolabile haemolysin (TLH) is another haemolysin of *V. parahaemolyticus* encoded by the *tlh* gene and causes the lysis of red blood cells. TLH is expressed by all clinical and environmental strains of *V. parahaemolyticus*, and the gene is significantly upregulated under simulated intestinal infection conditions [72].

Transmission Routes

Among seafood, shellfish is regarded as a high-risk food because it is infested with large populations of bacteria, including *V. parahaemolyticus*, to levels higher than those in the surrounding water [72]. The degree of *V. parahaemolyticus* contamination in raw shellfish is also known to relate to the water temperatures. *V. parahaemolyticus* is more likely to be detected in oysters harvested in the spring and summer than in the winter [73].

Symptoms

Clinical signs generally appear within 2–10 days. The acute gastroenteritis phase is characterised by diarrhoea, headache, vomiting, nausea, abdominal cramps and low fever. The distinct pathological changes in patients include mild erosion of the jejunum and ileum, gastric inflammation and internal organ damage (liver, spleen, lung congestion, etc.). Although the gastroenteritis caused by *V. parahaemolyticus* infection is often self-limited, the infection may cause life-threatening septicaemia in people with underlying medical conditions such as liver disease or immune disorders.

Isolation and Identification

For isolation, test samples are incubated in two enrichment media (salt polymyxin B broth and alkaline saline peptone water or saline glucose culture medium with sodium dodecyl sulfate) at

35 °C for 7–8 hours. The enriched samples are then plated on selective media (e.g. TCBS and triphenyltetrazolium chloride soya tryptone agar [TSAT]). After incubation, colonies that are smooth, green and 2–3 mm in diameter on TCBS or smooth, flat, dark red and 2–3 mm in diameter on TSAT are considered as characteristic colonies which need further confirmation by biochemical or molecular tests. A chromogenic medium (Bio-Chrome Vibrio medium) has been developed to allow differentiation of *V. parahaemolyticus* from other *Vibrio* spp. based on the formation of unique purple colonies on the medium.

TDH contributes to the formation of a distinct haemolytic ring on blood cell agar plates with high concentrations of salt and D-mannitol as the carbon source. This process is known as the Kanagawa phenomenon (KP). In past, the KP was regarded as an important indicator in the identification of pathogenic and non-pathogenic *V. parahaemolyticus* strains. However, the detection of *V. parahaemolyticus* based on KP is time-consuming, labour-intensive and unreliable, and involves the evaluation of large numbers of samples. Therefore, this method has been replaced with more specific, sensitive and rapid novel molecular tools such as PCR using the DNA primers targeting *tdh* and *trh* genes.

Immunological methods such as ELISA based on monoclonal antibodies directed against TDH, TLH and TRH have been used to identify these proteins in pathogenic isolates of *V. parahaemolyticus*.

Prevention and Control

The ubiquitous nature of *Vibrio* species in marine and estuarine environments makes it difficult to harvest seafood free from these species. Shellfish harvested for consumption need to be cooled down to 10 °C (50 °F). Thermal processes such as cold storage, freezing and low-temperature pasteurisation have been reported to achieve certain reductions of *Vibrio* species in oysters. The harvesting of oysters should be avoided during the warmer summer months in high-risk areas. Relaying and depuration are common approaches for reducing bacterial contaminants in shellfish.

- In the relaying process, shellfish are transferred before harvest from polluted areas to an unpolluted waterway for natural biological purification.
- Depuration is a controlled process that allows shellfish to purge sand and grit from the gut into clean sea water. The process usually leads to a reduction of microbial contaminants in shellfish and therefore increases the shelf-life of refrigerated products.

Consumer-level prevention includes the following.

- Keep raw seafood separate from other foods.
- Most infections caused by *V. parahaemolyticus* can be prevented by thorough cooking of seafood, especially oysters.
- Proper washing of hands, cutting boards, cutlery and utensils after handling raw seafood.

Vibrio vulnificus

Vibrio vulnificus is an emerging and enigmatic human pathogen that is considered as part of the normal microbiota of estuarine waters. The organism has been isolated from different environmental sources, including water, sediment and seafood (mainly molluscan shellfish) around the world [74].

Organism Characteristics

Three biotypes of *V. vulnificus* have been recognised. Biotype 1 is almost exclusively associated with human disease and is of great public health concern. Biotype 2 is associated primarily with infection in eels. In 1999, the third biotype of *V. vulnificus* was reported in Israel from persons who had received puncture wounds following contact with *Tilapia* [75]. *V. vulnificus* is an obligate halophile, requiring a minimum of 0.5% (wt/vol) NaCl for growth. This organism possesses a wide array of virulence factors, including acid neutralisation, capsular polysaccharide expression, iron acquisition, cytotoxicity, motility and expression of proteins involved in attachment and adhesion.

Epidemiology and Transmission Routes

Vibrio vulnificus occurs in estuarine environments worldwide; however, due to the effect of global climate change, there is an increasing incidence and geographic distribution of the pathogen [76]. The common sources of human infections are associated with the consumption of raw/undercooked molluscan shellfish, primarily oysters (mainly responsible for primary septicaemias) and/or exposure to seawater or seafood products (responsible for wound infections, mainly associated with recreational activities such as swimming, fishing and handling seafood).

Symptoms

Vibrio vulnificus is a serious human pathogen that carries the highest fatality rate of any food-borne pathogen [77]. *V. vulnificus* infections are characterised by a short incubation period typically within 24 hours of exposure [78]. Clinical signs range from relatively mild gastroenteritis with diarrhoea and abdominal cramps to the lethal septicemic form. Primary septicaemia is the most lethal infection caused by *V. vulnificus*, with an average mortality rate exceeding 50% [78]. In addition to septicaemia, *V. vulnificus* can produce serious wound infections that typically result from exposure of open wounds to water harbouring the bacteria. Severe wound infections are often characterised by necrotising skin and soft tissue infection, including fasciitis and gangrene. Most cases occur in immunocompromised patients with underlying conditions that result in elevated serum iron levels (e.g. alcohol-associated liver cirrhosis) [74].

Isolation and Identification

Vibrio vulnificus is known to enter a 'VBNC' state at temperatures below 13 °C, thus the inability to culture the organism at low temperatures does not necessarily mean the absence of the organism [74]. Most studies on the distribution of *V. vulnificus* in marine environments employ colistin-polymyxin B-cellobiose agar or its modifications for isolation of the organism. Due to significant phenotypic variation exhibited by *V. vulnificus*, molecular methods are commonly used to characterise the organism, including the use of DNA probes, PCR assays and immunological methods.

Prevention and Control

Proper cooking of oysters eliminates *V. vulnificus* cells and thus avoids infection. Other methods for post-harvest treatment of oysters to minimise the load of *V. vulnificus* include low-temperature pasteurisation, quick freezing, high hydrostatic pressure and irradiation (0.75–1.0 kGy). However, proper hygiene at the consumer level is paramount to avoid cross-contamination of food products.

Yersiniosis

Yersinia enterocolitica is the causative agent of yersiniosis. The organism is widespread, and habitats include the intestinal tracts of mammals, birds, cold-blooded animals and aquatic niches. Mostly, the isolates recovered from porcine sources contain human pathogenic serogroups. However, other animals like dogs, sheep and wild rodents may also harbour pathogenic *Y. enterocolitica* strains. Most of the environmental isolates are avirulent. *Y. enterocolitica* is mainly associated with gastrointestinal tract infections in humans.

Aetiology

The *Yersinia* genus belongs to the Enterobacteriaceae family and has 17 species. The three species that are pathogenic for humans are *Y. pestis* (transmitted by fleas which cause plague), *Y. pseudotuberculosis* (causative agent of rodentiosis) and *Y. enterocolitica* (causative agent of yersiniosis). Based on biochemical reactions, a total of six different biotypes of *Y. enterocolitica* have been reported: 1A, 1B, 2, 3, 4 and 5. The serotypes of *Y. enterocolitica* are classified based on lipopolysaccharide O-antigen. Eleven of the serotypes belonging to these six biotypes are associated with the development of yersiniosis in humans. The most pathogenic bioserotypes are: 1B/O:8, 2/O:5,27, 2/O:9, 3/O:3 and 4/O:3 [53]. Serotype O:3 of biotype 4 is considered to be responsible for the high incidence of yersiniosis among humans in Europe, Canada, Japan and China [79]. *Y. enterocolitica* biotype 1B with serotype O:8 is highly pathogenic and mainly associated with clinical settings. However, serogroups 4/O:3 and 2/O:9 are the most common causes of yersiniosis worldwide but are less destructive in clinical outcomes [80].

Organism Characteristics

Yersinia enterocolitica is a Gram-negative, facultatively anaerobic, non-sporulating and psychrophilic enteropathogen. These microbes are motile in temperatures ranging between 22 and 30 °C, due to a flagellum positioned on a pole of the bacterial surface. However, they are not mobile at 37 °C [80]. The bacteria can grow at temperatures ranging between 0 and 45 °C, whereas their optimum growth temperature ranges between 25 and 32 °C [81]. *Y. enterocolitica* can survive under the VBNC condition and can proliferate and produce a thermostable toxin under cooling conditions (4–8 °C). The organism grows at an environmental pH <9, and the water activity (a_w) must not be lower than 0.96. Low pH and the presence of organic acids, including acetic acid, lactic acid and citric acid, may inhibit the growth of *Y. enterocolitica*.

The plasmid of *Yersinia* virulence (pYV) with a size of 64–75 kb is the most important virulence marker of *Y. enterocolitica*. Important virulence factors include adhesion/invasion factors, lipopolysaccharides, Ysa T3SS, high pathogenicity island (HPI) genes and thermostable enterotoxin (a protein encoded by the chromosomal gene *yst*). Iron appears to play a crucial role in the pathogenesis of *Yersinia*, as one of the major differences between low- and high-pathogenicity strains is their ability to capture iron molecules.

Transmission Routes

Raw or undercooked pork is an important source of the organism, but raw milk and dairy products, meat and seafood, and contaminated drinking water can also be the source of infection. Food may be contaminated by contact with an infected animal, surface or equipment. Although pigs are considered as the main reservoir of *Y. enterocolitica*, the organism is abundant in the environment and has been isolated from other animals including poultry, ruminants, wild animals, rodents, cats and dogs. Pigs and other animals can harbour *Y. enterocolitica* asymptomatically. In pigs, the pathogen can occupy tongues, oral cavity, tonsils, lymph nodes and intestines, where it can shed through faeces. During slaughter and processing of meat, *Y. enterocolitica* may be transferred from infected tissues of the animal onto the meat and meat products.

Symptoms

Yersinia enterocolitica is primarily a gastrointestinal tract pathogen, but it has a strong propensity for extraintestinal spread. The clinical manifestations of the infection depend on the underlying immune status of the host and the bioserotype of the organism. The most frequent outcomes in children are enteritis, accompanied by fever, vomiting and watery, occasionally bloody diarrhoea.

The illness usually lasts from 3 to 28 days. In rare cases, the infection can cause erythema nodosum or joint pain that appears a month after the initial symptoms. In young adults, symptoms include acute terminal ileitis and mesenteric lymphadenitis with fever, diarrhoea and abdominal pain. The abdominal pain is usually localised in the right lower quadrant, thus mimicking appendicitis. This clinical syndrome usually lasts for 1–2 weeks. In severe cases, fatal NEC as well as a 'pseudo-tumorigenic' form of suppurative mesenteric adenitis may occur.

Sepsis is a rare complication of *Y. enterocolitica* infection which has been reported among immunocompromised patients or those who have a predisposing underlying disease or are in an iron-overloaded state. The clinical course of septicaemia may include liver and spleen abscess, pharyngitis, pneumonia, septic arthritis, meningitis, cellulitis, empyema and osteomyelitis, and may evolve into endocarditis. Unfortunately, *Y. enterocolitica* has emerged as a significant cause of blood transfusion-associated bacteraemia, associated with its ability to survive and replicate at low temperatures, even at 4 °C [79].

Isolation and Identification

The isolation of *Y. enterocolitica* strains from stool samples can be achieved on CIN agar (Cefsulodin, Irgasan, Novobiocin). CIN agar is a selective medium that inhibits the growth of normal enteric organisms and improves the recovery of *Y. enterocolitica* from faeces. The characteristic translucent and sharp-bordered colonies with a deep red centre (due to mannitol fermentation) are usually referred to as 'bull's eye' colonies. This allows easy identification of the organism on CIN agar. Serogroup analysis can be performed using specific antisera for typing pathogenic strains. This methodology is particularly important to detect serogroups O:3 and O:9 which are associated with most of the outbreaks. Molecular tools like PCR and MALDI-TOF mass spectrometry analysis can be used for rapid and accurate identification of the organism.

Prevention and Control

Like other food-borne pathogens, prevention and control measures are based on hygienic maintenance of the food chain. Some important considerations include the following.

- Avoid eating raw or undercooked pork. Thoroughly cook raw meat and poultry to destroy the bacteria.
- Keep raw pork and other meat separate from fresh produce and other foods.
- Wash raw fruits and vegetables before eating.
- Proper washing of hands, cutting boards, cutlery and utensils after handling uncooked pork.
- Always wash hands after contact with farm animals, pets, animal faeces and animal environments.

References

1 Cheng, A.C. and Currie, B.J. (2005). Melioidosis: epidemiology, pathophysiology, and management. *Clinical Microbiology Reviews* 18 (2): 383–416.
2 Centers for Disease Control and Prevention (2017). Federal Select Agent Program. www.selectagents.gov/
3 CFSPH Technical Fact Sheets. Melioidosis (2016). www.cfsph.iastate.edu/diseaseinfo/disease/?disease=melioidosis&lang=en
4 Lau, S.K., Sridhar, S., Ho, C.C. et al. (2015). Laboratory diagnosis of melioidosis: past, present and future. *Experimental Biology and Medicine 240* (6): 742–751.

5 Currie, B.J. (2015). Melioidosis: evolving concepts in epidemiology, pathogenesis, and treatment. *Seminars in Respiratory and Critical Care Medicine* 36: 111–125.

6 Popoff, M.R. (2020). Tetanus in animals. *Journal of Veterinary Diagnostic Investigation 32* (2): 184–191.

7 Afshar, M., Raju, M., Ansell, D., and Bleck, T.P. (2011). Narrative review: tetanus – a health threat after natural disasters in developing countries. *Annals of Internal Medicine 154* (5): 329–335.

8 Centers for Disease Control and Prevention (2019). Prevention of tetanus. www.cdc.gov/tetanus/about/prevention.html

9 Damborg, P., Broens, E.M., Chomel, B.B. et al. (2016). Bacterial zoonoses transmitted by household pets: state-of-the-art and future perspectives for targeted research and policy actions. *Journal of Comparative Pathology 155* (1): S27–S40.

10 Centers for Disease Control and Prevention Pets and *Capnocytophaga* germs (2018). www.cdc.gov/capnocytophaga/pets/index.html

11 Glaser, C., Lewis, P., and Wong, S. (2000). Pet-, animal-, and vector-borne infections. *Pediatrics in Review 21*, 7: 219.

12 Krauss, H., Weber, A., Appel, M. et al. (2003). *Zoonoses: Infectious Diseases Transmissible from Animals to Humans*, 456. Washington, DC: ASM Press.

13 Centre for Food Security and Public Health (2013). Rat bite fever. www.cfsph.iastate.edu/Factsheets/pdfs/rat_bite_fever.pdf

14 Fukushima, K., Yanagisawa, N., Imaoka, K. et al. (2018). Rat-bite fever due to *Streptobacillus notomytis* isolated from a human specimen. *Journal of Infection and Chemotherapy 24* (4): 302–304.

15 Elliott, S.P. (2007). Rat bite fever and *Streptobacillus moniliformis*. *Clinical Microbiology Reviews 20* (1): 13–22.

16 Jessberger, N., Dietrich, R., Granum, P.E., and Märtlbauer, E. (2020). The *Bacillus cereus* food infection as multifactorial process. *Toxins 12* (11): 701.

17 U.S. Food and Drug Administration (FDA) (2012). *Bacillus cereus* and other *Bacillus* s. In: *Bad Bug Book: Foodborne Pathogenic Microorganisms and Natural Toxins Handbook* (ed. Center for Food Safety and Applied Nutrition), 92–95. Silver Spring, MD: U.S. Food and Drug Administration.

18 Wijnands, L.M., Dufrenne, J.B., Zwietering, M.H., and Van Leusden, F.M. (2006). Spores from mesophilic *Bacillus cereus* strains germinate better and grow faster in simulated gastro-intestinal conditions than spores from psychrotrophic strains. *International Journal of Food Microbiology 112* (2): 120–128.

19 Tuipulotu, D.E., Mathur, A., Ngo, C., and Man, S.M. (2021). *Bacillus cereus*: epidemiology, virulence factors, and host–pathogen interactions. *Trends in Microbiology* 29 (5): 458–471.

20 Messelhäußer, U. and Ehling-Schulz, M. (2018). *Bacillus cereus* – a multifaceted opportunistic pathogen. *Current Clinical Microbiology Reports 5* (2): 120–125.

21 Ichikawa, K., Gakumazawa, M., Inaba, A. et al. (2010). Acute encephalopathy of *Bacillus cereus* mimicking Reye syndrome. *Brain and Development 32* (8): 688–690.

22 Hansson, I., Sandberg, M., Habib, I. et al. (2018). Knowledge gaps in control of *Campylobacter* for prevention of campylobacteriosis. *Transboundary and Emerging Diseases 65*: 30–48.

23 Soro, A.B., Whyte, P., Bolton, D.J., and Tiwari, B.K. (2020). Strategies and novel technologies to control *Campylobacter* in the poultry chain: a review. *Comprehensive Reviews in Food Science and Food Safety 19* (4): 1353–1377.

24 Hsieh, Y.H., Simpson, S., Kerdahi, K., and Sulaiman, I.M. (2018). A comparative evaluation study of growth conditions for culturing the isolates of *Campylobacter* spp. *Current Microbiology 75* (1): 71–78.

25 Axelrad, J.E. and Sauk, J.S. (2020). Gastrointestinal infections in IBD flares: can PCR-based stool tests differentiate the smoke from the fire? *Digestive Diseases and Sciences* 65: 3064–3065.

26 Yuki, N., Susuki, K., Koga, M. et al. (2004). Carbohydrate mimicry between human ganglioside GM1 and *Campylobacter jejuni* lipooligosaccharide causes Guillain–Barré syndrome. *Proceedings of the National Academy of Sciences 101* (31): 11404–11409.

27 Murphy, C., Carroll, C., and Jordan, K.N. (2003). Induction of an adaptive tolerance response in the foodborne pathogen, *Campylobacter jejuni. FEMS Microbiology Letters 223* (1): 89–93.

28 Rood, J.I., Adams, V., Lacey, J. et al. (2018). Expansion of the *Clostridium perfringens* toxin-based typing scheme. *Anaerobe 53*: 5–10.

29 Kiu, R. and Hall, L.J. (2018). An update on the human and animal enteric pathogen *Clostridium perfringens. Emerging Microbes & Infections 7* (1): 1–15.

30 Collie, R.E. and McClane, B.A. (1998). Evidence that the enterotoxin gene can be episomal in *Clostridium perfringens* isolates associated with non-food-borne human gastrointestinal diseases. *Journal of Clinical Microbiology 36* (1): 30–36.

31 Pedersen, P.V., Halveg, A.B., Hansen, F.H. et al. (1976). Necrotising enterocolitis of the newborn – is it gas-gangrene of the bowel? *Lancet 308* (7988): 715–716.

32 Bhunia, A.K. (ed.) (2018). *Clostridium botulinum, Clostridium perfringens, Clostridium difficile*. In: *Foodborne Microbial Pathogens: Mechanisms and Patholgenesis*, 209–228. New York: Springer.

33 World Health Organization (2018). Botulism: fact sheet. www.who.int/news-room/fact-sheets/detail/botulism

34 Gill, D.M. (1982). Bacterial toxins: a table of lethal amounts. *Microbiological Reviews 46* (1): 86–94.

35 Lindstrom, M. and Korkeala, H. (2006). Laboratory diagnostics of botulism. *Clinical Microbiology Reviews 19* (2): 298–314.

36 Nataro, J.P. and Kaper, J.B. (1998). Diarrheagenic *Escherichia coli. Clinical Microbiology Reviews 11* (1): 142–201.

37 Gomes, T.A., Elias, W.P., Scaletsky, I.C. et al. (2016). Diarrheagenic *Escherichia coli. Brazilian Journal of Microbiology 47*: 3–30.

38 Croxen, M.A., Law, R.J., Scholz, R. et al. (2013). Recent advances in understanding enteric pathogenic *Escherichia coli. Clinical Microbiology Reviews 26* (4): 822–880.

39 Fleckenstein, J.M., Hardwidge, P.R., Munson, G.P. et al. (2010). Molecular mechanisms of enterotoxigenic *Escherichia coli* infection. *Microbes and Infection 12* (2): 89–98.

40 Moura, R.A., Sircili, M.P., Leomil, L. et al. (2009). Clonal relationship among atypical enteropathogenic *Escherichia coli* strains isolated from different animal species and humans. *Applied and Environmental Microbiology 75* (23): 7399–7408.

41 U.S. Food and Drug Administration (FDA) (2012). Pathogenic *Escherichia coli* Group. In: *Bad Bug Book: Foodborne Pathogenic Microorganisms and Natural Toxins Handbook* (ed. Center for Food Safety and Applied Nutrition), 68–81. Silver Spring, MD: U.S. Food and Drug Administration.

42 Estrada-Garcia, T., Perez-Martinez, I., Bernal-Reynaga, R., and Zaidi, M.B. (2014). Enteroaggregative *Escherichia coli*: a pathogen bridging the north and south. *Current Tropical Medicine Reports 1* (2): 88–96.

43 Kaper, J.B., Nataro, J.P., and Mobley, H.L. (2004). Pathogenic *Escherichia coli. Nature Reviews Microbiology 2* (2): 123–140.

44 Paduro, C., Montero, D.A., Chamorro, N. et al. (2020). Ten years of molecular epidemiology surveillance of *Listeria monocytogenes* in Chile 2008–2017. *Food Microbiology 85*: 103280.

45 Ferreira, V., Wiedmann, M., Teixeira, P., and Stasiewicz, M.J. (2014). *Listeria monocytogenes* persistence in food-associated environments: epidemiology, strain characteristics, and implications for public health. *Journal of Food Protection 77* (1): 150–170.

46 Ooi, S.T. and Lorber, B. (2005). Gastroenteritis due to *Listeria monocytogenes. Clinical Infectious Diseases 40* (9): 1327–1332.

47 Cossart, P., Vicente, M.F., Mengaud, J. et al. (1989). Listeriolysin O is essential for virulence of *Listeria monocytogenes*: direct evidence obtained by gene complementation. *Infection and Immunity 57* (11): 3629–3636.

48 Zhang, T., Abel, S., Zur Wiesch, P.A. et al. (2017). Deciphering the landscape of host barriers to *Listeria monocytogenes* infection. *Proceedings of the National Academy of Sciences 114* (24): 6334–6339.

49 Schlech, W.F. III, Lavigne, P.M., Bortolussi, R.A. et al. (1983). Epidemic listeriosis – evidence for transmission by food. *New England Journal of Medicine 308* (4): 203–206.

50 Lecuit, M. (2020). *Listeria monocytogenes*, a model in infection biology. *Cellular Microbiology 22* (4): e13186.

51 Allerberger, F. and Wagner, M. (2010). Listeriosis: a resurgent foodborne infection. *Clinical Microbiology and Infection 16* (1): 16–23.

52 Buchanan, R.L., Gorris, L.G., Hayman, M.M. et al. (2017). A review of *Listeria monocytogenes*: an update on outbreaks, virulence, dose-response, ecology, and risk assessments. *Food Control 75*: 1–13.

53 Chlebicz, A. and Śliżewska, K. (2018). Campylobacteriosis, salmonellosis, yersiniosis, and listeriosis as zoonotic foodborne diseases: a review. *International Journal of Environmental Research and Public Health 15* (5): 863.

54 Brenner, F.W., Villar, R.G., Angulo, F.J. et al. (2000). Salmonella nomenclature. *Journal of Clinical Microbiology 38* (7): 2465–2467.

55 Kurtz, J.R., Goggins, J.A., and McLachlan, J.B. (2017). Salmonella infection: interplay between the bacteria and host immune system. *Immunology Letters 190*: 42–50.

56 Fàbrega, A. and Vila, J. (2013). Salmonella enterica serovar Typhimurium skills to succeed in the host: virulence and regulation. *Clinical Microbiology Reviews 26* (2): 308–341.

57 Chen, H.M., Wang, Y., Su, L.H., and Chiu, C.H. (2013). Nontyphoid Salmonella infection: microbiology, clinical features, and antimicrobial therapy. *Pediatrics and Neonatology 54* (3): 147–152.

58 Liang, L., Juarez, S., Nga, T.V. et al. (2013). Immune profiling with a Salmonella Typhi antigen microarray identifies new diagnostic biomarkers of human typhoid. *Science Reports* 3: 1043.

59 Beyene, T., Hayishe, H., Gizaw, F. et al. (2017). Prevalence and antimicrobial resistance profile of Staphylococcus in dairy farms, abattoir and humans in Addis Ababa, Ethiopia. *BMC Research Notes 10* (1): 1–9.

60 Craft, K.M., Nguyen, J.M., Berg, L.J., and Townsend, S.D. (2019). Methicillin-resistant *Staphylococcus aureus* (MRSA): antibiotic-resistance and the biofilm phenotype. *MedChemComm 10* (8): 1231–1241.

61 Kadariya, J., Smith, T.C., and Thapaliya, D. (2014). *Staphylococcus aureus* and staphylococcal food-borne disease: an ongoing challenge in public health. *BioMed Research International* 2014: 827965.

62 U.S. Food and Drug Administration (FDA) (2012). *Staphylococcus aureus*. In: *Bad Bug Book: Foodborne Pathogenic Microorganisms and Natural Toxins* (ed. Center for Food Safety and Applied Nutrition), 87–91. Silver Spring, MD: U.S. Food and Drug Administration.

63 Argudín, M.Á., Mendoza, M.C., and Rodicio, M.R. (2010). Food poisoning and *Staphylococcus aureus* enterotoxins. *Toxins 2* (7): 1751–1773.

64 Pinchuk, I.V., Beswick, E.J., and Reyes, V.E. (2010). Staphylococcal enterotoxins. *Toxins 2* (8): 2177–2197.

65 Domman, D., Quilici, M.L., Dorman, M.J. et al. (2017). Integrated view of *Vibrio cholerae* in the Americas. *Science 358* (6364): 789–793.

66 Silva, A.J. and Benitez, J.A. (2016). *Vibrio cholerae* biofilms and cholera pathogenesis. *PLoS Neglected Tropical Diseases 10* (2): e0004330.

67 Azman, A.S., Rudolph, K.E., Cummings, D.A., and Lessler, J. (2013). The incubation period of cholera: a systematic review. *Journal of Infection 66* (5): 432–438.

68 Harris, J., LaRocque, R.C., Ryan, F.E., and Calderwood, S.B. (2012). Cholera. *Lancet 379*: 2466–2476.

69 Su, Y.C. and Liu, C. (2007). *Vibrio parahaemolyticus*: a concern of seafood safety. *Food Microbiology 24* (6): 549–558.

70 Jones, J.L., Lüdeke, C.H., Bowers, J.C. et al. (2012). Biochemical, serological, and virulence characterization of clinical and oyster *Vibrio parahaemolyticus* isolates. *Journal of Clinical Microbiology 50* (7): 2343–2352.

71 Martinez-Urtaza, J., Simental, L., Velasco, D. et al. (2005). Pandemic *Vibrio parahaemolyticus* O3: K6, Europe. *Emerging Infectious Diseases 11* (8): 1319.

72 Wang, R., Zhong, Y., Gu, X. et al. (2015). The pathogenesis, detection, and prevention of *Vibrio parahaemolyticus. Frontiers in Microbiology 6*: 144.

73 DePaola, A., Kaysner, C.A., Bowers, J., and Cook, D.W. (2000). Environmental investigations of Vibrio parahaemolyticus in oysters after outbreaks in Washington, Texas, and New York (1997 and 1998). *Applied and Environmental Microbiology 66* (11): 4649–4654.

74 Baker-Austin, C. and Oliver, J.D. (2018). *Vibrio vulnificus*: new insights into a deadly opportunistic pathogen. *Environmental Microbiology 20* (2): 423–430.

75 Bisharat, N., Agmon, V., Finkelstein, R. et al. (1999). Clinical, epidemiological, and microbiological features of *Vibrio vulnificus* biogroup 3 causing outbreaks of wound infection and bacteraemia in Israel. *Lancet 354* (9188): 1421–1424.

76 Baker-Austin, C., Trinanes, J.A., Taylor, N.G. et al. (2013). Emerging Vibrio risk at high latitudes in response to ocean warming. *Nature Climate Change 3* (1): 73–77.

77 Rippey, S.R. (1994). Infectious diseases associated with molluscan shellfish consumption. *Clinical Microbiology Reviews 7* (4): 419–425.

78 Jones, M.K. and Oliver, J.D. (2009). *Vibrio vulnificus*: disease and pathogenesis. *Infection and Immunity 77* (5): 1723–1733.

79 Rahman, A., Bonny, T.S., Stonsaovapak, S., and Ananchaipattana, C. (2011). *Yersinia enterocolitica*: epidemiological studies and outbreaks. *Journal of Pathogens* 2011: 239391.

80 Fàbrega, A. and Vila, J. (2012). *Yersinia enterocolitica*: pathogenesis, virulence and antimicrobial resistance. *Enfermedades Infecciosas y Microbiología Clínica 30* (1): 24–32.

81 Dekker, J.P. and Frank, K.M. (2015). *Salmonella, Shigella,* and *Yersinia*. *Clinics in Laboratory Medicine 35* (2): 225–246.

Section 2

Viral Zoonoses

Introduction

Viruses are obligate intracellular parasites that can replicate only within a living host cell since they cannot carry out metabolic processes on their own. Viruses are very small, having a diameter of fewer than 200 nanometres (nm), and based on genetic material, they can be divided into RNA viruses and DNA viruses. The DNA viruses probably have been present in and have co-evolved with humans for long periods; however, the RNA viruses are different, and a majority of these viruses that infect humans are derived from animal sources. Therefore, RNA viruses are of great interest in the context of emerging infectious diseases and are considered to have the potential to cause pandemics [1].

Out of more than 1400 human pathogens, around 61% are considered zoonotic [2]. Among the various aetiological agents, viruses account for a small fraction (less than 15%) of the total number of human pathogens. However, zoonotic viruses constitute over 65% of pathogens discovered since 1980 [2]. In a study, Woolhouse and co-workers listed 87 novel pathogens which were reported to be pathogenic to humans during the period 1980–2005. They found that two-thirds of these were viruses and 85% of them had a single-stranded RNA (ssRNA) genome [2]. The predominance of RNA viruses among the emerging pathogens is mostly due to the following characteristics [3].

1) The error rate during RNA replication (i.e. $\sim10^{-4}$) is greater than that of DNA (i.e. $\sim10^{-5}$) due to the lack of proofreading abilities of DNA polymerase or postreplication mismatch repair. Therefore, the potential for mutation per replication cycle is high and the lack of fidelity might have limited the size of RNA genomes, many of which are in the range of 10 000–15 000 nucleotides.
2) Most RNA viruses are zoonotic as they are capable of species jump. Even some of the viruses that are transmitting exclusively between humans (e.g. HIV and hepatitis C) are likely to have animal origins. All arthropod-borne viruses (arboviruses) are zoonotic, although some, like dengue, yellow fever and chikungunya, have adapted to efficient vector-borne transmission between humans.

Factors Responsible for the Emergence of Viral Zoonoses

In accordance with other emerging zoonoses, the emergence of most viral zoonoses is associated with population growth-related unsustainable urbanisation, deforestation, biodiversity loss and globalisation which accelerate the movement of humans, livestock and commodities, leading to the transfer of exotic pathogens and vectors to new geographical areas [4]. Examples of emerging viruses of human health importance along with the natural reservoir hosts from

Textbook of Zoonoses, First Edition. Jasbir Singh Bedi, Deepthi Vijay, and Pankaj Dhaka.

which they originated are described in Table 1 [5]. It is important to note that this is an ever-expanding list; many of the anthropogenic activities listed above have opened a Pandora's box allowing new diseases to emerge.

Table 1 Examples of emerging viral diseases in humans.

Sl. No.	Virus (Family)	Genome	Pathogenesis in humans	Natural host
1	Chikungunya (Togaviridae)	+ssRNA	High fever, skin rash, arthralgia	African primates
2	Crimean-Congo hemorrhagic fever (Bunyaviridae)	−ssRNA	Haemorrhagic fever	Hares, large herbivores?
3	Ebola (Filoviridae)	−ssRNA	Haemorrhagic fever	Fruit bats
4	Hanta (Bunyaviridae)	−ssRNA	Haemorrhagic fever with renal syndrome, cardiopulmonary syndrome	Rodents, shrews, and bats
5	Hendra and Nipah (Paramyxoviridae)	−ssRNA	Severe acute encephalitis, respiratory disease, systemic vasculitis	Fruit bats
6	Hepatitis E (Hepeviridae)	+ssRNA	Hepatitis	Pigs
7	HIV (Retroviridae)	−ssRNA	Acquired immunodeficiency syndrome (AIDS)	African primates
8	Influenza A (Orthomyxoviridae)	−ssRNA	Respiratory symptoms	Aquatic birds
9	Lassa (Arenaviridae)	−ssRNA	Mild febrile illness but can result in haemorrhagic fever	Rodents
10	Lymphocytic choriomeningitis (Arenaviridae)	−ssRNA	Mild febrile illness to meningoencephalitis	Rodents
11	Menangle (Paramyxoviridae)	−ssRNA	Influenza-like illness and rash	Fruit bats
12	MERS coronavirus (Coronaviridae)	+ssRNA	Acute pneumonia, renal failure	Bats, camels
13	SARS coronavirus (Coronaviridae)	+ssRNA	Progressive atypical pneumonia	Horseshoe bats
14	SARS-CoV-2 (Coronaviridae)	+ssRNA	Progressive atypical pneumonia	Bats?
15	Rabies (Rhabdoviridae)	−ssRNA	Neurological disease	Bats
16	Rift Valley fever (Bunyaviridae)	−ssRNA	Haemorrhagic fever	?
17	West Nile (Flaviviridae)	+ssRNA	Fever, meningoencephalitis	Birds?
18	Yellow fever (Flaviviridae)	+ssRNA	Haemorrhagic fever, jaundice	African primates

Notable Zoonotic Viral Outbreaks During the Twenty-First Century

Historically, viral pathogens caused outbreaks with epidemic and pandemic potential. The breach of the human–animal/human–wildlife interface due to anthropogenic activities (e.g. road building, deforestation, dam construction, agricultural development, etc.) can be the main factor(s) in spillover of zoonotic pathogens. Some of the recent outbreaks due to viruses affecting a huge proportion of the human population are described below.

1) **Severe acute respiratory syndrome (SARS):** coronaviruses are a large family of RNA viruses that are common in different species of animals (e.g. camels, cattle, cats, bats, etc.) and humans. The first pandemic of the twenty-first century was the outbreak of SARS caused by SARS-CoV in 2003, which affected 26 countries. According to the World Health Organization (WHO), the outbreak resulted in 8098 cases globally, and of these, 774 died [6].
2) **2009 H1N1 pandemic (H1N1pdm09 virus):** historically, the influenza viruses posed a high potential for pandemics. After early outbreaks in North America during April 2009, the new influenza virus (H1N1pdm09) spread rapidly around the world in 74 countries and the WHO declared it as a pandemic in June 2009. To date, most countries in the world have confirmed infections from the new virus with seasonal outbreaks.
3) **Middle East respiratory syndrome coronavirus (MERS-CoV)**: the Middle East respiratory syndrome (MERS) emerged in 2012 in Saudi Arabia. It is believed that MERS-CoV, like many other coronaviruses, originated in bats. However, dromedary camels seem to be the only animal host responsible for the spillover of infections to humans. According to the WHO, since its first detection in 2012, MERS-CoV continues to cause sporadic and localised outbreaks, where 27 countries have reported cases of MERS. From 2012 to 31 January 2020, the total number of laboratory-confirmed MERS-CoV cases reported to WHO was 2519, with 866 deaths. Many of the human cases of MERS-CoV infections have been attributed to human-to-human transmission in healthcare settings.
4) **Ebola virus epidemic (2013–2016) in West Africa:** the deadliest epidemic of the haemorrhagic Ebola fever was reported in West Africa during December 2013. The epidemic lasted more than 2 years and led to the death of more than 11 300 people, mainly in Guinea, Liberia and Sierra Leone. On 8 August 2014, the WHO declared the epidemic in West Africa a 'Public Health Emergency of International Concern' (PHEIC). The outbreak was caused by the Zaire strain of the Ebola virus and the factors responsible for the epidemic were attributed to the unprecedented circulation of the virus into crowded urban areas, increased mobilisation across borders, unregulated key infection control practices, and prevailing cultural and traditional practices in West African countries.
5) **Zika virus outbreak:** Zika virus was first isolated in 1947 from the Zika Forest of Uganda. The disease is spread predominantly by the bite of infected *Aedes* species mosquito (*Ae. aegypti* and *Ae. albopictus*). Before 2007, the virus was rarely reported in humans and was not considered a major public health concern. However, new clinical findings after outbreaks in the Federated States of Micronesia (2007), French Polynesia (2013) and Brazil (2015–2016) changed the insights on the pathophysiology of the disease; an increased risk of neurological complications was found to be associated with Zika virus infection in adults and children, which includes Guillain–Barré syndrome, neuropathy and myelitis. On 1 February 2016, the WHO declared the Zika virus epidemic a PHEIC. A total of 86 countries and territories have reported evidence of mosquito-transmitted Zika infection [7].

6) **Coronavirus disease 2019 (COVID-19):** the initial outbreak of novel coronavirus disease was reported from Wuhan in China in December 2019. The virus was later named SARS-CoV-2 and the disease it causes was named 'coronavirus disease 2019' (abbreviated 'COVID-19'). On 30 January 2020, the WHO declared COVID-19 a PHEIC. This pandemic forced the scientific community to reassess the zoonotic potential of RNA viruses. The main source of the pandemic is still debatable, but some studies suggest bats as the reservoir host [8]. The ongoing outbreak has influenced human life across the globe due to huge socio-economic disruption with millions of cases and deaths.

In conclusion, emerging and re-emerging pathogens present a huge challenge to human and animal health. Proactive approaches integrated with a robust surveillance system are considered as a key defence against emerging pathogens that need effective co-ordination on regional, national and global scales for early diagnosis and reporting of these emerging zoonoses. Better management of emerging diseases demands a multidisciplinary research effort within the One Health framework [5].

References

1 Olival, K.J., Hosseini, P.R., Zambrana-Torrelio, C. et al. (2017). Host and viral traits predict zoonotic spillover from mammals. *Nature* 546 (7660): 646–650.

2 Woolhouse, M. and Gaunt, E. (2007). Ecological origins of novel human pathogens. *Critical Reviews in Microbiology* 33 (4): 231–242.

3 Rosenberg, R. (2015). Detecting the emergence of novel, zoonotic viruses pathogenic to humans. *Cellular and Molecular Life Sciences 72* (6): 1115–1125.

4 Jones, B.A., Grace, D., Kock, R. et al. (2013). Zoonosis emergence linked to agricultural intensification and environmental change. *Proceedings of the National Academy of Sciences 110* (21): 8399–8404.

5 Woolhouse, M.E. (2002). Population biology of emerging and re-emerging pathogens. *Trends in Microbiology 10* (10): s3–s7.

6 Peiris, J.S.M., Lai, S.T., Poon, L.L.M. et al. (2003). Coronavirus as a possible cause of severe acute respiratory syndrome. *Lancet* 361 (9366): 1319–1325.

7 World Health Organization (2018). Zika Virus. www.who.int/news-room/fact-sheets/detail/zika-virus

8 Zhou, P., Yang, X.L., Wang, X.G. et al. (2020). A pneumonia outbreak associated with a new coronavirus of probable bat origin. *Nature* 579 (7798): 270–273.

13

Crimean-Congo Haemorrhagic Fever (CCHF)

Crimean-Congo haemorrhagic fever (CCHF) is a tick-borne viral zoonosis caused by CCHF virus, belonging to the family Bunyaviridae of genus *Nairovirus* [1]. The pathogen is transmitted to people either by tick bites or through contact with the blood or tissue of infected animals during slaughter operations. The majority of cases are reported in people associated with livestock, such as agricultural workers, slaughterhouse workers, and veterinarians. Human-to-human transmission can occur due to close contact with the blood, organs, or other body fluids of the infected person. As per the Centers for Disease Control and Prevention (CDC), the CCHF virus is considered a Biological Safety Level (BSL)-4 pathogen. The high fatality rate (up to 40%) and secondary attack rate make this virus a potential bioterrorism agent [2].

Historical Context

Crimean-Congo haemorrhagic fever was first traced as a haemorrhagic syndrome in the early twelfth century in Tadzhikistan. However, the disease was first described in the Crimean Peninsula in 1944–1945, when it infected 200 Soviet military personnel who were exposed to tick bites due to outdoor sleeping, and thus the disease was named Crimean haemorrhagic fever (CHF) [3]. A similar disease virus was isolated in 1956 from a febrile patient in the Belgian Congo, named as Congo virus. In 1968, it was conclusively proved that both viruses were antigenically identical, so the two names were combined to describe the disease as Crimean-Congo haemorrhagic fever [4].

Epidemiology and Transmission

Crimean-Congo haemorrhagic fever is considered one of the most widely distributed arboviral diseases in the world. The widespread prevalence is mainly associated with the ubiquitous nature of its principal vector, i.e. *Hyalomma* species of ticks. The disease is considered an emerging zoonotic viral disease because of its rapid transmission potential and the recently reported sporadic outbreaks in non-endemic countries. These outbreaks are associated with unsustainable human interventions into forest ecosystems. The human–wildlife interface has exposed multiple channels for spillover to humans of this infection previously confined to wild animals. The major prevalence of the disease is reported from Africa, Asia, South Eastern Europe, and the Middle East countries. In addition, the transboundary transmission potential of the disease is attributed to the dissemination of ticks and viruses through the annual migration of the birds in the North–South

Textbook of Zoonoses, First Edition. Jasbir Singh Bedi, Deepthi Vijay, and Pankaj Dhaka.

axis. The ticks can also be dispersed between continents by the movement and trade of animals. The high incidences of human infection in resource-limited countries are due to the increased interaction with livestock coupled with poor healthcare settings [5].

Hosts

The major hosts for the CCHF virus are various species of animals (e.g. cattle, sheep, goats, pigs, horses) and humans. Many species of birds are resistant to infection, but ostriches are susceptible and may show a high prevalence of infection in endemic areas. The clinical symptoms of the disease are mainly exhibited by humans only whereas animals remain as asymptomatic carriers [1].

Vectors

Crimean-Congo haemorrhagic fever virus has been isolated from at least 31 species of ticks and one species of biting midges (*Culicoides* spp.). Among these possible vectors, *Hyalomma* species of tick act as the main vector for the virus [6].

Reservoirs

Small mammals like hares, hedgehogs and rodents act as a reservoir for the CCHF virus. Birds generally act as mechanical carriers of the virus with no reported viraemia or antibody titres [1].

Transmission Cycles

The virus circulates in nature through the enzootic cycle and epizootic-epidemic cycle [7]. An outline of the transmission cycle of CCHF is presented in Figure 13.1.

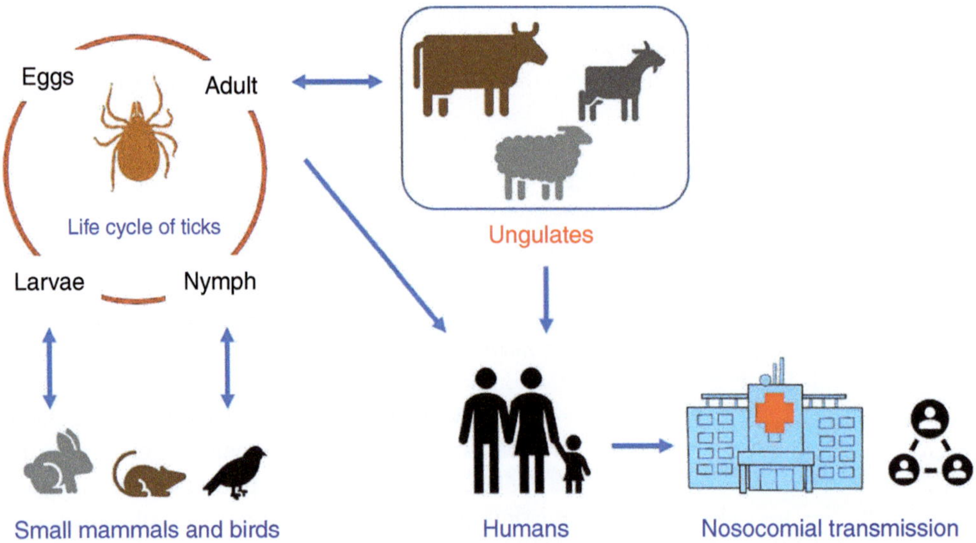

Figure 13.1 Transmission cycle of CCHF involving ticks, small mammals and birds, ungulates and humans.

- In the enzootic cycle, the *Ixodid* (hard) ticks (mainly *Hyalomma* spp.) act as a reservoir as well as a vector for the virus. The virus is maintained in nature by transovarial, trans-stadial and venereal transmission in ticks.
- In the epizootic-epidemic cycle, wild as well as domestic animals such as cattle, goats, sheep and hare acts as amplifying hosts and *Hyalomma* spp. of ticks as vectors. Humans become infected either through tick bites or when they come in direct contact with the blood or tissue of infected animals and/or persons. High-risk groups involve veterinarians, slaughterhouse personnel, butchers and hospital workers. Human-to-human transmission can occur from close contact with the blood, secretions, organs or other body fluids of infected persons, especially in healthcare settings.

Risk Factors for Disease Occurrence

The important risk factors responsible for the occurrence of CCHF are described below [8].

- In endemic areas, the farming community is at risk as they are involved in livestock and agricultural practices and handle animals and animal products without following necessary precautions.
- The vector (*Hyalomma* spp.) of the disease has a wide geographical distribution and it is difficult to control the transboundary migration of animals harbouring infected ticks due to the lack of robust surveillance measures in many countries.
- Changes in climate and agricultural practices have made many of the previously naïve habitats suitable for *Hyalomma* spp. of ticks, consequently increasing the incidence of disease in humans.
- Migrating birds act as mechanical carriers of the disease and may transmit the virus and/or infected ticks from one area to another.
- Insufficient medical preparedness, including the unavailability of an effective vaccine and specific treatment protocol, are responsible for the emerging cases and associated high case fatality rate (up to 40%) in resource-limited countries.

Pathogenesis

Similar to other haemorrhagic viruses, viraemia develops in infected humans and the organism multiplies in the endothelial layer of blood vessels. During replication, it causes a proinflammatory response by the release of cytokines like tumour necrosis factor (TNF)-α and interleukin (IL)-6 in blood, which further aggravates the endothelial damage, resulting in endothelial toxicosis. The aggregation and degranulation of platelets on damaged endothelial surfaces lead to the activation of the intrinsic coagulation cascade which results in disseminated intravascular coagulation (DIC) and multiorgan failure [9].

Disease in Animals and Humans

The clinical symptoms of the disease are mainly associated with humans whereas animals show no apparent disease manifestation and act as asymptomatic carriers.

In humans, the clinical course of the disease occurs in four phases: incubation period, prehaemorrhagic period, haemorrhagic period, and convalescent period [10].

- The incubation period ranges from 3 to 7 days, which mainly depends on the route of infection. Infection acquired through tick bite becomes apparent in 1–3 days, while it takes 5–6 days when the entry of virus is through direct contact with infected blood or tissue. Viraemia usually occurs in this phase.
- The prehaemorrhagic period of disease ranges from 1 to 7 days. The characteristic clinical signs of this period are fever, nausea, vomiting, diarrhoea, myalgia, arthralgia, dizziness and photophobia. Subsequently, platelet and white blood cell (WBC) counts decrease and aspartate aminotransferase (AST) and alanine aminotransferase (ALT) levels increase.
- The fatal haemorrhagic period usually ranges from 2 to 3 days. The initial symptoms of this phase include petechial rashes followed by ecchymoses in the internal mucous membranes like mouth and throat and on the skin. In the later phase, bleeding from different natural orifices, including epistaxis, melaena, haematemesis, haemoptysis and haematuria, occurs. The patients feel prolonged and pronounced sleepiness. In some patients, hepatomegaly and splenomegaly are also observed. There is a high mortality rate (10–40%) during this period (second week from starting of infection) mainly due to DIC, multiorgan failure and cardiovascular arrest [1].
- If the patient gets through the first three phases due to prompt treatment and management, then the convalescent period starts which ranges from 10 to 20 days and in some cases can extend up to years. In this phase, the patient feels prolonged and pronounced weakness and weak pulse and experiences temporary or permanent hair loss. In severe cases, laboured breathing, dizziness, polyneuritis, loss of vision, hearing loss and loss of memory have been reported [3].

Diagnosis

Diagnostic techniques including virus isolation, immunological assays and molecular diagnostic assays can be used to detect CCHF infection. All the diagnostic procedures for suspected CCHF infections should be performed in a BSL-4 facility. The virus isolation technique is a relatively less sensitive method, which needs a high concentration of the virus. The virus can be cultured and isolated from infected blood and tissue suspensions in various cell lines such as LLC-MK2, Vero, BHK-21 and SW-13 cells after 4–7 days of inoculation. Cytopathic effect (CPE) produced by the virus varies with the cell line and strain of the virus used and may even develop as a non-cytopathic persistent infection.

Serological methods such as immunofluorescence assay (IFA) and enzyme-linked immunosorbent assay (ELISA) based on IgM and IgG detection are used for the detection of antibodies against the exposure of the virus. Rapid detection of the virus is possible by reverse transcriptase-polymerase chain reaction (RT-PCR) with high sensitivity and specificity [1].

Treatment

There is no effective vaccine for CCHF infection for either humans or animals [1]. However, a formalin-inactivated suckling mouse brain-derived human vaccine is used in some parts of the world including Bulgaria, the Soviet Union and Eastern Europe.

There is no approved drug for the treatment of CCHF. General supportive care with symptomatic treatment is the main approach for managing CCHF in humans. The antiviral drug ribavirin has been used to treat CCHF infection with apparent benefit, but no randomised controlled trials (RCTs) have been performed. In later haemorrhagic phases, blood and plasma transfusion and infusion of plasma volume extenders such as polyglutin and hemodes are carried out. Platelet transfusion is done in case of severe thrombocytopenia [11].

Prevention and Control

The important strategy for the reduction of CCHF occurrence is the control of disease in animals and ticks. However, the disease remains asymptomatic in animals, so it is difficult to control the natural tick–animal–tick cycle in endemic areas. Furthermore, the tick vectors are numerous and widespread, so tick control with acaricides is only the realistic option for well-managed livestock production facilities [1]. Some practical approaches for prevention and control of disease in humans include the following.

- Visits to endemic areas should be avoided especially in the spring and summer seasons when tick activity is high.
- Avoid tick bites by following basic precautions like wearing light-coloured long-sleeves clothes, long trousers and shoes in tick endemic areas. The use of tick repellents such as DEET (N-N-diethyl meta-toluamide) on skin and clothes is also a viable option.
- To reduce the risk of the animal–human transmission cycle, practices such as wearing gloves and protective clothing while handling animals, animal tissues or products should be followed. Since the lifespan of the CCHF virus in the animal body is less (7–10 days), quarantine of the animal is an effective strategy.
- The risk of human-to-human transmission in the community can be managed by avoiding close physical contact with CCHF-infected people and wearing suitable personal protective equipment while taking care of cases. Reports of nosocomial transmission warrant the use of personal protection equipment by health workers. Regular hand washing must be carried out after caring for or visiting ill people.
- Avoiding the consumption of unpasteurised milk and uncooked meat is important to prevent food-associated transmission.
- Awareness and education are necessary in endemic areas, especially for high-risk groups (farmers, veterinarians, abattoir workers, etc.). Surveillance and early warning systems should be implemented in high-risk regions.

References

1 World Health Organization (2013). Fact-Sheet: Crimean-Congo haemorrhagic fever. www.who.int/news-room/fact-sheets/detail/crimean-congo-haemorrhagic-fever (accessed 7 December 2021).

2 Borio, L., Inglesby, T., Peters, C.J. et al. (2002). Hemorrhagic fever viruses as biological weapons: medical and public health management. *Journal of the American Medical Association* 287: 2391–2405.

3 Hoogstraal, H. (1979). The epidemiology of tick-borne Crimean-Congo hemorrhagic fever in Asia, Europe and Africa. *Journal of Medical Entomology* 15: 307–417.

4 Casals, J. (1969). Antigenic similarity between the virus causing Crimean hemorrhagic fever and Congo virus. *Proceedings of the Society for Experimental Biology and Medicine* 131: 233–236.

5 Goodman, L.J., Dennis, T.D., and Sonenshine, E. (ed.) (2005). *Tick-Borne Disease of Humans.* Washington, D.C.: ASM Press.

6 Linthicum, K.J. and Bailey, C.L. (1994). Ecology of Crimean–Congo hemorrhagic fever. In: *Ecological Dynamics of Tick-Borne Zoonoses* (ed. D.E. Sonenshine and T.N. Mather), 392–437. New York: Oxford University Press.

7 Dohm, D.J., Logan, T.M., Linthicum, K.J. et al. (1996). Transmission of Crimean-Congo hemorrhagic fever virus by Hyalomma impeltatum (Acari: Ixodidae) after experimental infection. *Journal of Medical Entomology* 33: 848–851.

8 Maltezou, H.C. and Papa, A. (2010). Crimean-Congo hemorrhagic fever: risk for emergence of new endemic foci in Europe? *Travel Medicine and Infectious Disease* 8: 139–143.

9 Hensley, L.E., Young, H.A., Jahrling, P.B., and Geisbert, T.W. (2002). Proinflammatory response during Ebola virus infection of primate models: possible involvement of the tumor necrosis factor receptor superfamily. *Immunology Letters* 80: 169–179.

10 Ergonul, O. (2013). Crimean-Congo hemorrhagic fever virus: new outbreaks, new discoveries. *Current Opinion in Virology* 2: 215–220.

11 Andersson, I., Bladh, L., Mousavi-Jazi, M. et al. (2004). Human MxA protein inhibits the replication of Crimean-Congo hemorrhagic fever virus. *Journal of Virology* 78: 4323–4329.

14

Ebola Virus

Ebola viruses are the causative agent of a severe form of viral haemorrhagic fever in humans, known as Ebola haemorrhagic fever or Ebola virus disease (EVD). Outbreaks of EVD constitute a significant public health threat in the African continent, and in the era of globalised trade and tourism, the virus may spill over to other regions. In addition, the misuse of the virus (Centers for Disease Control and Prevention [CDC]'s category-A organism) as an agent for biological terrorism also remains a point of concern.

The virus was initially presumed to be transmitted to the human population through contact with an infected animal, such as a fruit bat or non-human primate (species spillover), which can later spread through human-to-human transmission in the community. The high case fatality rates with Ebola outbreaks makes it one of the deadliest viral zoonotic diseases. The average EVD case fatality rate is around 50%, but rates have varied from 25% to 90% in past outbreaks [1]. The high case fatality rate combined with the absence of standard treatment and vaccination makes the Ebola virus a deadly zoonotic pathogen [2].

Aetiological Agent

The Ebola virus belongs to the family Filoviridae and order Mononegavirales. Filoviruses comprise Ebola, Marburg and Cueva virus, which are enveloped, non-segmented, negative-stranded RNA viruses of varying morphology. These viruses have characteristic filamentous particles that give the virus family its name. Within the genus *Ebolavirus*, six species have been identified: *zaire*, *bundibugyo*, *sudan*, *taï forest*, *reston* and *bombali* [1]. Of these, only four (Zaire, Sudan, Taï Forest and Bundibugyo viruses) are known to cause disease in humans. Reston virus is predominantly found in the Philippines, and is known to cause disease in non-human primates and pigs, but not in humans. The status of infection of the Bombali virus (identified in bats) in animals and humans is unknown.

Historical Context

Ebola virus disease was first investigated in 1976 in two simultaneous outbreaks: one in Nzara (a town in south Sudan) and the other in Yambuku (Democratic Republic of the Congo), a village near the Ebola River, from which the disease takes its name. Since 1976, there have been more than 20 EVD outbreaks across Central Africa, the majority of them caused by the Ebola virus (species *zaire*) [1]. The EVD epidemic in West Africa (2014–2016) evolved rapidly from a small outbreak in Guinea into

Textbook of Zoonoses, First Edition. Jasbir Singh Bedi, Deepthi Vijay, and Pankaj Dhaka.

the largest outbreak of EVD declared as a global public health emergency, which resulted in 28616 cases and 11310 deaths [2].

Epidemiology and Disease Transmission

Fruit bats of the Pteropodidae family are considered natural hosts or reservoir hosts for the Ebola virus. Chimpanzees, gorillas and duikers have all been suggested to serve as intermediate hosts for the transmission of the virus to humans. However, non-human primates are not considered natural hosts because of their high sensitivity to the virus and associated high mortality rate.

Ebola virus can be transmitted to humans through contact with tissue or fluids (e.g. saliva, blood) of infected animals. Additionally, droplet aerosol transmission has also been observed in animal models. Animal-to-human transmission may occur during hunting and consumption of the reservoir species or infected non-human primates.

Ebola outbreaks are sustained by secondary human-to-human transmission that occurs through exposure to blood and body excretions and fluids such as urine, faeces, saliva, sweat, vomit, breast milk, semen and vaginal fluids. In hospital settings, nosocomial transmission remains a significant concern. The virus can survive in immunologically privileged sites of the body after acute infection, which includes testes, the interior of the eyes, placenta and central nervous system, particularly cerebrospinal fluid. Pregnant women who recover from acute Ebola infection may still carry the virus in breast milk or pregnancy-related fluids and tissues. The virus can remain in the semen of a patient who has recovered from EVD, even if they no longer have symptoms of severe illness [3]. A brief overview of the Ebola transmission cycle is presented in Figure 14.1.

Pathogenesis

Ebola virus infections are characterised by immune suppression, causing lymphocyte apoptosis and attenuation of the protective effects of interferon and systemic inflammatory response causing impairment of the vascular, coagulation and immune systems. These sequences of events ultimately lead to multiorgan failure and shock.

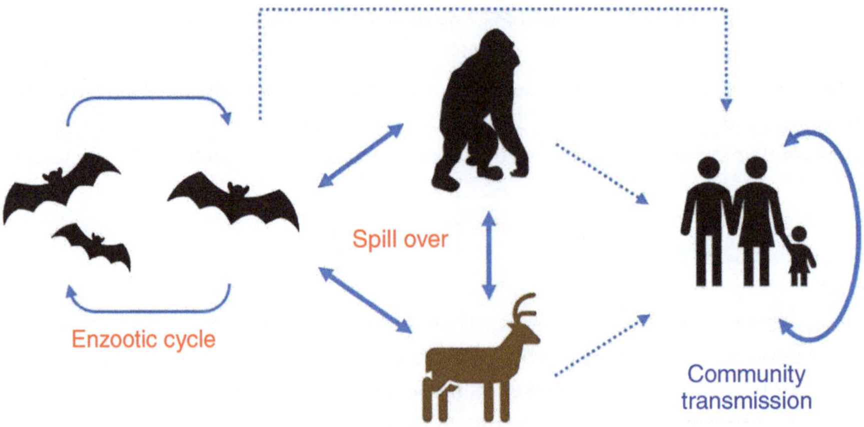

Figure 14.1 Transmission cycle of Ebola virus among bats, non-human primates, other animals and humans.

During the initial infection, preferred sites of the virus replication include monocytes, macrophages and dendritic cells. The infected cells migrate to the regional lymph nodes, liver and spleen, thereby disseminating the infection. Progression to severe disease occurs when the virus triggers the expression of proinflammatory cytokines, including interferons, interleukins (ILs) such as IL-2, IL-6, IL-8 and IL-10, and tumour necrosis factor (TNF)-α. This causes endothelial activation, reduced vascular integrity, release of tissue factor (with the associated onset of coagulopathy) and increased nitric oxide levels (with associated hypotension). Thrombocytopenia is most commonly caused by loss of platelets from damaged tissue or more generalised virus-induced disseminated intravascular coagulation, where coagulation factors are depleted. Disseminated intravascular coagulation, along with acute hepatic impairment, predisposes the patient for bleeding complications. Other complications of severe disease include acute kidney damage, hepatitis and pancreatitis [4].

Disease in Animals and Humans

Animals

The Ebola epidemics have had critical effects on non-human primates. The incubation period of their infection is 2–14 days, and clinical signs include, anorexia, cough and bleeding with a high mortality rate (usually 100%). Fruit bats can be infected with the Ebola virus but do not exhibit any clinical signs, and are considered as the main reservoir species [5].

Humans

The incubation period of EVD can be as long as 21 days. The initial presentation is non-specific, which makes early detection of cases difficult. The symptoms include fever, fatigue, muscle pain, headache and sore throat followed by vomiting, diarrhoea, rash and symptoms of impaired kidney and liver function. Haemorrhages, both internal and external, occur in 30–80% of patients, mostly at the end of the illness, expressed by purpura, epistaxis, gingival bleeding, gastrointestinal bleeding, etc., and appear to be associated with severity of infection. In acute EVD, hepatic and renal involvement is indicated by elevated levels of serum transaminases (aspartate transaminase [AST] and alanine transaminase [ALT]), blood urea nitrogen (BUN) and creatinine as well as proteinuria. Thrombocytopenia, longer prothrombin times and high D-dimer levels are indicators of disseminated intravascular coagulation and can contribute to multiple organ failure and shock, which can be fatal in more than 50% of cases [3].

Diagnosis

For any haemorrhagic fever, which is difficult to manage clinically even with early diagnosis, delays can increase fatalities. The initial non-specific symptoms of EVD are difficult to distinguish clinically from other infectious diseases such as malaria, dengue, leptospirosis, typhoid fever, Lassa fever, meningitis, etc. The clinical samples (e.g. blood, body fluids, semen, etc.) collected from patients are biohazards so laboratory testing on non-inactivated samples should be conducted under maximum containment Biological Safety Level (BSL)-4 laboratory conditions. Apart from human samples, the epidemiological surveillance programme may include fruit bats and non-human primates (apes or monkeys) for testing. All biological specimens should be packaged using the triple packaging system when transporting nationally and internationally.

The commonly used diagnostic tests for Ebola fall into three basic categories.

- **Molecular tests that detect viral RNA sequences:** The gold standard for Ebola diagnosis is viral genome detection by reverse transcriptase-polymerase chain reaction (RT-PCR).
- **Serological tests that detect host antibodies generated against the virus:** For example, indirect fluorescent antibody detection test (IFAT), Enzyme-linked immunosorbent assay (ELISA).
- **Antigen tests that detect viral proteins:** For example, ELISA, real-time RT-PCR, lateral flow immunoassays (LFIs).

The WHO recommends automated or semi-automated nucleic acid tests for routine diagnostic management. Rapid antigen detection tests can be used in remote settings where nucleic acid tests are not readily available. These tests are recommended for screening purposes as part of surveillance activities but reactive tests should be confirmed with nucleic acid tests.

Cell Culture

The traditional gold standard method to confirm the presence of the Ebola virus is viral isolation in cell culture, typically using Vero E6 African Green monkey kidney cells. The propagated virus can be directly visualised under electron microscopy or indirectly visualised by immunofluorescence microscopy within 1–5 days of inoculation. While detection of the virus by these methods is definitive, these methods require BSL-4 containment and are typically restricted to research and public health laboratories.

Treatment

There is currently no approved antiviral drug licensed to treat EVD in people. Therefore, supportive care, including rehydration with oral or intravenous fluids and symptomatic treatment, is used. A range of potential treatments such as immune therapies and drug therapies are currently being evaluated for EVD. During the 2018 Eastern Democratic Republic of the Congo outbreak, four therapies were initially investigated to treat patients with confirmed Ebola. Two of these treatments were found to increase the survival chances of cases: Regeneron's Antibody Cocktail (REGN-EB3, a cocktail of three monoclonal Ebola antibodies) and mAb114 (a single monoclonal antibody) [2, 6].

Vaccine

An experimental Ebola vaccine (rVSV-ZEBOV) showed significant protection against EVD in a trial in Guinea during 2015. The trial involved 11841 people, where 5837 people received the vaccine, and no Ebola cases were recorded 10 days or more after vaccination [1]. However, the safety and efficacy of the rVSV-ZEBOV vaccine have been evaluated against only the *zaire* species [7].

Prevention and Control

Good outbreak control practices rely on applying a package of interventions, including case management, surveillance, contact tracing, a good laboratory service, safe burials and controlled social mobilisation. Community engagement is the key to successful control of EVD outbreaks. Raising awareness of risk factors for Ebola infection and protective measures that individuals can adopt is an effective way to reduce human transmission.

The risk reduction procedures should focus on several factors including the following.

- **Reducing the risk of wildlife-to-human transmission:** Contact with infected fruit bats, monkeys, apes, forest antelope or porcupines should be avoided. Animals should be handled with gloves and other appropriate protective clothing. Animal products (blood and meat) should be thoroughly cooked before consumption.
- **Reducing the risk of human-to-human transmission:** Direct or close contact with infected people and their contaminated body fluids should be avoided. Personal protective equipment (e.g. impermeable gown or coverall, N95 mask, face shield, double gloves, boot covers, etc.) and barrier nursing protocols need to be strictly observed while handling suspected cases. Regular hand washing is required after visiting patients in hospital, as well as after taking care of patients at home. In epidemic areas, the patient's home should be sprayed with 0.5% chlorine solution. The patient's home and any personal belongings that might have been contaminated should be disinfected or disposed of (usually by incineration). Safe burial practices must be followed to eliminate transmission that would otherwise occur during ritual burial rites that include washing of the corpse [3].
- **Outbreak containment measures:** Keys for controlling EVD outbreaks include (i) active case identification and isolation of patients from the community to prevent continued virus spread; (ii) identifying contacts of ill or deceased persons and tracking the contacts daily for the entire incubation period of 21 days; (iii) investigation of retrospective and current cases to document all historical and ongoing chains of virus transmission; (iv) identifying deaths in the community and using safe burial practices; and (v) daily reporting of cases.
- **Reducing the risk of possible sexual transmission:** The WHO recommends that male survivors of EVD practise safer sex and hygiene for 12 months from the onset of symptoms or until their semen tests are negative twice for the Ebola virus. Contact with body fluids should be avoided and washing with soap and water is recommended.
- **Reducing the risk of transmission from pregnancy-related fluids and tissue:** Pregnant women who have survived Ebola disease need community support to enable them to attend frequent antenatal care (ANC) visits, to handle any pregnancy complications, and meet their need for sexual and reproductive care and delivery in a safe way.
- **Controlling infection in healthcare settings:** Healthcare workers should always take standard precautions when caring for patients that can lead to contact with blood and body fluids (such as urine, faeces, saliva, sweat, vomit, breast milk, semen and vaginal fluids). These include basic hand hygiene, respiratory hygiene, use of personal protective equipment, safe injection practices and safe burial practices.

References

1 World Health Organization (2020). Ebola virus disease. www.who.int/news-room/fact-sheets/detail/ebola-virus-disease (accessed 7 December 2021).

2 Centers for Disease Control and Prevention. (2019). Ebola (Ebola Virus Disease). www.cdc.gov/vhf/ebola (accessed 7 December 2021).

3 Boisen, M.L., Hartnett, J.N., Goba, A. et al. (2016). Epidemiology and management of the 2013–16 West African Ebola outbreak. *Annual Review of Virology 3*: 147–171.

4 Beeching, N.J., Fenech, M., and Houlihan, C.F. (2014). Ebola virus disease. *BMJ* 349: 7348.

5 Gumusova, S., Sunbul, M., and Leblebicioglu, H. (2015). Ebola virus disease and the veterinary perspective. *Annals of Clinical Microbiology and Antimicrobials 14* (1): 30.

6 Mulangu, S., Dodd, L.E., Davey, R.T. Jr. et al. (2019). A randomized, controlled trial of Ebola virus disease therapeutics. *New England Journal of Medicine 381* (24): 2293–2303.

7 Henao-Restrepo, A.M., Camacho, A., Longini, I.M. et al. (2017). Efficacy and effectiveness of an rVSV-vectored vaccine in preventing Ebola virus disease: final results from the Guinea ring vaccination, open-label, cluster-randomised trial (Ebola Ça Suffit!). *Lancet 389* (10068): 505–518.

15

Hantavirus

Hantaviruses are rodent-borne viruses identified around the world which cause clinical illness in humans of varying severity, ranging from acute renal failure to pulmonary oedema and severe haemorrhagic illness. Hantaviruses are members of the genus *Orthohantavirus* in the family Hantaviridae and order Bunyavirales. They are enveloped single-stranded RNA viruses with a negative-sense, trisegmented genome. Each hantavirus is specific to one or more rodent hosts. In contrast to other Bunyaviruses, hantaviruses are not transmitted by an arthropod vector but are carried and transmitted to humans by persistently infected rodents or insectivore hosts and even bats.

There are various hantaviruses with different geographical distribution and causing different clinical forms of diseases. Apart from the 41 known species of hantaviruses, there are additional viruses that have been discovered but not yet classified [1]. Hantaan, Seoul, Puumala, Dobrava-Belgrade, Sin Nombre and Andes viruses are predominant zoonotic viruses of the family Hantaviridae. Tula virus and the shrew-borne Thottapalayam viruses have been implicated in a few clinical cases [1].

Hantaviruses in the Americas are known as 'New World' hantaviruses and cause hantavirus pulmonary syndrome (HPS) which represents the prototype of hantavirus infection occurring in the Western hemisphere, characterised by pneumonia and cardiovascular dysfunction. Other hantaviruses, known as 'Old World' hantaviruses, are found mostly in Europe and Asia and may cause haemorrhagic fever with renal syndrome (HFRS), characterised by renal failure and haemorrhagic manifestations.

Historical Context

First described in Chinese writings 900 years ago, the disease resembling hantavirus infection came to global attention during the Korean conflict (1950–1953). More than 3000 United Nations and US soldiers experienced an acute febrile illness with acute renal failure and shock; these cases were observed near the River Hantaan in South Korea, so the disease was then called Korean haemorrhagic fever and later referred to as HFRS [2]. Until the early 1980s, the causative agent of the disease remained unknown, and then Hantaan virus was isolated from the lungs of its natural reservoir, the striped field mouse (*Apodemus agrarius*) by Ho Wang Lee and co-workers [3]. Although the milder form of HFRS, nephropathia epidemica (NE), has been known since the early 1930s, its aetiological agent Puumala virus (PUUV) was only discovered in bank voles (*Myodes glareolus*) in Finland in 1980 [4]. HPS, another variant of hantavirus infection, was first recognized

Textbook of Zoonoses, First Edition. Jasbir Singh Bedi, Deepthi Vijay, and Pankaj Dhaka.

in 1993 when an outbreak of severe respiratory disease struck in the Four Corners region of the US. The hantavirus responsible for this disease, Sin Nombre virus (SNV), is harboured by the deer mouse (*Peromyscus maniculatus*) [5].

Epidemiology and Transmission

Hantaviruses occur worldwide but the distribution of each virus is limited by the geographic range of its reservoir host(s). The hantaviruses in the Eastern Hemisphere are usually associated with HFRS. These include pathogenic Old World hantaviruses like Hantaan (epidemiologically most important species with mortality rates up to 15% in Asia), Dobrava-Belgrade, Seoul, Tula and PUUV. HFRS caused by Hantaan and Dobrava-Belgrade virus is more severe with mortality rates ranging from 5% to 15%, whereas Seoul virus causes moderate forms and PUUV causes mild forms of the disease with mortality rates of less than 1%. The Hantaan virus predominantly circulates in Asia. Seoul virus and Tula virus are found in both Europe and Asia, while Dobrava-Belgrade and PUUV circulate in Europe.

From the early 1990s, numerous pathogenic New World hantaviruses were identified and characterised in numerous reservoir hosts. New World hantaviruses are the causative agent of HPS in North and South America, with lethality rates up to 50%. Most clinical cases are caused by SNV in North America and Andes virus in South America. Cases of HPS have been confirmed elsewhere in the Americas, including Canada, Argentina, Bolivia, Brazil, Chile, Panama, Paraguay and Uruguay. Several novel hantaviruses with unknown pathogenic potential have been identified in Africa in a variety of insectivore hosts [6].

Hosts

Hantaviruses are hosted by persistently infected rodents, shrews and bats. Each hantavirus serotype appears to have a predominant natural mammal reservoir, suggesting long-term co-evolution of the host and microbe [7]. The important natural reservoirs of hantaviruses are mammals of families Muridae (subfamily Murinae including Old World rats and mice) and Crecetidae (subfamilies Arvicolinae, Neotominae and Sigmodontinae including voles, lemmings and New World rats and mice, respectively). Each virus is thought to be adapted to one or a few species, but spillover in other rodents, insectivore hosts and bats is possible. The distribution of single hantavirus species correlates with the geographic extension of their hosts and hantavirus genotypes of the same geographic area are phylogenetically related. The important genotype of Hantaan virus, with its associated disease, host and geographic distribution, is described in Table 15.1.

In rodents, hantaviruses are thought to be transmitted by aerosols and through intense close contact such as biting, grooming and sharing of food. Rodents can shed hantaviruses in saliva, faeces and urine. Transplacental transmission does not seem to occur. However, infected rodents can carry hantaviruses for weeks to years, and they may remain infected for their entire life. Dogs and cats are not known to carry hantavirus but they may bring infected rodents into contact with humans if they catch such animals and carry them home.

Transmission Cycles

The transmission of the virus to humans occurs through the contact and/or inhalation of infected urine, droppings or saliva of the rodents. When fresh rodent urine, droppings or nesting materials

Table 15.1 Various genotypes of Hantan virus along with their host and geographic distribution.

Genotype	Disease	Geographic distribution	Rodent(s) involved in transmission
Hantaan	HFRS	Asia, east Russia, south China	*Apodemus agrarius*
Seoul	HFRS	Worldwide	*Rattus norvegicus*
Puumula	Nephropathia epidemica (mild form of HFRS)	Europe, Russia, Korea	*Myodes glareolus*
Dobrava-Belgrade	HFRS	Balkans countries	*Apodemus flavicollis*, *A. ponticus*
Tula	Low pathogenic	Europe, Russia	*Microtus arvalis*, *M. levis*
Sin Nombre	HPS	North America	*Peromyscus maniculatus*
Andes	HPS	Argentina, Chile	*Oligoryzomys longicaudatus*

HFRS: haemorrhagic fever with renal syndrome; HPS: hantavirus pulmonary syndrome.

are stirred up, tiny droplets containing the virus get into the air and lead to air-borne transmission. There are several other routes through which the rodents can spread hantavirus to people.

- If a rodent with the virus bites someone, the virus may spread to that person.
- If people touch something that has been contaminated with rodent urine, droppings or saliva, and then touch their nose or mouth.
- If they eat food contaminated by urine, droppings or saliva from an infected rodent

Human hantavirus infections are assumed to occur accidentally, and humans are considered dead-end hosts. Transmission of the virus from infected to healthy people normally does not occur except for the Andes hantavirus, a South American strain in Chile and Argentina, of which sporadic cases of human-to-human transmissions have been reported [8].

Pathogenesis

The complex pathogenesis of hantavirus infection suggests that immune mechanisms might play an important role instead of direct viral cytopathology. Viraemia occurs after the initial infection of alveolar macrophages and the life-threatening acute-phase symptoms are induced primarily by infection of vascular endothelial cells of the lung and kidneys with concomitant loss of barrier function, which results in a severe increase in endothelial permeability.

Disease in Animals and Humans

Antibodies against hantavirus have been reported in various animal species other than rodents, e.g. cattle, moose, cat, dog, primates, etc. [1]. However, in natural conditions, there are limited reports of infection in animals.

Humans are not considered as the natural host of hantaviruses, and the infection occurs accidentally via virus-containing aerosolised rodent excretions such as urine, faeces or saliva. People who live or work in close contact with infected rodents are at high risk of infection. Risk factors for infection include involvement in outdoor activities, such as rural- and forest-related activities like camping and hiking, peridomestic rodent presence, exposure to potentially infected dust and outdoor military training. Wild rodents kept as pets or for laboratory research purposes can pose significant risks. High-risk activities also include opening and cleaning previously unused buildings including barns, garages and storage facilities, work related to construction, and pest control workers who can be exposed to rodent population. Ecological and climatic factors related to the increase in rodent populations can be associated with human outbreaks.

The three syndromes seen in humans along with their clinical manifestations are described below.

HFRS

This form of the disease is mainly observed in Europe and Asia. The incubation period of HFRS is 7–36 days, where 10–15% of cases have a severe course, with lethality rates between 6% and 15%. The clinical presentation of HFRS varies from subclinical mild and moderate to severe, depending on the causative agent of the disease. It induces various haemorrhagic manifestations by the systemic involvement of capillaries and venules. Renal involvement is characterised by acute renal failure as a result of interstitial haemorrhage and interstitial infiltrates.The clinical course is subdivided into five phases: febrile, hypotensive, oliguric, diuretic and convalescent. The onset of HFRS starts with high fever, backache, abdominal pain, chills, myalgia, malaise and bradycardia. On the initial 3–5 days, petechia develops on the palate, conjunctival haemorrhages may appear and temporary impairment of visual function has been reported. The urinary sediment reveals haematuria and atypical gross proteinuria. The hypotensive phase ranges from 3 to 6 days after the onset of fever which is characterised by shock or hypotension. The oliguric phase starts at approximately day 8, in which haemorrhagic manifestations become more prominent. The diuretic phase starts at approximately day 11, and the convalescent phase lasts approximately 3 weeks to 6 months.

The sequelae of the disease are rare but include chronic renal failure and hypertension. Extrarenal manifestations include acute impairment of visual function, acute myopia, CNS complications, sometimes myocarditis and severe gastrointestinal haemorrhages. Lung involvement may occur but to a lesser extent than in HPS.

Nephropathia Epidemica (NE)

In Europe, the hantavirus serotype Puumala is associated with NE, which is considered as a milder variant of HFRS, with mortality rates of 0.1%. NE is characterised by sudden onset with high fever, headache, backache, abdominal pain and haemorrhages. The renal involvement results in transient massive proteinuria, haematuria and impairment of renal function. Acute renal failure is present in many of the hospital-treated patients and transient haemodialysis is needed in a minority of the cases. However, the syndrome is associated with a low mortality rate.

HPS

This form of the disease is mainly reported in the USA. The onset of HPS is characterised by general flu-like symptoms such as high fever, fatigue, myalgia and headache. Almost half of HPS cases experience headaches, dizziness, chills and abdominal complications, such as nausea, vomiting, diarrhoea and abdominal pain. After 4–10 days of the initial phase of illness, the late symptoms of HPS include coughing and shortness of breath due to acute non-cardiac pulmonary oedema and hypotension. Mortality rates among HPS cases are approximately 50%. Patients who survive the acute phase of the disease recover normally within 5–7 days without any sequelae. The secondary complication is acute renal failure which occurs as a result of shock and respiratory failure.

Diagnosis

The diagnosis of hantavirus infection in humans is based on clinical and epidemiological information as well as laboratory testing. Hantavirus should be suspected in a patient with fever, lumbago, renal failure and recent outdoor activities in endemic regions. The correlation of history of potential rodent exposure and clinical signs like fever, fatigue and shortness of breath is strongly suggestive of HPS. Laboratory diagnosis of hantavirus infection is based on four primary categories of tests: serology, reverse transcription polymerase chain reaction (RT)-PCR, immunochemistry and virus culture.

Serological diagnosis is considered the most practical approach to detect exposure to hantavirus infection. A high level of IgM antibodies in acute cases and IgG antibodies in chronic infections or convalescent stage can be detected by employing enzyme-linked immunosorbent assays and immunoblot tests.

Molecular diagnostic assays based on RT-PCR are widely in use, as the hantavirus RNA is detectable 7–10 days after onset of symptoms. Further, the PCR product may be sequenced to identify the virus genotype and conduct phylogenetic analysis [9]. Virus isolation from human samples is tedious and requires specialised laboratory facilities, so it is not considered an option in the routine diagnosis of human hantavirus infection. However, isolation of hantaviruses for research purposes can be achieved by inoculation of infected clinical materials onto Vero E-6 cell cultures.

Treatment

There is no specific treatment or vaccine available for hantavirus infection. However, early detection of cases and proper medical care help in the clinical improvement of patients. The treatment regime is mostly symptomatic, and patients can be intubated and given oxygen therapy to alleviate the phases of severe respiratory distress.

Prevention and Control

The key to disease prevention is to avoid close contact with rodents and areas contaminated by rodent droppings. Any activity associated with contact with rodent droppings, urine, saliva or nesting materials increases the risk of infection. There should be efforts to control rodents which include elimination of rodent food sources inside and around the home, measures to prevent rodents from entering the home and elimination of possible nesting sites. When cleaning up potentially rodent-infested areas and rooms, appropriate precautions should be taken, such as proper ventilation of the room before entering, use of gloves and disinfectant, avoidance of stirring up and breathing dust, etc. The use of gloves and masks is recommended during the manipulation of rodent traps and handling of dead rodents.

References

1 Center for Food Security and Public Health (2018). Hanta Virus Disease. www.cfsph.iastate.edu/Factsheets/pdfs/hantavirus.pdf (accessed 7 December 2021).

2 Johnson, K.M. (2001). Hantaviruses: history and overview. In: *Hantaviruses: History and Overview.*, 1–14. Berlin.: Springer.

3 Lee, H.W., Lee, P.W., and Johnson, K.M. (1978). Isolation of the etiologic agent of Korean hemorrhagic fever. *Journal of Infectious Diseases* 137: 298–308.

4 Brummer-Korvenkontio, M., Vaheri, A., Hovi, T. et al. (1980). Nephropathia epidemica: detection of antigen in bank voles and serologic diagnosis of human infection. *Journal of Infectious Diseases* 141 (2): 131–134.

5 Nichol, S.T., Spiropoulou, C.F., Morzunov, S. et al. (1993). Genetic identification of a hantavirus associated with an outbreak of acute respiratory illness. *Science* 262 (5135): 914–917.

6 Klempa, B. (2009). Hantaviruses and climate change. *Clinical Microbiology and Infection 15* (6): 518–523.

7 Maes, P., Clement, J., Gavrilovskaya, I., and van Ranst, M. (2004). Hantaviruses: immunology, treatment, and prevention. *Viral Immunology 17* (4): 481–497.

8 Pinna, D.M., Martinez, V.P., Bellomo, C.M. et al. (2004). New epidemiologic and molecular evidence of person to person transmission of hantavirus Andes Sout. *Medicina 64* (1): 43–46.

9 Avšič-Županc, T., Saksida, A., and Korva, M. (2019). Hantavirus infections. *Clinical Microbiology and Infection 21*: e6–e16.

16

Influenza Viruses

Aetiological Agent

Influenza viruses belong to the family Orthomyxoviridae which includes enveloped negative-strand RNA viruses with segmented genomes (7–8 gene segments) [1, 2]. The family Orthomyxoviridae consists of four genera: Alphainfluenzavirus (species: influenza A virus), Betainfluenzavirus (species: influenza B virus), Gammainfluenzavirus (species: influenza C virus), and Deltainfluenzavirus (species: influenza D virus) [3]. All the species of these four genera are of human and/or animal health significance. The influenza A and B viruses have a similar structure and contain eight discrete single-stranded RNA segments, whereas influenza C and influenza D are more divergent and have a seven-segmented RNA genome.

Among these four genera, the influenza A virus can infect a wide variety of warm-blooded animals, including birds, swine, horses and humans. Therefore, it poses a significant risk of zoonotic infection where the pathogen can switch hosts and is capable of generation of epidemics. The influenza B and C viruses are mainly adapted to humans; however, influenza B viruses have been isolated from seals, and influenza C viruses have been isolated from pigs and dogs [2]. The novel species influenza D virus was isolated in 2011 from pigs with influenza-like symptoms and subsequently from cattle (the main reservoir of the virus). The influenza D virus is not known to infect or cause illness in humans [3].

Subtypes of Influenza A Viruses

Based on antigenic properties of the surface glycoproteins, i.e. haemagglutinin (HA) and neuraminidase (NA), the influenza A viruses are further divided into 18 HA (H1–H18) and 11 NA (N1–N11) subtypes. Thereby, the combination of HA and NA in a virus defines its subtype (e.g. H1N1, H1N2, H3N2, etc.) [4].

Nomenclature of Influenza Viruses

The internationally accepted naming convention for influenza viruses was accepted by the World Health Organization (WHO) in 1979 and published in 1980 in the Bulletin of the WHO. The nomenclature approach uses the following components [3].

Textbook of Zoonoses, First Edition. Jasbir Singh Bedi, Deepthi Vijay, and Pankaj Dhaka.

1) Antigenic type (e.g. A, B, C, D).
2) Host of origin (e.g. swine, equine, chicken, etc.). For human-origin viruses, no host of origin designation is given. Examples:
   - For the duck: avian influenza A(H1N1), A/duck/Alberta/35/76
   - For humans: seasonal influenza A(H3N2), A/Perth/16/2019.
3) For influenza A viruses: the haemagglutinin and neuraminidase antigen descriptions are provided in parentheses (e.g. influenza A[H1N1] virus, influenza A[H5N1] virus).
4) Geographical origin (e.g. Denver, Taiwan, etc.).
5) Strain number (e.g. 7, 15, etc.).
6) Year of collection (e.g. 57, 2009, etc.).

Role of Haemagglutinin and Neuraminidase Glycoproteins

The HA viral glycoprotein mediates attachment to sialic acid-containing receptors on the host cell and is the principal target for induction of neutralising antibodies. At the molecular level, sialic acids are attached to galactose residues by α-2,3 or α-2,6 linkages. In binding assays, human influenza viruses prefer to bind to α-2,6-linked (human-type) receptors, whereas avian viruses prefer α-2,3-linked (avian-type) receptors. The sialic acid binding is also responsible for the agglutination of red blood cells, and this property is used for diagnostic applications in haemagglutination and haemagglutination inhibition assays. The NA viral glycoprotein enables virus release from the infected cell by breaking the bonds between sialic acids and adjacent sugar residues [5].

Genetic Reassortment

The replication of the influenza RNA genome lacks effective exonuclease proofreading capability, so there are chances of introducing base mutations at relatively high rates which can lead to antigenic 'drift'. In addition, the segmented nature of the influenza genome allows two viruses (within the same genera) co-infecting the same host to exchange RNA segments during viral replication, a process known as genetic 'reassortment'. From the co-infection with two influenza A viruses, each carrying eight segments, a total of 256 ($2^8 = 256$) different progeny genotypes are possible. This high diversity can facilitate the rapid evolution of the virus under selective pressure, including adaptation to new host environments, evasion of host immune responses and acquisition of resistance to antiviral drugs [6].

The high mutation rates in influenza A viruses allow the evasion of immunity. The mutations that change amino acids in the antigenic portions of the surface glycoproteins (HA and NA) may produce selective advantages for viral strains by allowing them to evade the pre-existing immunity. The pandemic strains of influenza A viruses must possess at least three properties for long-term transmission in the population [1].

- The strain should be able to infect humans.
- It should be able to spread person to person.
- It should be able to evade immunity in the human population.

Historical Context

Influenza viruses have raised global public health concerns due to their potential to cause pandemics in humans as well as animals, especially in the poultry population, and outbreaks are associated with high socio-economic impact [1]. Most of the influenza virus pandemics have been initiated by the introduction and successful adaptation of a novel HA subtype to humans from an animal source, resulting in antigenic shift. In the twentieth century, the following three strains of the influenza virus were responsible for the major pandemics in humans:

- 1918 Spanish influenza virus (H1N1)
- 1957 Asian influenza virus (H2N2)
- 1968 Hong Kong influenza virus (H3N2).

The 1918 Spanish influenza pandemic remains one of the worst pandemics in recorded history, which was estimated to claim 50 million human lives worldwide. The influenza pandemics of 1957 and 1968 have been estimated to claim 500 000–20 00 000 human lives [7].

In 2009, a novel H1N1 virus lineage (A/H1N1/2009), known as the H1N1pdm09 virus, emerged in Mexico and the United States. This lineage was antigenically divergent from the seasonal H1N1 virus, as most of the human population were immunologically naive for this strain. The H1N1pdm09 virus probably arose through 'intercontinental' reassortment between swine influenza A viruses of North American and Eurasian lineages, followed by transmission from pigs to humans and then human-to-human transmission. Within the short span of its emergence, the virus has swept across the world and resulted in the first influenza pandemic of the twenty-first century. As per an epidemiological modelling study, the estimated range of global deaths from 2009 H1N1 virus infection during the first year of circulation was between 1 51 700 and 5 75 400 people [8].

Epidemiology and Disease Transmission

Reservoir Hosts

The genetically diverse influenza A viruses are widely distributed in wild avian species around the world. Wild waterfowl are believed to be the natural reservoir of influenza A viruses. They are maintained predominantly by asymptomatic infections among aquatic birds of the orders Anseriformes (ducks, geese, swans, etc.) and Charadriiformes (gulls, terns, etc.), which are termed 'low pathogenic avian influenza' (LPAI). The viruses in wild aquatic birds replicate predominantly in the intestinal tract and tend to be mainly transmitted via the faecal–oral route. These aquatic bird species remain the ultimate source of influenza virus for numerous other species, primarily poultry, pigs and humans.

Interspecies Transmission

Interspecies transmission of influenza viruses occurs frequently between wild and domestic waterfowl. In reservoir species (aquatic wild birds), the influenza virus subtypes are low pathogenic (LP) and mostly are not associated with any apparent symptoms. Two of the 16 subtypes (i.e. subtypes having H5 and H7) can evolve into 'highly pathogenic' (HP) viruses. The exchange of strains of influenza viruses can occur between various species of waterfowls (both wild and domestic), terrestrial poultry, backyard poultry and in live poultry markets that provide optimal conditions for the genetic mixing of influenza viruses and their interspecies transmission.

In humans, mainly the viruses of H1N1, H2N2 and H3N2 subtypes have circulated in different geographical regions for extended periods. However, in the recent past, the avian influenza viruses of the H5N1 and H7N9 subtypes have been found to spill over the species barrier and infect humans since their emergence in 1997 and 2013, respectively; however, none of the human outbreaks from these strains have increased to reach to epidemic level.

Pathogenesis

In humans, influenza viruses mainly infect the respiratory epithelium. The HA proteins of influenza A virus and influenza B virus, or the haemagglutinin-esterase-fusion (HEF) proteins of influenza C virus, bind to sialic acid and cause endocytosis. The viral genome replicates in the nucleus. The new viruses assemble at the cell surface and are released by the receptor-cleaving NA proteins of influenza A virus and influenza B virus or the HEF protein of influenza C virus [9].

Disease in Humans and Animals

The worldwide outbreaks due to influenza viruses have been associated with considerable socio-economic losses. In addition to the impact on human health, the influenza viruses also cause considerable losses to the poultry, swine and equine industries. The relentless growth of domestic swine and poultry populations in recent decades has contributed to the increased genetic diversity of influenza viruses circulating in domestic animals, thus expanding the pool of influenza viruses with pandemic potential. Some of the important clinical manifestations of influenza viruses in humans and animals are described below.

Humans

Pandemics of influenza viruses in humans are characterised by high attack rates, morbidity and mortality burdens. The various strains of the virus can infect a large proportion of the population, especially when the population exhibits low pre-existing immunity against these strain(s). A population with naive or immature immune responses, e.g. infants, elderly and individuals with co-morbidities, are at risk of severe clinical manifestations that may be further complicated by secondary bacterial infections. The seasonal influenza A viruses are associated with annual winter epidemics that infect around 5–15% of the world population, resulting in 3–5 million severe cases and 250000–500 000 deaths every year [10].

Highly Pathogenic Avian Influenza

Avian influenza is also known as fowl plague due to its devastating effect on the poultry industry. The viruses usually infect migratory waterfowl that can carry the LPAI viruses without showing any clinical signs. These LPAI virus strains can be occasionally introduced into domestic poultry flocks with no clinical signs or with mild clinical consequences; however, the strains carrying H5 or H7 gene can mutate into 'highly pathogenic avian influenza' (HPAI) strains that are associated with high mortality in domestic poultry. Due to the devastating effect of HPAI outbreaks in commercial poultry, all outbreaks caused by H5 and H7 subtypes are notifiable.

The HPAI virus strain of subtype H5N1 has circulated in many countries of Eurasia and Africa, associated with high mortality in poultry. Millions of domestic birds died from the effects of the disease or from culling efforts to control the spread of the virus. The virus was first detected in 1996 in geese in China and was first detected in humans in 1997 during a poultry outbreak in Hong Kong. Since then, the virus strain has been detected in poultry and wild birds in more than 50 countries in Africa, Asia, Europe and the Middle East. Migratory birds are considered to be responsible for the long-distance dispersal of the virus.

The incubation period for HPAI ranges from 3 to 14 days in naturally infected chickens. Depending on host species, age, characteristics of the viral strain and environmental factors, HPAI in susceptible birds may lead to clinical outcomes ranging from sudden death with no overt clinical signs to characteristic clinical presentations including respiratory signs, such as ocular and nasal discharges, coughing, difficulty in breathing, blood-tinged discharge from nostrils, swelling of the sinuses, reduced vocalisation, cyanosis of the skin, wattles and comb, inco-ordination, nervous signs, marked reduction in feed and water intake, and diarrhoea. In laying birds, additional clinical features include a drop in egg production. Typically, high morbidity is accompanied by high and rapidly escalating mortality [11].

Postmortem lesions may include swelling of the face and clear straw-coloured fluid in the subcutaneous tissues. The blood vessels are usually engorged and extensive haemorrhages may be seen in the trachea, proventriculus and throughout the intestine [11].

Zoonotic Potential of HPAI

Avian influenza is primarily considered as a disease of birds; however, sporadic cases have been periodically reported in humans, which reflects the potential of the virus to breach species barriers. Two commonly reported avian influenza strains from human clinical cases are Asian lineage H5N1 HPAI viruses and H7N9 LPAI viruses (in China).

The first reported case of the H5N1 virus in humans was in 1997 in a 3-year-old boy in Hong Kong, who subsequently died of respiratory failure. Globally, from 2003 to 2021, a total of 863 cases of human infection with avian influenza A (H5N1) virus have been reported from 18 countries. Of these 863 cases, 456 were fatal with a case fatality rate of 52.8% [12].

The human-type receptor for avian influenza A (H5N1) virus is found throughout the upper and lower respiratory tract of humans, as well as in pigs, whereas the avian-type receptor is almost exclusively found in the lungs of both species. The scarcity of avian-type receptors in the nose and trachea of humans is believed to hamper the transmission of avian viruses to and between humans. While H5N1 has not yet demonstrated the ability to transmit efficiently from person to person, the high case fatality associated with infection and the immense potential for influenza viruses to mutate and adapt to other hosts mean that H5N1 remains a persistent public health concern. An overview of disease transmission among reservoir birds, pigs and humans is depicted in Figure 16.1.

The symptoms of H5N1 infection in humans include fever, malaise, cough and muscle aches. Other early symptoms may include abdominal pain, chest pain and diarrhoea. The infection may

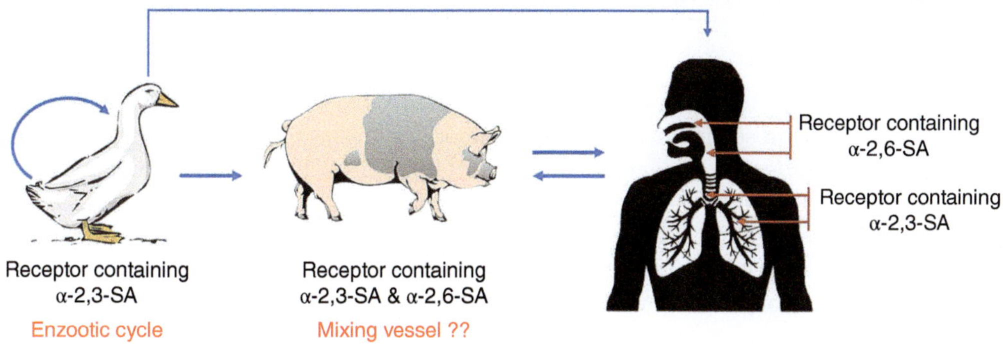

Figure 16.1 Transmission cycle of avian influenza virus among reservoir birds, pigs and humans.

progress to severe respiratory illness with symptoms including difficulty in breathing or shortness of breath, pneumonia, acute respiratory distress syndrome and neurological changes involving altered mental status or seizures.

In 2013, human infections with the avian influenza A (H7N9) virus were reported for the first time in China. Since then, virus outbreaks have been observed in the poultry population across the country, and also resulted in more than 1500 reported human cases [13].

Swine Influenza

Swine are considered important mammalian influenza virus reservoirs. Influenza viruses are widespread in swine and multiple lineages circulate in the pig population. The predominant virus subtypes H1N1, H3N2 and H1N2 have been associated with the majority of outbreaks. Most of these strains are highly contagious where morbidity rates can reach 100%, while mortality rates are generally low. Some strains can circulate in pigs with few or no clinical signs. The primary economic impact is related to decrease in weight gain which increases the number of days to reach market weight. The clinical discourse may include an acute upper respiratory infection characterised by fever, lethargy, anorexia, weight loss, nasal discharge and laboured breathing. Coughing, sneezing and nasal discharge are commonly seen. Complications may include secondary bacterial or viral infections. A decrease in semen production in boars and abortions in sows may also occur due to secondary effects of the infection. Severe, potentially fatal bronchopneumonia is occasionally seen.

Zoonotic Potential of Swine Influenza

Swine influenza viruses do not normally infect humans. However, sporadic human infections with influenza viruses normally circulating in swine have been reported with the 'variant viruses' of H1N1, H3N2 and H1N2. The major risk factors for most human cases include proximity to infected pigs or visiting locations where pigs are exhibited. In limited cases, human-to-human transmission has been reported. The illnesses associated with these variant viruses are mostly mild with symptoms similar to those of seasonal flu.

Further, pigs are also susceptible to infection with the strains adapted to humans and birds, due to the presence of both α 2,6- and α 2,3-linked sialic acid receptors on the epithelia of their upper respiratory tracts. Thereby, pigs can act as a 'mixing vessel' for influenza viruses, where the viruses that normally circulate in distinct host species (i.e. birds, humans, swine) can meet and interact, which can result in the genesis of novel strains [14].

Equine Influenza

Equine influenza A viruses are the common respiratory pathogens of horses, where the involvement of two subtypes is predominant (i.e. H7N7 and H3N8). Clinical signs include fever and harsh dry cough followed by nasal discharge. Further, depression, loss of appetite, muscle pain and weakness are frequently observed. The clinical signs generally abate within a few days, but complications due to secondary infections are common. While most animals recover in 2 weeks, the cough may continue longer and it may take as much as 6 months for some horses to regain their full health [15].

Diagnosis

Diagnosis in Humans

The diagnostic tests available for influenza virus include viral culture, serological tests (e.g. immunofluorescence assays, lateral flow assays, etc.) and rapid molecular assays (e.g. reverse transcription-polymerase chain reaction [RT-PCR]). The preferred samples for influenza testing are nasopharyngeal or nasal swab, and nasal wash or aspirate. As with any diagnostic test, the results should be evaluated in the context of other clinical and epidemiological information available to healthcare providers.

Viral culture is restricted to specialised laboratories and allows for genetic characterisation of influenza viruses. The procedure is time-consuming and the culture results do not yield timely results to be used for clinical management. Shell-vial tissue culture results may take 1–3 days, while traditional tissue-cell viral culture results may take 3–10 days. However, the collection of representative respiratory samples for viral culture is essential for surveillance and antigenic characterisation of new seasonal influenza strains that may need to be included in the ongoing influenza vaccine schedule [11]. Routine serological testing requires paired sera samples (acute and convalescent sera), so it is not particularly relevant for clinical decision making and is mainly carried out for research and public health investigations.

For quick diagnosis, rapid influenza diagnostic tests (RIDTs) can be performed, where the antigen-based assays can detect influenza viruses within minutes with low to moderate sensitivity and high specificity. However, it is advised to confirm these results with a more reliable molecular assay (e.g. RT-PCR) before arriving at any confirmatory conclusions.

Diagnosis in Poultry

During poultry outbreaks, oropharyngeal and cloacal swabs (or faeces) from live birds, and the faeces and pooled samples of organs from dead birds, should be taken in appropriate antibiotic solution to inhibit bacterial contamination. Virus isolation can be useful for virus characterisation. The isolation can be carried out in embryonated eggs and/or cell culture. The virus can be detected by various methods, including agar gel immunodiffusion (AGID), antigen detection enzyme-linked immunosorbent assay (ELISA) or other immunoassays, or using a molecular test such as RT-PCR. They can be subtyped with specific antisera through HA and NA inhibition tests, or by RT-PCR, or by using sequence analysis of the viral HA and NA genes. Genetic tests to identify characteristic patterns in the HA (at its cleavage site) and/or virulence tests in young chickens are used to distinguish LPAI from HPAI viruses [11].

The World Organisation for Animal Health (OIE) recommends antigen detection tests to identify avian influenza only in flocks and not in individual birds. RT-PCR assay can detect influenza viruses directly in clinical samples, and remains the diagnostic method of choice in many laboratories. Serological tests targeting antibodies used in poultry include AGID, haemagglutination inhibition (HI) and ELISAs. Serodiagnosis can be valuable for surveillance purposes and to demonstrate freedom from infection. However, it is not useful in diagnosing HPAI infections among highly susceptible birds, as they usually die before the development of antibodies. Moreover, cross-reactivity between influenza viruses can pose additional ambiguity for the interpretation of serological tests. Therefore, specific diagnostic tests that can distinguish infected from vaccinated birds (DIVA tests) should be used in surveillance when vaccination is a part of the disease control programme [11].

Treatment

In Animals and Poultry

There is no specific treatment for influenza virus infections in animals and poultry. Poultry flocks infected with HPAI viruses are generally depopulated (and this is mandatory in HPAI-free countries).

Influenza viruses may be subject to antigenic drift and antigenic shift which impose major challenges in vaccine development. Inactivated whole-virus and subunit influenza virus vaccines are available for humans, horses, birds and pigs. However, due to recurrent mutations in the HA and NA genes through antigenic drift, these vaccines need to be revised annually [11].

Given the global spread of the H5N1 virus, effective control exclusively by culling is not feasible. Therefore, vaccination strategies need to be implemented as part of comprehensive disease control programmes in affected countries. In most endemic countries, the vaccine is used in emergency vaccination programmes or as a preventive measure when the risk of an H5N1 virus is high. Avian influenza vaccines include both traditional inactivated whole-virus vaccines and novel recombinant vectored vaccines. Most vaccines are produced for chickens and their effectiveness can differ in other species. In addition to suppressing clinical signs, some vaccines are capable of increasing resistance to infection and thereby decreasing virus excretion and further transmission. In different countries, vaccines may be used routinely to protect poultry flocks, as an adjunct control measure during an outbreak or to protect valuable species such as zoo birds from severe clinical consequences.

For pigs, the currently available vaccines are either whole virus or split virus, and are adjuvanted, inactivated, prepared typically from virus propagated in embryonated hen eggs or cell lines. These vaccines have a major drawback in that they do not consistently confer cross-protection against new subtypes of the virus [11].

In Humans

The treatment for avian influenza in humans depends on the severity of the case. Along with symptomatic treatment, treatment with antivirals might be needed for severe cases. Two groups of antiviral drugs, adamantanes (e.g. amantadine, rimantadine) and neuraminidase inhibitors (e.g. zanamivir, oseltamivir, peramivir, laninamivir), are effective against some influenza A viruses. Oseltamivir is the most widely used antiviral drug which appears to increase the chance of survival in patients infected with Asian lineage H5N1 and H7N9 viruses. Recently, antiviral resistance against these drugs has been a point of concern as it can develop rapidly in influenza viruses, and may even emerge during treatment. At present, Asian lineage H5N1 HPAI viruses are usually sensitive to oseltamivir, and they are often (though not always) resistant to adamantanes [13].

Prevention and Control

There is no 'one size fits all' control strategy for the influenza virus. Various factors like the presence or absence of virus, the pathogenicity of the virus strain, HA subtype of the virus, species of birds at risk or infected, the type of ecosystem, available logistics, veterinary and medical infrastructure, political will and existing control programmes by government and non-government organisations affect the formulation and implementation of prevention and control programmes. Some of the important considerations are highlighted below.

In Poultry

During outbreaks, HPAI viruses are normally eradicated by depopulation of infected flocks, combined with other measures such as movement controls, quarantines and emergency vaccination. Insect and rodent control, disposal of contaminated material and thorough cleaning and disinfection are also important to prevent the further spread of the virus. International and/or national guidelines must be followed to contain the ongoing outbreak and prevent future outbreaks.

In Swine and Equines

A robust biosecurity plan for influenza virus must identify potential pathways for the introduction and spread of disease. Once influenza is established on a farm, it can be very difficult to eradicate the virus without complete depopulation. Disease control methods like partial depopulation, segregation of early-weaned animals, all-in all-out systems, along with good hygiene practices, can be implemented to control the disease incidence and minimise the economic impact on affected farms. In equines, vaccination is practised in most countries. However, due to the difficulty in matching the vaccine strain to the strains of the virus in circulation, vaccination does not always prevent infection, although it is found to reduce the severity of the disease.

The cross-species transmission of influenza viruses has been reported between humans and pigs; therefore, biosecurity measures must also take into account factors like human–pig interactions, particularly the exposure of pigs to persons with influenza-like illnesses.

In Humans

H5N1 vaccines for humans have been developed but are not in routine use. Protective measures for zoonotic avian influenza viruses include the following [11, 13].

- Controlling the source of the virus (e.g. depopulation of infected birds, closing infected poultry markets).
- Avoiding contact with sick animals and their environments.
- Employing good sanitation and hygiene (e.g. hand washing).
- Use of personal protective equipment (PPE), where appropriate. This may include respiratory and eye protection such as respirators and goggles, as well as protective clothing including gloves.
- HPAI viruses have been found in the meat and eggs of several avian species; therefore, careful food handling practices are important when working with raw poultry or wild game bird products in endemic areas. All poultry products should be completely cooked before eating.
- Wild birds may be the carriers of various viruses. Therefore, these birds should not be handled or eaten without proper cooking.
- Individuals working with swine should practise good hygiene measures and the use of proper PPE. Isolation of sick or infected pigs and other farm biosecurity measures would help to prevent the transmission of the influenza virus.

References

1 Taubenberger, J.K. and Kash, J.C. (2010). Influenza virus evolution, host adaptation, and pandemic formation. *Cell Host & Microbe* 7 (6): 440–451.

2 Wright, P.F., Neumann, G., and Kawaoka, Y. (2007). Orthomyxoviruses. In: *Fields Virology* (ed. D.M. Knipe and P.M. Howley), 1691–1740. Philadelphia: Lippincott, Williams & Wilkins.

3 Centers for Disease Control and Prevention (2021). Types of influenza viruses. www.cdc.gov/flu/about/viruses/types.htm (accessed 7 December 2021).

4 Schrauwen, E.J. and Fouchier, R.A. (2014). Host adaptation and transmission of influenza A viruses in mammals. *Emerging Microbes & Infections* 3 (1): 1–10.

5 Ramos, I., Bernal-Rubio, D., Durham, N. et al. (2011). Effects of receptor binding specificity of avian influenza virus on the human innate immune response. *Journal of Virology* 85 (9): 4421–4431.

6 Steel, J. and Lowen, A.C. (2014). Influenza A virus reassortment. In: *Influenza Pathogenesis and Control, Volume I* (ed. R. Compans and M. Oldstone), 377–401. Berlin: Springer.

7 Guan, Y., Vijaykrishna, D., Bahl, J. et al. (2010). The emergence of pandemic influenza viruses. *Protein & Cell* 1 (1): 9–13.

8 Dawood, F.S., Iuliano, A.D., Reed, C. et al. (2012). Estimated global mortality associated with the first 12 months of 2009 pandemic influenza A H1N1 virus circulation: a modelling study. *Lancet Infectious Diseases* 12 (9): 687–695.

9 Hutchinson, E.C. (2018). Influenza virus. *Trends in Microbiology* 26 (9): 809–810.

10 World Health Organization (2014). Influenza (seasonal). Fact sheet no. 211. www.who.int/mediacentre/factsheets/fs211/en/ (accessed 7 December 2021).

11 World Organisation for Animal Health (2016). Avian influenza. www.oie.int/fileadmin/Home/eng/Animal_Health_in_the_World/docs/pdf/Disease_cards/HPAI.pdf (accessed 7 December 2021).

12 World Health Organization (2021). Cumulative number of confirmed human cases for avian influenza A(H5N1) reported to WHO, 2003–2021. https://cdn.who.int/media/docs/default-source/influenza/human-animal-interface-risk-assessments/2021_oct_tableh5n1.pdf?sfvrsn=e678d3f7_7&download=true (accessed 7 December 2021). (accessed 7 December 2021).

13 World Health Organization (2018). Influenza (avian and other zoonotic). www.who.int/news-room/fact-sheets/detail/influenza-(avian-and-other-zoonotic) (accessed 7 December 2021).

14 Yoon, S.W., Webby, R.J., and Webster, R.G. (2014). Evolution and ecology of influenza A viruses. In: *Influenza Pathogenesis and Control, Volume I* (ed. R. Compans and M. Oldstone), 359–375. Berlin: Springer.

15 World Organisation for Animal Health (2019). Equine influenza. www.oie.int/en/disease/equine-influenza/ (accessed 7 December 2021).

17

Japanese Encephalitis

Japanese encephalitis (JE) is a vector-borne viral encephalitis that occurs mainly in South-East Asia and the Western Pacific region. The aetiological agent is the Japanese encephalitis virus (JEV) which is an enveloped single-stranded RNA virus of the genus *Flavivirus*, family Flaviviridae, and placed in the same antigenic complex as the West Nile virus [1]. The World Organisation for Animal Health (OIE) considers JEV in livestock as a notifiable disease that could affect trade between the countries.

Historical Context

Japanese encephalitis was first described in 1871 in Japan. In 1924, the organism was isolated from human brain tissue and around 10 years later, it was proven to be JEV by inducing infection in monkey brains. In 1935, the prototype Nakayama strain was isolated from the brain of a patient with encephalitis. Thereafter, the virus has been classified as a 'group B arbovirus' in the family Togaviridae. In 1938, the involvement of ardeids and pigs as reservoir hosts, and the role of *Culex tritaeniorhynchus* as a vector, were established. In 1985, JEV was designated under the separate family Flaviviridae, as a member of the genus *Flavivirus* [2].

Epidemiology and Transmission

Japanese encephalitis is considered an epidemic disease in South-East Asia and the Western Pacific region. The JEV is extending its horizon to new Asian and Australian regions, thus it is considered as an emerging and/or re-emerging disease [2].

JEV Ecology

More than 30 mosquito species belonging to different genera, including *Aedes*, *Anopheles*, *Armigeres*, *Culex* and *Mansonia*, are recognised as potential vectors of JEV; however, these all are not equally competent for virus transmission. In tropical and subtropical regions of Asia, the virus is primarily transmitted by *Culex* species, particularly *Culex tritaeniorhynchus*. This species mainly feeds on birds and the natural ecological cycle involves circulation of the virus between mosquitoes and avian species. *Cx. tritaeniorhynchus* also feeds on mammals, so it acts as a 'bridge vector' that causes infection in livestock and humans.

Textbook of Zoonoses, First Edition. Jasbir Singh Bedi, Deepthi Vijay, and Pankaj Dhaka.

The larval habitat of *Cx. tritaeniorhynchus* primarily consists of low-lying flooded areas such as fallow rice fields, but can also be found in wells, ponds, ditches and urban environments in proximity to the human population (e.g. water storage containers in houses).

Vector Horizon

Although *Cx. tritaeniorhynchus* is a native of northern Asia, it has a wider distribution, including areas of Africa (north east and sub-Saharan) and the Middle East. It can be found in locations where the annual mean temperature ranges between 8.2 °C and 28.9 °C, with elevations of a maximum of 838 m above sea level [3]. Apart from endemic zones, the emergence of mosquito vectors in non-endemic areas such as European countries (e.g. Greece, Turkey, etc.) increases the risk of the introduction of JEV in these regions [4].

Transmission Cycle

The virus is maintained through the enzootic transmission cycle among mosquitoes and sylvatic avian reservoirs, primarily large ardeid water birds (family Ardeidae) such as the cattle egret (*Bubulcus ibis*) and pond herons (*Ardeola grayii*). Domestic and feral pigs act as amplifying hosts for the virus. Other domesticated animals (e.g. cows, goats, horses, dogs, poultry) and wild species such as flying foxes, ducks, snakes and frogs have been identified as host species for JEV. However, these are considered dead-end hosts as they rarely develop sufficient viraemia to infect mosquitoes that feed post infection. Irrigated rice fields provide a suitable breeding ground for mosquitoes and also attract migratory wading birds which contribute to maintenance of the sylvatic transmission cycle. The zoophilic habits of *Cx. tritaeniorhynchus* persuade them to access nearby pig farms for a blood meal. As soon as the number of mosquitoes explodes, they start biting humans which act as a dead-end host for the infection. An overview of the transmission of JEV is depicted in Figure 17.1.

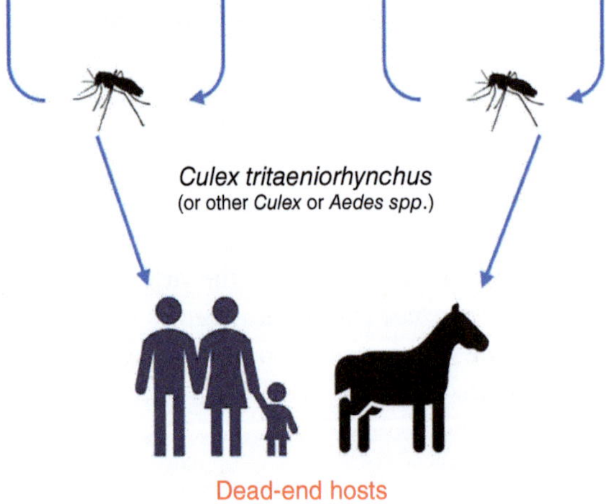

Figure 17.1 The natural and amplification transmission cycle of Japanese encephalitis virus (JEV).

Disease in Animals and Humans

In Animals

Several livestock species can act as amplifying hosts of the virus, and transmission from several species has been reported, including pigs, horses and cattle. Of these, pigs are considered the most significant host in transmission of the virus to feeding mosquitoes. Most pigs remain asymptomatic, but in some cases, pyrexia and anorexia have been reported. During large-scale outbreaks, JEV infection was found to be associated with a high risk of stillbirth and congenital deformity. Moreover, in non-endemic areas, the infection can have a significant effect on the reproductive performance of pigs. Under experimental conditions, the vector-free transmission of JEV between pigs has been described [5]. The experimentally infected pigs were found to shed the virus through oronasal emissions and transmit it to co-housed uninfected pigs. This has not been demonstrated under natural conditions but could provide a mechanism for the rapid spread of JEV among intensively farmed pig herds, which can enable the transmission of disease during vector-free periods.

The disease in horses is rare and most of the infections are subclinical. The seroconversion of unvaccinated horses in response to infection without any clinical signs of the disease is common, and is associated with long-term immunity in infected animals. Sometimes, the infected horse can present with pyrexia, loss of appetite and early signs of depression with neurological involvement, including ataxia. A similar clinical picture is observed for JEV infection in cattle [6]. Other species of domestic animals such as goats, dogs and cats can be subclinically infected. These animals do not act as a reservoir but can be used as sentinel species to provide early warning for seasonal occurrence of the disease. Domestic poultry is not thought to play a significant role in the transmission of JEV.

In Humans

Most human infections remain asymptomatic, with less than 1% of infected people developing the clinical form of the disease. The complex JEV cycle persists among young infants hailing from rural regions with unhygienic surroundings and malnourishment. Acute encephalitis in children is considered the most commonly recognised clinical manifestation, so the disease is also known as 'brain fever' in endemic areas. It has been estimated that only 1 in 250 infections end with encephalitis.

The incubation period of the disease is generally 5–15 days. The clinical symptoms usually begin with sudden onset of fever, frontal headache and malaise. In severe cases, neck rigidity, weakness, mental status changes, focal neurological deficits and movement disorders with mental retardation may develop throughout infection. The classic description of the disease includes a parkinsonian syndrome with symptoms of tremor, cogwheel rigidity and choreoathetosis movements. Acute flaccid paralysis with symptoms similar to those of poliomyelitis has also been associated with JEV infection. Seizures and mental retardation are noticed especially among children. The case fatality rate is approximately 20–30% in children. Among survivors, 30–50% have serious neurological sequelae [7].

Diagnosis

In Animals

Detection of the virus in the infected animals is challenging due to the short viraemic period and limited diagnostic facilities available in many of the endemic countries. Therefore, serological detection of JEV-specific immunoglobulin (IgM and IgG) is considered the most effective means of confirming infection.

Serological assays are useful for large-scale assessment of the prevalence of infection in the animal population, and the level of antibody protection following vaccination. The assays are used to detect markers of the immune response in cerebrospinal fluid (CSF) or serum samples. These assays include enzyme-linked immunosorbent assay (ELISA), virus neutralisation tests (VNT), haemagglutination inhibition tests (HI) and complement fixation tests (CFT) [8]. However, diagnosis using serological methods may be challenging in endemic areas, as the suspected animal might have previously been exposed to the virus or may have been vaccinated for the JEV. Additionally, the specificity of each assay needs to be considered due to cross-reactivity between other flaviviruses, particularly with the serologically related West Nile virus. The plaque reduction neutralisation test (PRNT) is considered the gold-standard assay for JEV diagnosis, with high specificity and minimal cross-reactivity with other flaviviruses [8]. ELISA for detection of antibodies specific for the JEV non-structural protein 1 (NS1) has demonstrated efficacy in differentiating antibodies induced by natural infection from those induced by vaccination; this enables differentiation between infected and vaccinated animals (DIVA) [8].

Several molecular methods have been described for the detection of JEV nucleic acid by reverse transcription-polymerase chain reaction (RT-PCR). These include a reverse transcription loop-mediated isothermal amplification (RT-LAMP) assay, which may be useful for testing in the field in locations with limited laboratory equipment.

Definitive diagnosis of JEV relies on isolation of the virus from central nervous system (CNS) tissue of infected or dead animals. Virus isolation can be carried out by tissue culture technique using primary cell cultures prepared from chicken embryos, porcine or hamster kidney cells, or with established cell lines such as Vero (African green monkey kidney), BHK (baby hamster kidney) or C6/36 (mosquito-*Aedes albopictus*). The *in vivo* isolation of the virus is carried out in 2–4-day-old mice by intracerebral inoculation with a homogenate of CNS tissue of the infected animal. If the diagnostic sample is positive for JEV, the mice will exhibit neurological signs and succumb within 14 days. All the laboratory work should be carried out under the Biological Safety Level 3 (BSL-3) protection.

In Humans

A patient with evidence of neurological infection (such as encephalitis, meningitis or acute flaccid paralysis) and a history of recent travel to or residence in an endemic area should be held under suspicion and must be recommended further laboratory diagnostic testing for confirmation of the disease.

During the initial phase of the infection, the JEV nucleic acid or antigens can be targeted using molecular tools such as RT-PCR and its variants. Along with detection of short fragments of nucleic acid, the application of whole-genome sequencing techniques can provide a more thorough analysis of the genetic identity of the virus, and is of particular use in identifying the geographical origin of a particular JEV strain.

Common serological methods for the diagnosis of JEV infection include the detection of IgM and IgG virus-specific antibodies using ELISA techniques [8]. Detection of IgM is useful for the identification of recent or acute cases of JEV infection, where the IgM is detectable in serum and CSF within 7 days after disease onset [1]. The recommended test is JE virus-specific IgM-capture ELISA using CSF or sera samples.

Treatment

In Animals

Vaccination of swine is considered a major preventive measure to reduce the impact of infection in endemic areas [2]. Some vaccines are commercially available in Asian countries for swine and horses but the cost of vaccination often outweighs the benefits of vaccine use or is constrained by the required logistics for vaccinating livestock during periods of vector activity. Vaccination of high-value racehorses that travel to JE-endemic regions is recommended. There is no antiviral prophylaxis available for treatment of the disease. Therapy mainly consists of supportive care and management of complications to reduce the symptoms of the disease.

In Humans

Inactivated human vaccines for JEV have been available since the 1930s. This inactivated mouse brain-derived (IMB) vaccine has been replaced with cell culture-based vaccines. The live attenuated vaccine based on the SA 14-14-2 strain of JEV is widely used in China and other Asian countries, including India, the Republic of Korea, Sri Lanka and Thailand. A Vero cell-derived inactivated and alum-adjuvanted JE vaccine based on the SA 14-14-2 strain was approved in 2009 in North America, Australia and various European countries [1]. All vaccine preparations can protect against all known isolates of JEV, and the cross-neutralisation of other flaviviruses has also been observed in vaccinated individuals. There is no antiviral treatment for patients with JE, but hospitalisation for supportive care and close observation is generally required. The mortality rate is high (20–30%) among patients who develop encephalitis [1].

Prevention and Control

A large number of cases go unreported due to the lack of surveillance and public awareness, so the actual threat of JE may be considerably higher in endemic regions. Control of the disease requires a strong surveillance system with integrated vector control, modified agricultural practices and the implementation of regular immunisation among young children, as well as in pigs. In many of the endemic regions, the lack of vaccination and disease control programmes accelerates the interaction of host, agent and environment which leads to enhancement of the activity of vector populations along with JEV maintenance, amplification and transmission to susceptible hosts.

Some of the important strategies for prevention and control of JE are described below.

- The control of mosquito vectors is the key to break down the transmission cycle of JEV. Animal housing must follow all the hygienic and sanitary protocols to avoid the breeding of mosquitoes. In endemic areas, adult mosquitoes can be targeted through the application of insecticides (e.g. fogging with chemicals such as pyrethrin) or by introducing mosquito-proof screens to animal housing to prevent vector access. The juvenile stages of the mosquitoes can be targeted with larvicides such as *Bacillus thuringiensis* toxin.
- During travel to endemic regions, it is recommended to use insect repellent and wear long-sleeved shirts and long trousers to avoid mosquito bites. Wherever possible, always try to get vaccinated before the visit.

- Pigs are considered the main amplifying host of the JEV. Therefore, in endemic regions, the pig population should not be in proximity to human habitats, and regular vaccination of the pigs should be carried out.
- There should be robust disease surveillance systems that include monitoring of factors influencing the transmission of JE. Capacity-building approaches for early recognition of impending outbreaks or epidemics should be established.

References

1 World Health Organization (2019). Japanese encephalitis www.who.int/news-room/fact-sheets/detail/japanese-encephalitis (accessed 7 December 2021).
2 Erlanger, T.E., Weiss, S., Keiser, J. et al. (2009). Past, present, and future of Japanese encephalitis. *Emerging Infectious Diseases* 15 (1): 1–7.
3 Miller, R.H., Masuoka, P., Klein, T.A. et al. (2012). Ecological niche modeling to estimate the distribution of Japanese encephalitis virus in Asia. *PLoS Neglected Tropical Diseases 6* (6): e1678.
4 Gunay, F., Alten, B., Simsek, F. et al. (2015). Barcoding Turkish Culex mosquitoes to facilitate arbovirus vector incrimination studies reveals hidden diversity and new potential vectors. *Acta Tropica 143*: 112–120.
5 Ricklin, M.E., Garcìa-Nicolàs, O., Brechbühl, D. et al. (2016). Japanese encephalitis virus tropism in experimentally infected pigs. *Veterinary Research 47* (1): 34.
6 Kako, N., Suzuki, S., Sugie, N. et al. (2014). Japanese encephalitis in a 114-month-old cow: pathological investigation of the affected cow and genetic characterization of Japanese encephalitis virus isolate. *BMC Veterinary Research 10* (1): 63.
7 Ghosh, D. and Basu, A. (2009). Japanese encephalitis – a pathological and clinical perspective. *PLoS Neglected Tropical Diseases* 3 (9): e437.
8 Mansfield, K.L., Hernández-Triana, L.M., Banyard, A.C. et al. (2017). Japanese encephalitis virus infection, diagnosis and control in domestic animals. *Veterinary Microbiology 201*: 85–92.

18

Nipah

Nipah is an emerging bat-borne zoonosis that causes sporadic outbreaks of fatal encephalitis in regions of South Asia. The Nipah virus is an enveloped, non-segmented, negative-sense, single-stranded RNA virus belonging to the family Paramyxoviridae. The family includes other important viruses affecting humans (e.g. measles, mumps, etc.) and animals (e.g. rinderpest, Newcastle disease, etc.) [1]. Various ecological and anthropogenic factors have led to the emergence of two highly pathogenic novel paramyxoviruses: Nipah virus and Hendra virus. Both of these viruses belong to the recently designated genus *Henipavirus* within the family Paramyxoviridae [2]. In past decades, outbreaks of the Nipah viruses were attributed to spillover from bats (considered as natural reservoirs) to other terrestrial mammals and humans in some of the populous regions of Asia. To date, human Nipah virus infections have been reported in Malaysia, Bangladesh, India, Singapore and the Philippines.

Transmission Cycle

Pteropid fruit bats are considered the reservoir of the Nipah virus. These bats can harbour the virus without any overt clinical signs and can directly or indirectly spill over to animals (e.g. pigs during the Malaysian outbreak) or humans. The reservoir frugivorous bats (*Pteropus*) are widely distributed throughout Asia, and the emergence of these viruses is probably due to increased agricultural encroachment into natural bat habitats such as fruit orchards.

Brief descriptions of three major Nipah outbreaks that have been reported with significant mortality rates and adverse socio-economic impacts are provided below.

Malaysian Outbreak

The first outbreak of Nipah was reported in 1998 in Malaysia. The virus was isolated from a fatal human case in the Sungai Nipah region of Malaysia, hence the name [3]. The epidemiology of the outbreak has been correlated with the slash-and-burn destruction of forest areas of Borneo and Sumatra, as well as the effect of El Niño, both of which eventually led to the mass exodus of fruit bats. These bats later settled in orchid plantations near intensively farmed piggeries, which resulted in spillover of the viruses to the pigs [4]. In due course, the rapid transportation of infected pigs to five states of Malaysia and Singapore resulted in 265 human cases with 105 deaths [5]. In March 1999, the Nipah virus caused febrile illness in 11 abattoir workers (including one death) in Singapore following close contact with pigs imported from Malaysia. Finally, the outbreak was contained by employing strict public health measures directed at the culling of more than 1 million pigs [6].

Textbook of Zoonoses, First Edition. Jasbir Singh Bedi, Deepthi Vijay, and Pankaj Dhaka.

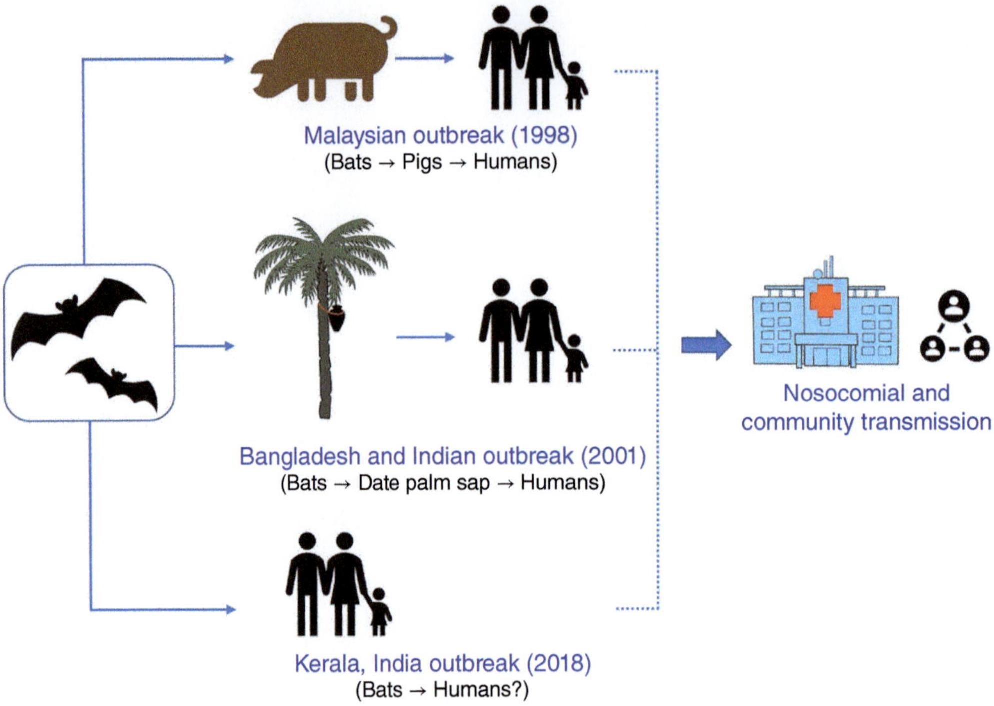

Figure 18.1 Transmission pathways of Nipah virus during past major outbreaks.

Outbreaks in Bangladesh and India

The second major outbreak of the Nipah virus occurred during 2001 in the Meherpur area of Bangladesh. However, the outbreak was not investigated till 2003, when another cluster of febrile illnesses with neurological features was reported in adjoining villages of the Naogaon district, resulting in eight deaths [7]. At the same time, the outbreak was also reported in Siliguri, India (adjoining area to Bangladesh). The primary route for the bat-to-human transmission of the virus was linked to the consumption of contaminated date palm sap. In addition, nosocomial transmissions of infection to healthcare workers were also reported during the outbreak [8].

Outbreak in Kerala, India

A Nipah outbreak was reported in the Indian state of Kerala during 2018. The index case contracted the virus from fruit bats and later the transmission of the disease was observed from person to person and to healthcare workers. The outbreak claimed 17 lives out of 19 cases [9].

The major pathways of virus spillover in these outbreaks are depicted in Figure 18.1.

Disease in Humans and Animals

Animals

The virus displays broad species tropism since it uses ephrin B2/B3 molecules as entry receptors, which are highly conserved amongst all mammals [10]. Pigs and other domestic animals (e.g. horses, goats, sheep, cats, dogs) were found to be seropositive during the Malaysian outbreak [11].

It should be noted that animals may incubate the virus for up to 18 days, and during this period the infected animals may be asymptomatic but are infectious. In the Malaysian outbreak, most of the pigs remained asymptomatic but some cases developed acute febrile illness, laboured breathing, loud non-productive cough (that named the disease as 'barking pig syndrome' and 'One-mile cough'), and neurological symptoms such as trembling, twitching and muscle spasms. The mortality among pigs was low, except in young piglets [12].

Humans

The incubation period of the disease varies from 4 days to 2 months (more than 90% of cases at 2 weeks or less) [13]. Mostly, the patient shows non-specific symptoms including mild fever, vomiting, headache and dizziness. A high incidence of acute respiratory distress syndrome was observed in the Bangladesh and Indian outbreaks (50–67% cases) compared to the Malaysian outbreaks (14–29% of cases) [14]. In severe cases, the clinical signs of encephalitis become prominent, which include reduced level of consciousness, brainstem dysfunction and diverse and multifocal neurological involvement. The high mortality rate among cases is due to encephalitis or respiratory involvement. In some cases, the development of relapse and late-onset encephalitis has been observed after months or years of acute illness.

Diagnosis

The Nipah infection in humans and animals can be confirmed by virus isolation, nucleic acid amplification tests and serological tests. As the Nipah virus is classified as a Biosafety Level-4 (BSL-4) agent, precautions and standard procedures must be undertaken during the collection, submission and processing of samples. The most commonly used serological assays are enzyme-linked immunosorbent assays (ELISAs) to target IgM and IgG antibodies against the infection, whereas polymerase chain reaction (PCR) assays can be applied for rapid diagnosis of the viruses, especially during the initial stages of infection.

Treatment

There are currently no antiviral drugs or vaccines available to treat Nipah virus infection in humans or animals. Therefore, supportive care is the mainstay for treatment protocols. The treatment regime may include anticonvulsants, treatment of secondary infection, mechanical ventilation and rehabilitation. In severe cases, the use of monoclonal antibodies and empirical treatment with ribavirin is advocated.

Prevention and Control

Early detection of outbreaks and implementation of preventive measures are important, as the treatment options for the disease are limited. The risk for spillover of the virus should be determined by carrying out surveillance activities for henipaviruses. For at-risk regions, it is important to characterise the genetic diversity of the viruses and to understand the determinants of Nipah virus transmissibility and pathogenicity among humans. Medical and veterinary professionals, along with ecologists and social scientists, should increase awareness of the disease, particularly regarding animal hosts and mode of transmission of the virus in the framework of the One Health approach. Some of the important prevention strategies include the following.

At Farm Level

- Suitable biosecurity interventions to prevent animal infection either by direct contact with bats or by feeding contaminated fruits to farm animals.
- Avoid construction of animal shelters near fruit trees which could attract bats.
- Reduce overcrowding in farms to avoid animal stress and rapid spread of the infection.

Prevent Food Contamination

- Use of physical barriers to prevent access of bats to date palm sap.
- Suspected bat-eaten fruits and contaminated date palm sap should be discarded.

Prevent Human-to-Human Spread

- It is difficult to diagnose the infection by assessing clinical signs, as many symptoms are similar to those of other common infections, such as Japanese encephalitis, malaria and measles. Therefore, always consult a physician in suspected cases.
- Avoid close contact with infected individuals.
- Use of proper personal protective equipment (PPE) while handling cases.
- Proper hand hygiene and sanitation.

References

1 Clayton, B.A., Wang, L.F., and Marsh, G.A. (2013). Henipaviruses: an updated review focusing on the pteropid reservoir and features of transmission. *Zoonoses and Public Health 60* (1): 69–83.

2 Eaton, B.T., Broder, C.C., Middleton, D., and Wang, L.F. (2006). Hendra and Nipah viruses: different and dangerous. *Nature Reviews Microbiology 4* (1): 23–35.

3 Field, H., Young, P., Yob, J.M. et al. (2001). The natural history of Hendra and Nipah viruses. *Microbes and Infection 3* (4): 307–314.

4 Chua, K.B., Chua, B.H., and Wang, C.W. (2002). Anthropogenic deforestation, El Nino and the emergence of Nipah virus in Malaysia. *Malaysian Journal of Pathology 24* (1): 15–21.

5 Parashar, U.D., Sunn, L.M., Ong, F. et al. (2000). Case-control study of risk factors for human infection with a new zoonotic paramyxovirus, Nipah virus, during a 1998–1999 outbreak of severe encephalitis in Malaysia. *Journal of Infectious Diseases* 181 (5): 1755–1759.

6 Lam, S.K. (2003). Nipah virus – a potential agent of bioterrorism? *Antiviral Research 57* (1–2): 113–119.

7 Hsu, V.P., Hossain, M.J., Parashar, U.D. et al. (2004). Nipah virus encephalitis reemergence, Bangladesh. *Emerging Infectious Diseases 10* (12): 2082.

8 Islam, M.S., Sazzad, H.M., Satter, S.M. et al. (2016). Nipah virus transmission from bats to humans associated with drinking traditional liquor made from date palm sap, Bangladesh, 2011–2014. *Emerging Infectious Diseases 22* (4): 664.

9 17 picked Nipah virus from first victim, finds Kerala govt. study (2018). *The Hindu*.www.thehindu.com/news/national/kerala/17-picked-nipah-virus-from-first-victim-finds-kerala-govt-study/article24428589.ece (accessed 7 December 2021).

10 Negrete, O.A., Wolf, M.C., Aguilar, H.C. et al. (2006). Two key residues in ephrinB3 are critical for its use as an alternative receptor for Nipah virus. *PLoS Pathogens 2* (2): e7.

11 Chua, K.B. (2003). Nipah virus outbreak in Malaysia. *Journal of Clinical Virology 26* (3): 265–275.

12 Looi, L.M. and Chua, K.B. (2007). Lessons from the Nipah virus outbreak in Malaysia. *Malaysian Journal of Pathology 29* (2): 63–67.

13 Goh, K.J., Tan, C.T., Chew, N.K. et al. (2000). Clinical features of Nipah virus encephalitis among pig farmers in Malaysia. *New England Journal of Medicine 342* (17): 1229–1235.

14 Ang, B.S., Lim, T.C., and Wang, L. (2018). Nipah virus infection. *Journal of Clinical Microbiology 56* (6): e01875–e01817.

19

Rabies

Rabies (Latin meaning 'rage' or 'madness') is one of the oldest known zoonoses and is considered the deadliest disease with nearly 100% mortality if treatment is not initiated immediately after exposure to the rabies virus.

Aetiology

The disease is invariably fatal with progressive encephalitis, caused by the virus belonging to the genus *Lyssavirus* of the Rhabdoviridae family. The viruses in this family have a distinct bullet-shaped structure, and the family includes three important genera of animal viruses: *Lyssavirus*, *Ephemerovirus* and *Vesiculovirus*. *Lyssavirus* is enveloped with a single-stranded, negative-sense RNA genome. The genome of the virus encodes five genes whose order is highly conserved, and these genes code for nucleoprotein (N), phosphoprotein (P), matrix protein (M), glycoprotein (G) and viral RNA polymerase (L) [1].

Historical Context

The first rabies vaccine was developed by Louis Pasteur and was administered on July 6, 1885, to Joseph Meister, a 9-year-old boy who had been attacked by a rabid dog. The boy survived and avoided contracting rabies. Due to this historical development, every year 6th July is marked as World Zoonoses Day.

Epidemiology and Transmission

Rabies is primarily a disease of terrestrial mammals, including dogs, wolves, foxes, jackals, cats, lions, mongooses, skunks, badgers, monkeys and humans. Rabies is present in all continents, except Antarctica. The disease is endemic in more than 150 countries and causes 40000–70000 deaths every year, most of which are in Asia and Africa [2, 3]. Rabies is considered a neglected disease of poor and vulnerable populations, where vaccines and immunoglobulin are not readily available or accessible, and cases are greatly under-reported. Countries predominantly affected by rabies often have poor diagnostic and reporting capacities, leading to the lack of accurate data and uncertainty around estimates of disease burden. Around 40% of people who are bitten by rabid

Textbook of Zoonoses, First Edition. Jasbir Singh Bedi, Deepthi Vijay, and Pankaj Dhaka.

animals are children under 15 years of age. The cases are mainly noticed among children of rural communities who are frequent victims because of their outdoor activities, during which they might be approaching dogs to play without any fear of attack. Many studies have revealed that children tend to hide dog bites from parents, which sometimes can be a life-threatening scenario if they have been bitten by a rabid animal [3].

Disease Transmission

The major burden of human rabies is attributed to dog-mediated transmission (around 99% of human rabies cases). However, the sylvatic cycle of rabies also exists, where wild animals (e.g. bats, raccoons, foxes) serve as the maintenance host for the virus. Human rabies cases following exposure to foxes, raccoons, skunks, jackals, mongooses and other carnivore host species are rarely reported [4].

When a rabid animal bites another warm-blooded mammal, the rabies virus is primarily transmitted through saliva. The infected animal drools excessive saliva which may also drip onto its claws. Scratches from an infected animal and contact of saliva with mucous membranes or abrasions or cuts can lead to exposure to the rabies virus.

Pathogenesis

On entry, the virus binds to cell receptors and replicates within striated muscle cells or can directly infect nerve cells. It then travels via retrograde axoplasmic transport mechanisms to the central nervous system (CNS), where both motor and sensory fibres can be involved, depending on the animal infected. Once it reaches the CNS, rapid replication of the virus can cause pathological effects on nerve cell physiology. The virus then moves from the CNS via anterograde axoplasmic flow within peripheral nerves and leads to the infection of adjacent non-nervous tissues (e.g. secretory tissues of salivary glands). Once clinical onset begins, the virus is widely disseminated throughout the body and leads to the shedding of virus in saliva, and this completes the infection cycle [5].

Disease in Animals and Humans

In Animals

The rabies virus causes acute encephalitis in all warm-blooded hosts with fatal clinical outcomes. The initial symptoms may be non-specific and include lethargy, fever, vomiting and anorexia. The clinical signs progress within days to cerebral dysfunction, cranial nerve dysfunction, ataxia, weakness, paralysis, seizures, difficulty in breathing and swallowing, excessive salivation, abnormal behaviour, aggression and self-mutilation [6]. In dogs, rabies is characterised by clinical manifestations, including unexplained paralysis and change in behaviour, such as:

- biting without provocation
- eating abnormal items such as sticks, nails, faeces, etc.
- aimless wandering
- vocal changes (e.g. hoarse barking and growling) or inability to produce sounds
- excessive salivation or foaming from the mouth.

There are other clinical signs that a rabid animal may or may not exhibit, such as anorexia, biting inanimate (non-food) objects, pawing at the mouth, having difficulty in swallowing, chewing at the site of the bite, seizures and exhibiting hypersensitivity to touch or sound, etc.

The two forms of rabies in mammals (including dogs and humans) are as follows [6].

- **Furious rabies:** Dogs with the furious form of rabies exhibit signs of hyperactivity, excited behaviour, hydrophobia (fear of water) and sometimes aerophobia (fear of flying). Death occurs via cardiorespiratory arrest in the infected animal after some days of infection.
- **Paralytic rabies:** The paralytic form runs a less dramatic and usually longer course than the furious form. The muscles of the infected animal gradually become paralysed, starting at the site of the bite or scratch. A coma slowly develops and eventually death occurs. This form of rabies is often misdiagnosed, contributing to the under-reporting of the disease.

In Humans

The average incubation period of rabies is 3–8 weeks. However, it can range from days to years depending on several factors, such as the dose of inoculum, severity of the wound, and length of the neural path from the wound to the brain (e.g. wounds on the face have a shorter incubation period than wounds on the leg). The initial symptoms of rabies may be similar to those of flu including general weakness, fever or headache. There may also be discomfort or prickling or itching sensation at the site of the bite, which can progress within days to acute symptoms of cerebral dysfunction, anxiety, confusion and agitation. The acute period of disease typically ends after 2–10 days. As the disease progresses, the patient may experience delirium, abnormal behaviour, hallucinations, hydrophobia and insomnia. Once the clinical signs of rabies appear, the disease is nearly always fatal (case fatality rate is nearly 100%), and only supportive treatment is possible [6].

Diagnosis

The clinical diagnosis of rabies is difficult unless the rabies-specific signs of hydrophobia or aerophobia are present. In most instances, rabies is fatal, and the testing of specimens is carried out in the postmortem state. The rabies diagnosis relies on laboratory tests for the detection of viral antigens. For diagnosis, an appropriate specimen is needed (e.g. brain tissue, cerebrospinal fluid, other specific specimens). Among diagnostic tests, the fluorescent antibody test (FAT) is considered the gold standard in postmortem rabies diagnosis. Alternative antigen detection methods such as the enzyme-linked immunosorbent assay (ELISA), direct rapid immunohistochemical test (DRIT) or indirect rapid immunohistochemistry test (IRIT) are also used [7].

Recently, molecular tools based on detection of the genetic information of rabies virus have been widely accepted for diagnosis. The development of reverse transcription-polymerase chain reaction (RT-PCR) techniques provided a valuable method for rapid postmortem and antemortem diagnosis of rabies [7].

For confirmation and virus isolation, the rabies tissue culture infection test (RTCIT) or the mouse inoculation test (MIT) are used, which are based on the propagation and isolation of the virus. The testing of suspected rabid dead animals or human samples does not pose a high risk for the further spread of the disease; therefore, Biosafety Level 2 (BSL-2) laboratory facilities are adequate.

Tests for Determination of Rabies Antibodies

Serum neutralisation assays are used to determine the potency of anti-rabies serum and immunoglobulins for postexposure treatment and to evaluate the immunogenicity of human and animal rabies vaccines. The standard methods recommended by the World Health Organization (WHO) are the mouse neutralisation test (MNT), plaque reduction assay and rapid fluorescent focus inhibition test (RFFIT). The RFFIT is considered the gold standard for assessing the viral neutralising antibodies. It is performed in cell culture to determine the rabies virus neutralising antibody level in human or animal sera. The assay is used to monitor antibody levels in persons who may have an occupational risk of rabies virus exposure (e.g. veterinarians, rabies virus laboratory workers, etc.). In some cases, such serological testing is used to check the immune response of a person undergoing rabies postexposure prophylaxis (PEP), when major deviations in the vaccination schedule occur, or there are concerns about a patient's immune status [8].

Treatment

Vaccination in Animals

Vaccination of dogs, ferrets and livestock can be started 3 months after birth and a booster vaccination should be administered 1 year later. The vaccination of at least 70% of the dog population in endemic regions is now accepted as the most effective way of preventing dog-mediated human rabies deaths [6].

In Humans

Initiation of an effective treatment schedule soon after exposure to rabies virus can prevent the onset of symptoms and death. Rabies is a 100% preventable zoonosis if proper prophylactic vaccination is provided as a part of preexposure prophylaxis (PrEP) or along with anti-rabies serum (rabies immunoglobins [RIGs]) as a part of PEP. PEP treatment of a bite victim should start immediately to prevent the virus entering the CNS. Just after the bite, thorough washing of the bite wound for a minimum of 15 minutes with soap or povidone-iodine or other effective disinfectant is recommended. After washing the bite wound, consult a physician for the course of effective rabies vaccination schedule as per WHO standards and administration of RIG (if indicated by the physician). The WHO promotes human rabies prevention through the use of the intradermal route for PEP which reduces the volume and thereby the cost of cell-culture vaccine by 60–80% [9]. Depending on the severity of the contact with a suspected rabid animal, the WHO recommends administration of a full PEP course as shown in the table below [6]/with permission of WHO.

Categories of contact with a suspected rabid animal	Postexposure prophylaxis measures
Category I: touching or feeding animals, animal licks on intact skin (no exposure)	Washing of exposed skin surfaces, no PEP required
Category II: nibbling of uncovered skin, minor scratches or abrasions without bleeding (exposure)	Wound washing and immediate vaccination
Category III: single or multiple transdermal bites or scratches, contamination of mucous membrane or broken skin with saliva from animal licks, and severe exposures due to direct contact with bats	Wound washing, immediate vaccination and administration of rabies immunoglobulin

Vaccination Schedule

Pre-exposure Vaccination

Pre-exposure vaccination is strongly recommended for occupational at-risk groups which include laboratory staff, veterinarians, animal health workers and wildlife officials. As per WHO guidelines, for the available modern cell-culture or embryonated-egg vaccines, three doses are required, one on each of days 0, 7 and 21 or 28 given intramuscular (1 or 0.5 mL/dose depending on the vaccine) or intradermal (0.1 mL/inoculation site).

Postexposure Vaccination Schedule [10]/BMJ Publishing Group Ltd.

For non-immunised or incompletely immunised people	
	Route: Intramuscular
Five-dose Essen regimen	• One intramuscular dose on each of days 0, 3, 7, 14 and 28 plus rabies immunoglobulin for category III exposures • In immunocompetent people, a reduced course with four vaccine doses on days 0, 3, 7 and 14 may be considered, provided they receive wound care plus rabies immunoglobulin for both categories II and III exposures and a WHO prequalified rabies vaccine is used
Four-dose Zagreb regimen	Two doses of vaccine on day 0, one dose on days 7 and 21
	Route: Intradermal[a]
Thai Red Cross regimen	Two intradermal doses of 0.1 mL vaccine at two different sites on days 0, 3, 7 and 28
For people with documented previous complete pre-exposure or postexposure prophylaxis with rabies CCEEVs[b]	
Intramuscular route	One intramuscular dose at one site on both days 0 and 3 (no rabies immunoglobulin required)[c]
Intradermal route	'One visit four-site' intradermal regimen: four injections of 0.1 mL equally distributed over left and right deltoids, thigh or suprascapular areas at one visit

CCEEVs, cell-culture and embryonated egg-based rabies vaccines.

[a] The WHO states that this regimen can be used for people with category II or III exposure in countries where the intradermal route has been endorsed by the national health authorities.

[b] People with category III exposure who have received complete pre-exposure or postexposure prophylaxis with a vaccine of unproved potency should be managed as if unvaccinated and receive a full postexposure vaccination course, including RIG.

[c] This regimen can also be given to people vaccinated against rabies who have detectable rabies virus-neutralising antibodies.

Prevention and Control

It is highly unfortunate that rabies, a zoonosis that can easily be prevented in humans and controlled in domestic animals, is still neglected and continues to cause significant mortality and socioeconomic burden on a global scale. In endemic regions, lack of awareness about the disease and access to appropriate PEP is still leading to thousands of human deaths per year [6]. The WHO, the World Organisation for Animal Health (OIE), the Food and Agriculture Organization of the

United Nations (FAO) and the Global Alliance for Rabies Control (GARC) have established a global 'United Against Rabies' collaboration to provide a common strategy to achieve 'Zero human rabies deaths by 2030'.

Some of the important strategies for prevention and control of rabies are as follows [6].

- **Management of rabies in dogs:** Dogs remain the major source of rabies in most endemic regions, so control measures should be primarily directed towards the control of canine rabies, which includes the following measures.
  - Dog vaccination is considered more cost-effective than human PEP. Vaccinating at least 70% of dogs can break the rabies transmission pathway in endemic regions.
  - Stay away from a suspected rabid dog and warn other people to keep away. Immediately contact the municipal authorities to manage the dog.
  - Establishment of proper quarantine facilities for import and export of pets.
  - Stray dog population control is important to reduce the contact of these dogs with humans and animals. Surgical sterilisation and compulsory vaccination of stray dogs are effective strategies for the control of rabies in stray dogs.
- **Management of rabies in wildlife.**
  - Prevent the spillover of infection by measures like parenteral vaccination of wildlife through 'trap–vaccinate–release' methods.
  - Oral vaccination and passive disease surveillance programmes among wildlife are required.
- **Management of rabies in humans.**
  - Vaccination of high-risk individuals (e.g. veterinarians, dog traders, etc.) is important.
  - Development of efficient laboratory diagnostic facilities for early diagnosis and treatment of rabies.
  - Easy access to modern tissue culture vaccines and anti-RIG.
- **Efforts by policymakers and community leaders.**
  - Setting up of reliable surveillance systems.
  - Education campaigns and public awareness about the disease.
  - Stress on evidence-based policies.
  - Collaborative efforts between multiple stakeholders.
- **International collaborations** with various global agencies to tackle the problem effectively.

References

1 Yousaf, M.Z., Qasim, M., Zia, S. et al. (2012). Rabies molecular virology, diagnosis, prevention and treatment. *Virology Journal 9* (1): 50.

2 World Health Organization (2005). *World Health Organization Expert Committee on Rabies, First report. 2005*, WHO Technical Report Series, vol. 931, 1–87. Geneva: WHO.

3 Hampson, K., Coudeville, L., Lembo, T. et al. (2015). Estimating the global burden of endemic canine rabies. *PLoS Neglected Tropical Diseases 9* (4): e0003709.

4 Singh, R., Singh, K.P., Cherian, S. et al. (2017). Rabies – epidemiology, pathogenesis, public health concerns and advances in diagnosis and control: a comprehensive review. *Veterinary Quarterly 37* (1): 212–251.

5 World Health Organization (2021). Rabies Bulletin Europe. Transmission and pathogenesis. www.who-rabies-bulletin.org/site-page/transmission-and-pathogenesis (accessed 7 December 2021).

6 World Health Organization (2018). Factsheet on rabies. www.who.int/en/news-room/fact-sheets/detail/rabies (accessed 7 December 2021).

7 Schlottau, K., Freuling, C.M., Müller, T. et al. (2017). Development of molecular confirmation tools for swift and easy rabies diagnostics. *Virology Journal 14* (1): 184.

8 World Health Organization (2019). Control of neglected tropical diseases. www.who.int/teams/control-of-neglected-tropical-diseases/rabies/diagnosis (accessed 7 December 2021).

9 World Health Organization (2012). Human dog-mediated-rabies: strengthening capacity and raising awareness are crucial for elimination. www.who.int/news/item/24-09-2012-human-dog-mediated-rabies-strengthening-capacity-and-raising-awareness-are-crucial-for-elimination (accessed 7 December 2021).

10 Crowcroft, N.S. and Thampi, N. (2015). The prevention and management of rabies. *BMJ 350*: 7827.

20

Rift Valley Fever

Rift Valley fever (RVF) is a mosquito-borne zoonotic viral disease of livestock and humans in Africa and the Middle East. Rift Valley fever virus (RVFV) is a significant haemorrhagic fever virus of humans that also causes high levels of mortality and morbidity in livestock, thereby posing a risk to both human and animal health [1].

Aetiology

Rift Valley fever virus is a negative-sense, trisegmented RNA virus of the order Bunyavirales and genus *Phlebovirus*. It is classified under 'category A' of the Centers for Disease Control and Prevention (CDC) bioterrorism agent list. The disease is also a World Organisation for Animal Health (OIE)-listed disease and any outbreak must be reported to the OIE. In RVFV enzootic or endemic regions, outbreaks occur during a wide interval of 3–17 years (average interepizootic/interepidemic interval of 7.9 years) [2]. Because of its long interepizootic intervals, it is also regarded as a re-emerging disease [1].

Historical Context

Rift Valley fever was first identified in 1931 during an epidemic investigation among sheep on a farm in the Rift Valley of Kenya. The most notable RVF epizootic occurred in Kenya during 1950–1951 when an estimated 1 000 000 sheep died and 500 000 aborted. In the past, a significant zoonotic impact of RVF has been reported, with 200 000 human cases and 600 deaths in Egypt during the outbreak in 1976, and 747 human cases with 230 deaths in Sudan during the outbreak in 2007–2008. Before 1977, outbreaks of RVF were reported only from sub-Saharan Africa but after that the virus continuously expanded its horizon to Egypt, Madagascar, the Comoros Islands and the Arabian Peninsula. To date, RVF has been reported from more than 30 countries. The potential spread of RVFV is facilitated by the presence of susceptible domestic animal hosts and mosquitoes in many parts of the world [3].

Textbook of Zoonoses, First Edition. Jasbir Singh Bedi, Deepthi Vijay, and Pankaj Dhaka.

Epidemiology and Transmission

Rift Valley fever outbreaks tend to be cyclical in endemic regions, where infections may persist for years at low prevalence in vectors and animals during an interepizootic period. Whenever the conditions are optimal (i.e. rainfall, vector density, population of susceptible livestock), a dramatic increase in the incidence of infections can be observed, which is also termed an 'epizootic period'. The transmission of RVFV is primarily by mosquitoes but could also be by direct contact with infected tissues and fluids of infected animals [4].

Vectors

Mosquito species of *Aedes*, *Culex* and *Mansonia* genera are considered the main vectors of RVFV. Irrigated areas (including rice fields) constitute favourable breeding sites for many of these mosquito species [1]. The mosquitoes of *Aedes* spp. are the important vectors involved in the vertical transmission of RVFV and are therefore termed 'reservoir or maintenance' vectors, whereas *Culex* spp. are considered as the important horizontal vectors of the virus, therefore termed as 'epidemic or amplifying' vectors.

Transmission Cycle

The accepted transmission paradigm involves the survival of RVFV in the eggs of *Aedes* spp. through transovarian transmission to their progeny during periods of drought. These mosquitoes perpetuate the virus by depositing virus-infected eggs at the edges of water-filled depressions (*dambos*) following flooding. At the end of flooding periods, these dambos dry out and the eggs may remain viable for long periods, waiting for the next cycle of inundating rains. When such habitats flood after rainfall, biological transmission of the virus occurs through infected mosquito saliva to domestic and wild herbivores which may be attracted to the water supply. The vertebrate hosts are typically viraemic for only 2–7 days, implying that chronic infection of the invertebrate vector is more important for the survival of RVFV from season to season.

Provided the larval habitats remain flooded for more than 2–3 weeks, the floodwater *Aedes* spp. are succeeded by *Culex* spp., which oviposit in small egg rafts on the surface of the water. The egg rafts lead to a population explosion of *Culex* mosquitoes, which become infected upon feeding on viraemic vertebrate hosts. While the floodwater *Aedes* spp. tend to remain near the larval habitats and only feed at dusk and dawn, the more nocturnal *Culex* spp. are more likely to disperse to find vertebrate hosts to feed on, which can lead to extensive dissemination of RVFV as a large-scale epidemic (Figure 20.1) [4, 5].

Other Transmission Routes

The virus can also be transmitted by direct contact with infected tissues and fluids. Aborted foetal materials and placental membranes of infected ruminants contain large numbers of virus particles (often exceeding 1.0×10^7 plaque-forming units [PFU]/g) which can either infect animals and humans in close contact or contaminate the local environment [4].

Transmission in Humans

Transmission in humans usually occurs through contact with blood, body fluids or tissues of infected animals [6]. Direct contact with infected animal(s) can occur during slaughter, while caring for sick animals, during veterinary procedures such as assisting animals during parturition,

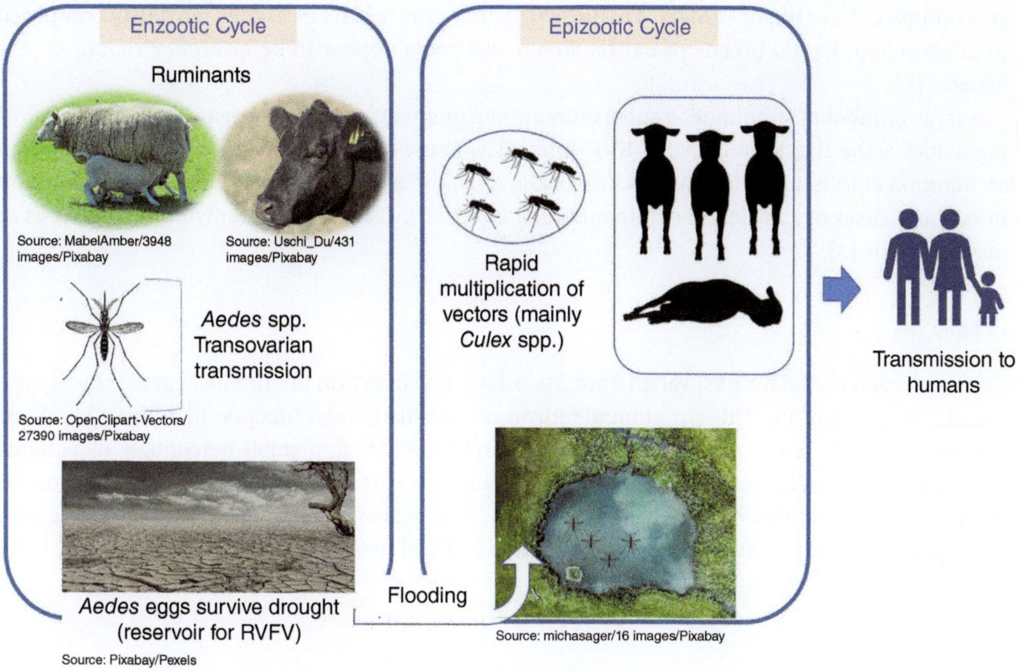

Figure 20.1 Transmission cycles of Rift Valley fever among *Aedes* spp. and *Culex* spp. mosquitoes.

and/or consuming raw or undercooked animal products. Humans can be infected with RVF through bites from infected mosquitoes. Aerosol transmission of RVFV has also been reported in laboratories. However, no human-to-human transmission of the RVFV has been documented [1, 4].

Pathogenesis

Like other arboviruses, inoculation of the virus by the bite of an infected mosquito leads to its spread to regional lymph nodes through the lymphatic system. Initial viral replication occurs in the lymph nodes, resulting in primary viraemia, and later the virus spreads to the target organs through the bloodstream. The major sites of viral replication include the liver, spleen and often the brain of animals dying from encephalitis [5]. During the acute phase, serum enzyme levels are often altered which indicates hepatocyte destruction. During the early phase of recovery, leucocytosis is often prominent. In severe cases, disseminated intravascular coagulation (DIC) may be observed which can lead to thrombocytopenia and fibrin thrombi in several organs of infected livestock [7]. Infection of pregnant animals often results in abortion of the foetus. Pathological outcomes of RVF in livestock and humans can vary considerably.

Disease in Animals and Humans

In Animals

During epizootics, ruminants infected with RVFV typically experience a high rate of abortions (almost 100% in ewes), foetal malformation and subclinical-to-fatal febrile illness. The newborn lambs usually die due to acute hepatitis. Sheep and goats appear to be more susceptible than cattle or camels. The infection in lambs results in higher mortality compared to adult sheep. Exotic breeds of cattle, sheep and goats appear to be at higher risk of severe disease [1].

A large number of simultaneous abortions among pregnant ruminants regardless of the stage of pregnancy is the classic hallmark of RVF epizootics. These massive abortion events are referred to as 'abortion storms' and high-rate abortions allow the differentiation of RVF from other common infectious causes of abortion in ruminants such as brucellosis, Q fever, chlamydiosis, listeriosis or toxoplasmosis [3].

In Humans

The incubation period for RVF varies from 2 to 6 days. The infection in humans is generally asymptomatic or self-limiting. The symptomatic forms are mostly benign (dengue-like illness) and last less than a week. While most human cases are relatively mild, a small percentage of patients (1–2%) develop a much more severe form of the disease. This usually appears as one or more of three distinct syndromes: ocular (eye) disease (0.5–2% of patients), meningoencephalitis (less than 1% of patients) or fatal haemorrhagic fever (less than 1% of patients) [4, 5].

Diagnosis

The diagnosis of RVF can be carried out by using antigen and antibody detection techniques and virus isolation. The various serological and virus antigen identification methods include IgG and IgM antibody-mediated enzyme-linked immunosorbent assays (ELISAs), virus neutralisation test (VNT), indirect immunofluorescent assays (IIFA), immunohistochemistry (IHC) and reverse transcription-polymerase chain reaction (RT-PCR) [1, 3]. Virus isolation capacity is restricted to a limited number of reference laboratories worldwide. The isolation and handling of RVFV require high biocontainment facilities of Biosafety Level 4 or enhanced Biosafety Level 3 laboratories. The laboratory procedures should be carried out by vaccinated laboratory staff.

Treatment

In Animals

Successfully implemented widespread livestock vaccination programmes could potentially save millions of animal lives and protect the economic livelihoods of thousands of herdsmen in endemic regions. Both modified live-attenuated virus and inactivated virus vaccines have been developed for veterinary use. The attenuated strain (known as the Smithburn strain) has been widely used to induce protection against RVFV among susceptible animals; however, its potential risk of inducing abortions, mainly in exotic breeds, has limited its use to areas threatened by an imminent outbreak. Other attenuated vaccine strains as well as novel DNA vaccine candidates have been developed to protect against RVF. It should be noted that if an epizootic is to be prevented, animal immunisation must be implemented before an outbreak. Once an outbreak has occurred, animal vaccination should not be implemented because there is a high risk of intensifying the outbreak [4].

In Humans

Most human cases of RVF are relatively mild and of short duration, so no specific treatment is required for these patients. For severe cases, general supportive therapy and symptomatic treatment is the only available option. An inactivated vaccine has been developed for human use; however, the vaccine is not licensed for commercial use.

Prevention and Control

The occupationally at-risk groups are those who remain in close contact with RVFV-infected animals and their meat products, which include pastoralists, farmers, shepherds, butchers, veterinarians, slaughterhouse workers, epidemiologists, entomologists, etc. There are various environmental, agricultural and anthropogenic factors implicated in the spread of RVF, so a multidisciplinary One Health approach is needed to prevent and control various drivers of RVF epidemics. The control measures can be boosted through a combination of RVF monitoring and targeted surveillance, animal vaccination and vector control programmes. The important preventive measures include the following [1–4].

- **Mosquito vector control:** Contact with RVFV-infected mosquitoes may be reduced by limiting mosquito populations. Various control measures such as habitat modification, use of larvicides, residual or aerosol adulticides, protecting individual hosts with repellents or physical barriers can be tailored to the local ecological demand. Individual protective measures for humans are challenging but attainable; however, it is difficult to keep mosquitoes away from livestock and nearly impossible to prevent mosquitoes from contacting wildlife hosts.
- **Restrictions on animal movements** in endemic regions can be effective in slowing the expansion of the virus from affected to disease-free regions.
- **Control of slaughter of infected ruminants to reduce the incidence of animal-to-human transmissions**: In epizootic regions, all animal products (blood, meat, milk) should be thoroughly cooked before eating to avoid food-borne transmission.
- **For at-risk groups**, public health awareness programmes for risk reduction should be focused on reducing the risk of animal-to-human transmission as a result of unsafe animal husbandry and slaughtering practices. Practising hand hygiene, wearing protective gloves and other appropriate personal protective equipment should be advocated while handling sick animals or their tissues or during animal slaughter.
- **Targeted surveillance** of animals, humans and vectors in endemic regions should be carried out to assess the effectiveness of ongoing disease control measures. As outbreaks of RVF in animals precede human cases, establishment of an active animal health surveillance system is required to detect new cases and provide early warning to the public health authorities.

References

1 Linthicum, K.J., Britch, S.C., and Anyamba, A. (2016). Rift valley fever: an emerging mosquito-borne disease. *Annual Review of Entomology 61*: 395–415.

2 Pepin, M., Bouloy, M., Bird, B.H. et al. (2010). Rift valley fever virus (Bunyaviridae: Phlebovirus): an update on pathogenesis, molecular epidemiology, vectors, diagnostics and prevention. *Veterinary Research 41* (6): 61.

3 Boshra, H., Lorenzo, G., Busquets, N., and Brun, A. (2011). Rift valley fever: recent insights into pathogenesis and prevention. *Journal of Virology 85* (13): 6098–6105.
4 Bird, B.H., Ksiazek, T.G., Nichol, S.T., and MacLachlan, N.J. (2009). Rift valley fever virus. *Journal of the American Veterinary Medical Association 234* (7): 883–893.
5 Anyangu, A.S., Gould, L.H., Sharif, S.K. et al. (2010). Risk factors for severe Rift valley fever infection in Kenya, 2007. *American Journal of Tropical Medicine and Hygiene* 83 (2_Suppl): 14–21.
6 Flick, R. and Bouloy, M. (2005). Rift valley fever virus. *Current Molecular Medicine 5*: 827–834.
7 Ikegami, T. and Makino, S. (2011). The pathogenesis of Rift valley fever. *Viruses 3* (5): 493–519.

21

West Nile Fever

West Nile fever is an arthropod-borne viral disease transmitted by mosquitoes of the genus *Culex*. West Nile virus (WNV) is a member of the family Flaviviridae. The virus is maintained in nature through a transmission cycle involving birds and mosquitoes. The virus can infect humans, horses, some birds and other mammals. It can cause fatal neurological outcomes in humans. The disease is listed by the World Organisation for Animal Health (OIE) requiring member countries to report its occurrence.

Aetiological Agent

The WNV is an enveloped, positive-sense, single-stranded RNA virus of the family Flaviviridae and the genus *Flavivirus*. The Flaviviridae family contains more than 70 species of virus that can be divided into tick-borne and mosquito-borne groups. The mosquito-borne viruses can be further subdivided into the 'encephalitic clade' (or Japanese encephalitis virus serocomplex), which includes WNV, St. Louis encephalitis virus and Japanese encephalitis virus, and the 'non-encephalitic or haemorrhagic fever clade' which includes the dengue virus, Zika virus and yellow fever virus.

Sequence analyses suggest that WNVs can be categorised into at least five phylogenetic lineages. Only lineage 1 and 2 WNVs have been associated with significant disease outbreaks in humans [1]. The lineage 1 viruses can be further subdivided into three sublineages (a–c). The isolates from the Western hemisphere, Africa, Middle East and Europe constitute lineage 1a, Kunjin virus from Australasia represents lineage 1b and lineage 1c consists of viruses from India. The lineage 1a viruses are the most widely dispersed and epidemiologically important, and have caused large outbreaks in Europe, Russia and North America during the past two decades [1].

Historical Context

In 1937, WNV was first isolated from a febrile woman in the West Nile district of Uganda. The first documented WNV epidemic occurred in Israel in 1951, where young children represented the majority of cases. The role of mosquitoes in viral transmission was delineated in Egypt during the 1950s. WNV was identified in birds (crows and columbiformes) in the Nile delta region in 1953. Previously, WNV was not considered pathogenic for birds but in 1997 in Israel, a virulent strain caused the death of various bird species such as geese, with signs of encephalitis and paralysis [2].

Textbook of Zoonoses, First Edition. Jasbir Singh Bedi, Deepthi Vijay, and Pankaj Dhaka.

Human infections attributable to WNV have been reported in many countries for over 50 years. In 1999, the disease appeared for the first time in the Western hemisphere, most likely through the importation of an infected bird, causing deaths in wild and zoo birds, horses and humans in the New York City area and spreading throughout the USA in the following years. Large outbreaks have occurred in Greece, Israel, Romania, Russia and the USA, where the outbreak sites usually overlapped with the major routes of migratory birds [2].

Epidemiology and Transmission

West Nile virus is commonly found in Africa, Europe, the Middle East, Australia, North America and west Asia [3]. The virus is maintained in nature in an enzootic cycle involving transmission between birds and mosquitoes. WNV has a broad host range. Mosquitoes are the primary vector and a variety of birds (e.g. crows, jays, sparrows) are known to serve as hosts, while some infected birds, especially crows and jays, are known to become sick and die from the infection. The virus replicates in birds, reptiles, amphibians, mammals, mosquitoes and ticks but most mammals do not develop enough virus in the bloodstream to spread the disease [3]. Humans and horses are the incidental hosts for the virus.

Transmission Cycles

Birds are the primary reservoir hosts for WNV, but the level and duration of viraemia vary with the species. Although more than 300 species of birds have been reported to be infected with WNV, the maintenance and amplification of the virus principally involve peridomestic passerine birds. WNV is transmitted to birds through the bite of infected mosquitoes of several genera, most importantly *Culex* spp.

Mosquitoes become infected while feeding on infected viraemic birds. The virus eventually enters the mosquito's salivary glands. During blood meals taken by mosquitoes, the virus may be injected into susceptible humans and animals, where it can multiply and possibly cause illness.

The virus may also be transmitted through contact with other infected animals, their blood or tissues. Some birds that are predators (such as hawks and owls) or scavengers (e.g. crows) can be infected after eating sick or dead birds infected with the WNV. A small proportion of human infections have occurred through organ transplants, blood transfusions and breast milk [2].

Pathogenesis

West Nile virus has a predilection for the central nervous system (CNS). Despite the neurotropism, less than 1% of infections result in natural infection of the CNS. Following inoculation by an infected mosquito vector, the virus replicates in the Langerhans and dendritic cells of the skin. From there, it spreads to the regional lymph nodes and to the bloodstream and peripheral organs such as the spleen and kidneys, where the second round of replication occurs. Viral replication in the host body is enhanced by the ability of the virus to negate the action of type I interferon and elude the antiviral activity of interferon-stimulated genes. The exact mechanism of the virus's ability to invade the CNS approximately 1 week after inoculation remains unclear, but the level of viraemia directly correlates with the probability of neuroinvasion [4].

Disease in Animals and Humans

In Animals

Most infected animals exhibit few signs of illness, but some of the infections may result in fatal neurological illnesses. In horses, clinical signs of the neurological disease caused by WNV include loss of appetite, depression, stumbling, muscle twitching, partial paralysis, impaired vision, head pressing, teeth grinding, aimless wandering, convulsions, circling and inability to swallow. The weakness, usually in hindlimbs, is sometimes followed by paralysis, coma and death of the animal.

Many species of birds are resistant to the disease. However, susceptible birds such as geese exhibit various signs of neurological involvement ranging from lying down to fatal wing paralysis. Such birds are either reluctant or unable to move when disturbed and may lose co-ordination. High mortality rates of 20–60% have been reported in geese [3].

In Humans

The incubation period ranges from 2 days to 2 weeks. Most human infections (around 80%) are asymptomatic. The symptomatic infections vary from flu-like malaise to serious neuroinvasive outcomes, where one in five patients develop fever, and 1 in 150 patients develop CNS disease [5]. The febrile illness is characterised by fever, fatigue, myalgias, headache, back pain, nausea, vomiting, diarrhoea, abdominal pain and maculopapular rash. The severe form of disease involving CNS manifestations (i.e. encephalitis, meningitis or meningoencephalitis) may present with fever, nausea, vomiting, headache, acute flaccid paralysis, seizures, coma and other cranial nerve abnormalities. Other rare outcomes include myocarditis, pancreatitis and hepatitis. Severe encephalitis and high mortality are associated with people of older age [5].

Diagnosis

West Nile virus infections can be diagnosed by isolating the virus, detecting viral antigens or RNA, or using appropriate serological methods [6].

Isolation of the Virus

West Nile virus is classified as a Biosafety Level 3 (BSL-3) agent by the Centers for Disease Control and Prevention (CDC). It is recommended that once the WNV is identified in a diagnostic specimen, all isolation procedures should be carried out in a BSL-3 laboratory with at least Class II biosafety cabinets. The virus is cultured in African green monkey kidney (Vero) cells or rabbit kidney (RK-13) cells. Mosquito cell lines and embryonated chicken eggs may also be used.

Serology

The laboratory diagnosis of WNV is generally accomplished by testing serum or cerebrospinal fluid (CSF) to detect WNV-specific antibodies. Immunoassays such as enzyme-linked immunosorbent assay (ELISA), haemagglutination inhibition (HI) and complement fixation (CF) are available commercially. The infection is confirmed by a fourfold or higher rise in plaque-reduction neutralising test (PRNT) antibody in paired sera. The close antigenic associations with other flaviviruses account for the serological cross-reactions that can lead to misdiagnosis of WNV.

Detecting Viral Antigens

Molecular tests to detect viral RNA (e.g. reverse transcription-polymerase chain reaction [RT-PCR]) can be performed on serum, CSF and tissue specimens collected during the early course of illness. In addition, immunohistochemistry (IHC) can detect WNV antigens in formalin-fixed tissue.

Treatment

Vaccines have been developed for horses. However, the available treatment is supportive and consistent with standard veterinary practices for animals infected with the viral agent.

For humans, there is no vaccine or specific antiviral treatment available for WNV infection. Most cases of WNV infection recover spontaneously. In severe cases, patients often need to be hospitalised to receive supportive treatment, such as intravenous fluids, pain medication and proper nursing care.

Prevention and Control

An integrated vector management approach and surveillance to monitor the level of risk to humans are crucial for preventing WNV infection. Some of the important strategies include the following [2, 6].

Control of Mosquito Bites

The most effective way to control WNV infection is to prevent infected mosquito bites. This can be accomplished by reducing mosquitoes using an integrated vector management approach and by use of personal protection measures such as the application of mosquito repellents, mosquito nets, etc.

Surveillance Programs in Birds and Horses

Outbreaks of WNV in animals precede human cases so the establishment of an animal health surveillance system to detect new cases in birds and horses is essential to provide early warning for public health authorities. Dead birds, especially of the crow family, are the most sensitive indicator of the presence of WNV, as these birds are highly susceptible to infection and are an indicator of early-season transmission. Thus, surveillance programmes often target dead crows and often encourage people to report such incidences. However, adequate care must be taken while disposing of the bird's carcass.

References

1 James, N. (2017). *Fenner's Veterinary Virology*. St Louis, MO: Elsevier Academic Press.
2 World Health Organization (2017). West Nile virus. www.who.int/news-room/fact-sheets/detail/west-nile-virus (accessed 7 December 2021).

3 World Organisation for Animal Health (2020). West Nile fever. www.oie.int/en/disease/west-nile-fever/ (accessed 7 December 2021).

4 Belgrave, R.L. (2015). West nile virus. In: *Robinson's Current Therapy in Equine Medicine* (ed. K. Sprayberry and N. Robinson), 152–154. Philadelphia, PA: WB Saunders.

5 Seybolt, L.M. (2007). West nile virus. In: *Pediatric Clinical Advisor* (ed. C. Garfunkel, J. Kaczorowski and C. Christy), 605. St Louis, MO: Elsevier.

6 Centers for Disease Control and Prevention (2018). West Nile virus. www.cdc.gov/westnile/transmission/index.html

22

Yellow Fever

Yellow fever is a mosquito-borne acute viral haemorrhagic disease affecting humans and non-human primates (NHPs). The disease is caused by the yellow fever virus (YFV) which is the prototype member of the genus *Flavivirus* and family Flaviviridae. The virus consists of single-stranded positive-sense RNA and has an envelope. Up to now, a single YFV serotype and seven genotypes have been described in Africa and South America. In Africa, five genotypes are described: West Africa I, West Africa II, East Africa, East/Central Africa and Angola [1]. YFV strains circulating in the Americas belong to two distinct genotypes (I and II), and these genotypes are derived from the West African genotype and diversified into several concurrent enzootic lineages [2].

Historical Context

Yellow fever was historically considered one of the most dangerous infectious diseases which was responsible for the deadliest epidemics during the fifteenth to nineteenth centuries. Large-scale outbreaks in port cities of North and South America, Africa and Europe caused devastating mortalities and helped to shape the expansion of colonial powers [3]. The disease was probably introduced to the Americas from Africa around 300–400 years ago, coinciding with the slave trade period, and causing numerous yellow fever urban epidemics [3].

The name of the disease was derived from yellowing of the skin (i.e. jaundice) caused by the destruction of the liver by the virus infection. In 1901, Walter Reed established that yellow fever was caused by a filterable agent found in the blood of infected patients and the disease was transmissible among humans via mosquitoes (*Aedes aegypti*) [4]. In 1927, Adrian Stokes isolated the YFV from an infected person in Ghana. The first vaccine against yellow fever, the 17D vaccine, was developed by Max Theiler in 1937 [5].

Epidemiology and Transmission

Yellow fever virus is endemic and intermittently epidemic in tropical and subtropical areas of Africa and South America, causing high morbidity and mortality in these regions. Africa accounts for nearly 90% of the global burden of YFV, where the sylvatic, savannah and urban cycles of the YFV exist [6]. Since 1950, the transmission of YFV in the Americas has been mostly maintained in a sylvatic cycle involving New World primates and mosquitoes of the genera *Haemagogus* and

Textbook of Zoonoses, First Edition. Jasbir Singh Bedi, Deepthi Vijay, and Pankaj Dhaka.

Sabethes. During recent decades, the virus has expanded its horizon and there have been several documented cases of the human importation of YFV to non-endemic areas.

Vectors and Hosts

Mosquitoes acquire the virus by feeding on infected primates (human or non-human) and then can transmit the virus to other susceptible primates. Mosquitoes are the true reservoir of yellow fever, as they remain infected throughout their life and can transmit the virus transovarially through infected eggs. Human and NHPs are temporary amplifiers of the virus available for mosquito infection. People infected with the YFV remain infectious to mosquitoes shortly before the onset of fever and up to 5 days after onset.

The primary wild hosts of YFV are NHPs in Africa and the Americas. However, NHPs exhibit different susceptibility to YFV. African monkeys are more resistant to the virus and seldom die from the infection. In contrast, New World primates can succumb to the virus, which makes them good sentinel animals for surveillance of the virus [7].

Transmission Cycles

Humans are considered incidental hosts for YFV. The virus is maintained by different cycles in tropical and subtropical regions of sub-Saharan Africa and South America via transmission among different species of mosquitoes and NHPs (Figure 22.1). There are three types of transmission cycles for yellow fever.

Sylvatic Cycle

The sylvatic cycle is reported in tropical rainforests. In this cycle, NHPs are the primary reservoir of yellow fever and are bitten by wild mosquitoes (*Aedes africanus* in Africa, and *Haemagogus* spp. and *Sabethes* spp. in South America) which pass the virus on to other susceptible NHPs. Occasionally, humans working or travelling in the forest are bitten by infected mosquitoes and develop yellow fever. In South America, YFV is endemic in the Amazon Basin (i.e. Brazil, Peru, Bolivia, Colombia, Ecuador, Venezuela, French Guiana, Suriname and Guyana) [8].

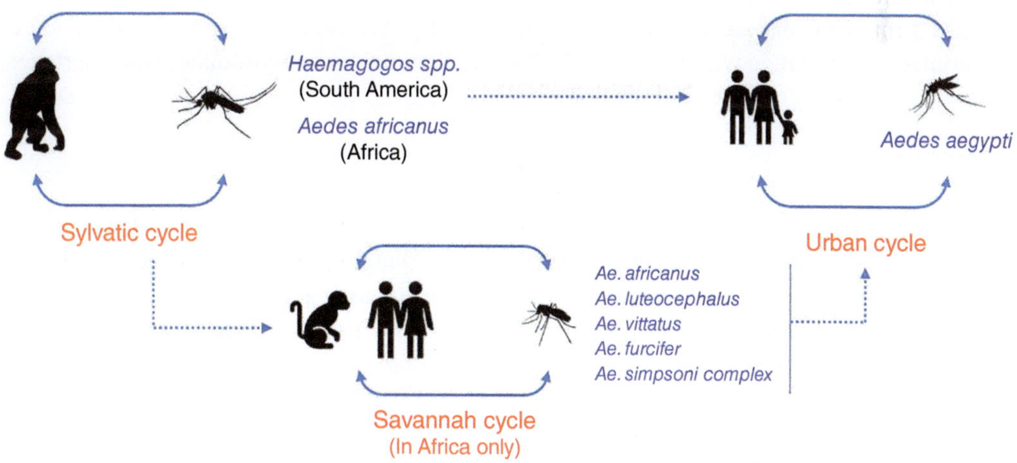

Figure 22.1 The sylvatic, savannah and urban transmission cycles of the yellow fever virus.

Intermediate Cycle

This is also called the savannah cycle which is the most common type of outbreak in Africa. In this type of transmission, semi-domestic mosquitoes (those that breed both in the wild and around households) infect both monkeys and humans. The forest-savannah ecotone has peridomestic anthropophilic *Aedes* spp. (e.g. *A. simpsoni*, *A. furcifer*, *A. taylori* and *A. luteocephalus*) as vectors for the virus.

Urban Cycle

The large epidemics of YFV occur when infected people introduce the virus into heavily populated areas where most of the people have little or no immunity (due to either lack of vaccination or no prior exposure to YFV), and the region has a high density of *Aedes* spp. mosquitoes (i.e. *A. aegypti* and *A. bromeliae*). In these conditions, infected mosquitoes transmit the virus from person to person and can cause large sustained epidemics [1].

Pathogenesis

The YFV is viscerotropic in humans and viral replication in the liver is critical to establishment of the severe form of the disease. YFV amplifies and primes the cellular immune response before spreading through the peripheral blood, and ultimately reaches the liver for active replication. In the liver, YFV induces hepatocyte apoptosis and lytic necrosis, which when combined with steatosis results in substantial liver damage. Significant lesions can also occur in the heart, thymus, kidney and spleen, where evidence of replication has been reported in humans. The early signs of infection are probably due to the innate immune response to the infection, which includes interferon-α, TNF-α and other acute-phase reactants. The systemic inflammatory response syndrome (SIRS, 'cytokine storm') contributes to the serious form of the disease, leading to mortality.

Disease in Animals and Humans

In Animals

The YFV infection in African monkeys is asymptomatic or mild. In contrast, the virus is lethal to Western hemisphere primates. NHPs, principally *Rhesus* and *Cynomolgus* macaques, develop the clinical form of the disease which is similar to human yellow fever after mosquito infection or experimental inoculation with wild-type YFV, except that the disease syndrome is foreshortened, with death occurring at the end of the first week.

In Humans

Following the bite of an infected mosquito, individuals typically experience an incubation period of 3–6 days. Most cases remain asymptomatic but when symptoms do appear, the common ones are fever, muscle pain with prominent backache, headache, loss of appetite, nausea and vomiting. In most cases, the symptoms disappear after 3–4 days. Some patients (20–60%) can enter into a more toxic second phase within 24 hours of recovering from the initial symptoms. In this phase, high fever returns and several body systems are affected, usually the liver and kidneys. The patients are likely to develop jaundice characterised by yellowing of skin and eyes (hence the name 'yellow fever'). Jaundice from excess bilirubin arises from liver cell damage, along with epistaxis, bleeding of the oral mucosa, haematemesis and petechial haemorrhage. Half of the patients who enter the toxic phase die within 7–10 days [9]. The terminal events that occur are characterised clinically by cardiovascular shock and multiorgan failure.

Diagnosis

In the early stages of yellow fever, the symptoms are similar to those of other tropical fevers such as malaria, leptospirosis or dengue, so it is difficult to confirm the disease clinically. The prioritised samples for epizootic investigation are blood, serum and tissues (liver, spleen, kidneys, heart, lung, brain). In the laboratory, viral isolation, serology, immunohistochemistry and genome detection are commonly attempted.

Virus Isolation

Yellow fever virus is a Risk Group 3 pathogen as per World Health Organization (WHO) classification and should be handled in a Biosafety Level 3 (BSL-3) laboratory. The virus can be propagated in a variety of cell lines, including monkey epithelial and kidney fibroblasts, rabbit and baby hamster-derived lines, and *Aedes pseudoscutellaris* (AP-61) and *A. albopictus* (C6/36) mosquito cells.

Serology

Serodiagnosis is usually established by blood tests showing the presence of antibodies to the virus. The detection of YFV-specific IgM in the absence of recent YF vaccination and negative diagnosis for other flaviviruses is considered confirmatory of YFV. A fourfold or greater increase in anti-YFV IgG antibody titres in acute and convalescent samples is considered a confirmatory diagnosis. However, the serodiagnosis can be complicated by cross-reactivity with other members of the genus *Flavivirus*, such as dengue virus, West Nile fever virus, St Louis encephalitis virus or Zika virus.

The plaque reduction neutralisation test (PRNT) assay or virus neutralisation test (VNT) is considered the most specific method for the detection of antibodies against YFV and the gold standard for flavivirus differential diagnosis. Other serological tests include indirect immunofluorescence methods, enzyme-linked immunosorbent assay (ELISA) and ELISA inhibition tests. Immunohistochemical detection of YFV antigens uses specific antibodies against YF and the avidin-biotin complex technique for diagnosis.

Immunohistochemistry

Histopathological analysis with immunohistochemistry performed on liver sections and other tissues is considered the gold standard assay for the diagnosis of yellow fever in fatal cases. Additionally, molecular detection can be performed in fresh or formalin-fixed (paraffin-embedded) tissue samples to confirm fatal cases.

Molecular Diagnosis

Viral RNA can be detected in serum samples during the first 10 days since the onset of symptoms (during the viraemic phase) or even longer than 10 days in severe cases. Genome detection can be carried out by real-time reverse transcription-polymerase chain reaction (RT-PCR) assays from blood or solid tissue samples.

Treatment

There is no treatment available for yellow fever, so mass vaccination with the highly potent live-attenuated YFV vaccine (i.e. YFV-17D) is the only weapon to fight the disease and prevent future outbreaks. There is currently no specific antiviral drug for yellow fever but supportive care to treat dehydration, fever, liver and kidney failure improves the outcome. The associated secondary bacterial infections can be treated with antibiotics.

Prevention and Control

The live-attenuated yellow fever 17D vaccine is one of the most potent vaccines ever developed. During the first half of the twentieth century, vaccination combined with mosquito control programmes eliminated YFV transmission in urban areas of many endemic regions. However, due to ecological and anthropogenic factors, the disease is considered as re-emerging in many parts of the world. Some of the important prevention and control measures include the following.

Vaccination

Yellow fever can be prevented by an extremely effective vaccine that is safe and affordable. A single dose of yellow fever vaccine is sufficient to confer sustained immunity and life-long protection against the disease. The effective vaccine immunity is achieved within 10 days for 80–100% of vaccinated individuals, and within 30 days for more than 99% of vaccinated people. The WHO recommends routine immunisation in all countries where the disease is present. This should typically occur between 9 and 12 months of age. People who are usually excluded from vaccination include infants aged less than 9 months, pregnant women, people with severe allergies to egg protein and people with severe immunodeficiency due to symptomatic HIV/AIDS or other causes, or who have thymus disorder.

Occasionally, travellers who visit yellow fever endemic countries may bring the disease to countries free from yellow fever. To prevent such importation of YFV, many countries require proof of vaccination against yellow fever before issuing a visa, particularly if travellers come from or have visited yellow fever endemic areas.

Vector Control

The risk of yellow fever transmission in urban areas can be reduced by eliminating potential mosquito breeding sites, which can be carried out by applying larvicides to water storage containers and other places where standing water collects. Personal preventive measures such as protective clothing minimising skin exposure and mosquito repellents are recommended to avoid mosquito bites. The use of insecticide-treated bed nets is limited by the fact that *Aedes* mosquitoes bite during the daytime.

Conclusion

In conclusion, prompt detection of yellow fever cases and rapid response through emergency vaccination campaigns are essential for controlling outbreaks. The use of NHPs as sentinels for early detection of the circulation of YFV is a useful surveillance tool to detect the presence of sylvatic activity of the virus. Early diagnosis can be helpful to prompt the activation of countermeasures like vector control and vaccination of the susceptible population.

References

1 Monath, T.P. and Vasconcelos, P.F. (2015). Yellow fever. *Journal of Clinical Virology 64*: 160–173.

2 Mir, D., Delatorre, E., Bonaldo, M. et al. (2017). Phylodynamics of yellow fever virus in the Americas: new insights into the origin of the 2017 Brazilian outbreak. *Scientific Reports 7* (1): 1–9.

3 Bryant, J.E., Holmes, E.C., and Barrett, A.D. (2007). Out of Africa: a molecular perspective on the introduction of yellow fever virus into the Americas. *PLoS Pathogens 3* (5): e75.

4 Reed, W., Carroll, J., and Agramonte, A. (2001). Experimental yellow fever. *Military Medicine 166* (9): 55.

5 Theiler, M. and Smith, H.H. (1937). The use of yellow fever virus modified by in vitro cultivation for human immunization. *Journal of Experimental Medicine 65* (6): 787–800.

6 Domingo, C., Charrel, R.N., Schmidt-Chanasit, J. et al. (2018). Yellow fever in the diagnostics laboratory. *Emerging Microbes & Infections 7* (1): 1–15.

7 Vasconcelos, P.F.D.C. (2003). Febre amarela. *Revista da Sociedade Brasileira de Medicina Tropical 36* (2): 275–293.

8 Espinoza Villar, J.C., Ronchail, J., Guyot, J.L. et al. (2009). Spatio-temporal rainfall variability in the Amazon basin countries (Brazil, Peru, Bolivia, Colombia, and Ecuador). *International Journal of Climatology 29* (11): 1574–1594.

9 Monath, T.P. (2008). Treatment of yellow fever. *Antiviral Research 78* (1): 116–124.

23

Zoonotic Coronaviruses

Coronaviruses (CoVs) are important pathogens for humans and vertebrate animals. These viruses can infect the respiratory, gastrointestinal, hepatic and central nervous system of humans, livestock, birds, bats and other wild animals [1]. In the past two decades, the world has faced three novel coronaviruses outbreaks/pandemics that have caused considerable public health concern and substantial socioeconomic losses. The outbreaks of the severe acute respiratory syndrome (SARS) in 2002–2003, the Middle East respiratory syndrome (MERS) in 2012 and the novel coronavirus disease 2019 (COVID-19) pandemic of December 2019 (still ongoing) have demonstrated the possibility of animal-to-human spillover and then adaptation to rapid human-to-human transmission by these newly emerging CoVs [1, 2].

Aetiology

Coronaviruses belong to the family Coronaviridae within the order Nidovirales, which comprises a group of enveloped, positive-sense, single-stranded RNA viruses. These viruses harbour the largest genome (26–32 kilobases) amongst the RNA viruses and were called 'coronaviruses' because of their crown-like morphology under the electron microscope [2]. Coronaviridae consists of two subfamilies: Letovirinae and Orthocoronavirinae. Based on the difference in protein sequences, the subfamily Orthocoronavirinae is classified into four genera: α-CoV, β-CoV, γ-CoV and δ-CoV. Among these, the genus β-CoV contains most human coronaviruses (HCoVs) and is subdivided into four lineages: A, B, C and D. The phylogenetic evidence has revealed that bats and rodents serve as the source for most of the α-CoVs and β-CoVs, while birds are the main reservoir of γ-CoVs and δ-CoVs [2].

Zoonotic Origin of Coronaviruses

The CoVs have frequently crossed species barriers and some have emerged as important human pathogens. There are multiple pieces of evidence to support that the evolutionary origin of all HCoVs is from bats, in which the viruses are well adapted and non-pathogenic but display great genetic diversity which enhances their spillover potential to other hosts.

Textbook of Zoonoses, First Edition. Jasbir Singh Bedi, Deepthi Vijay, and Pankaj Dhaka.

Bat as a Reservoir for CoVs

In addition to rapid mutation and genetic recombination, the diversity of bat CoVs provides ample opportunities for the emergence of novel HCoVs. Thereby, bat CoVs can serve as a vast gene pool for the emergence of HCoVs. Bats are well adapted anatomically and physiologically to CoVs. For example, inactivation of the proinflammatory response in bats efficiently reduces the pathology triggered by CoVs [3]. The natural killer cell activity in bats is suppressed due to upregulation of inhibitory natural killer cell receptor NKG2/CD94 and low expression of major histocompatibility complex class I molecules. Moreover, the high level of reactive oxygen species (ROS) generated from the high metabolic activity of bats could suppress CoVs replication and also affects the proofreading activity of exoribonuclease, and thus can exert selection pressure for the generation of mutated virus strains, which may be pathogenic when introduced into a new host species, including humans. Further, more pathogenic CoV strains might also evolve by recombination in the hosts, leading to the acquisition of novel proteins or protein features for host adaptation [3].

Emerging Zoonotic Coronaviruses

During the twenty-first century, the world has witnessed two pandemics of coronaviruses (SARS-CoV and SARS-CoV-2) and fatal sporadic outbreaks due to the emerging MERS-CoV [4, 5].

SARS

Severe acute respiratory syndrome was the first well-documented HCoV-caused pandemic in human history. The aetiological agent for the SARS is SARS-CoV and the disease is characterised by 'atypical pneumonia'. The virus was found to originate from bats of the Hipposideridae family, and palm civets were the intermediary host for the virus before dissemination to humans.

The first case of SARS was reported during late 2002 in Guangdong Province, China. The epidemic spread across many countries and continents and resulted in 8096 cases with 774 deaths (with a case fatality rate of 9.5%) [4].

Symptoms: Patients infected with SARS-CoV initially presented with myalgia, headache, fever, malaise and chills, followed by dyspnoea, cough and respiratory distress. Lymphopenia, altered liver function tests and elevated creatine kinase were common laboratory abnormalities of SARS. Around 20–30% of patients required intensive care and mechanical ventilation for recovery. In addition to the lower respiratory tract, multiple organs including the gastrointestinal tract, liver and kidney were also infected in severe cases, which are usually accompanied by cytokine storms that might be lethal particularly in immunocompromised patients.

MERS

Middle East respiratory syndrome-CoV was first isolated in 2012 from the lung of a 60-year-old patient who developed acute pneumonia and renal failure in Saudi Arabia. Most of the laboratory-confirmed cases of MERS originate from the Middle East, but imported cases with occasional secondary spread to close contacts have been reported in various European countries. A secondary outbreak was observed in South Korea in 2015 with 186 confirmed cases [4].

MERS-CoV is a β-coronavirus that is phylogenetically related to CoVs identified in bat species of the Vespertilionidae family, which are considered as natural hosts for the virus. Based on epidemiological studies, it has been observed that MERS-CoV mainly infects dromedary camels, which serve as a reservoir host for spillover of the virus to humans through close contacts. In camels experimentally infected with MERS-CoV, massive virus shedding has been observed. Notably, infected camels shed viruses not only through the respiratory route but also through the faecal–oral route, which is also the main route for virus shedding from bats [4].

Symptoms: Clinical manifestations of MERS resemble those of SARS, which is characterised by progressive acute pneumonia. Unlike SARS, many patients with MERS also developed acute renal failure, which is unique for MERS among the HCoV-caused infections. More than 30% of patients present with gastrointestinal symptoms, such as diarrhoea and vomiting. As per the MERS situation report of August 2021 (World Health Organization [WHO]), over 2578 laboratory-confirmed cases were reported, including 888 associated deaths with a high case fatality of 34.4% [6].

COVID-19

In December 2019, clusters of pneumonia patients, retrospectively known to be associated with SARS-CoV-2 infection, were detected in Wuhan, China. The initial cases had a history of contact with the wholesale seafood market, suggesting animal-to-human spillover of the virus. However, in subsequent cases, the development of effective human-to-human transmission of the virus was established.

On 30 January 2020, following the recommendations of the Emergency Committee, the WHO declared that the outbreak constituted a Public Health Emergency of International Concern (PHEIC).

On genomic analysis, the SARS-CoV-2 virus was found to be phylogenetically related to SARS-like bat viruses, so bats could be the possible primary reservoir for the initial outbreaks. Though SARS-CoV and SARS-CoV-2 are very similar due to a high nucleotide sequence homology of 82%, they cluster into different branches in phylogenetic analysis. SARS-CoV-2 is less pathogenic but more transmissible compared to SARS-CoV and MERS-CoV. Asymptomatic cases of SARS-CoV-2 have been reported during the rapid spread of the virus around the world. As of February, 2022, the disease has claimed more than 5.85 million lives and infected more than 415 million people.

Symptoms: SARS-CoV-2 causes severe respiratory infections like SARS-CoV and MERS-CoV, and cases initially present with fever, cough and dyspnoea. Symptoms of diarrhoea have also been reported among patients. Pneumonia is one of the most severe symptoms and critical patients may progress rapidly to acute respiratory distress syndrome (ARDS), septic shock, metabolic acidosis, coagulation dysfunction and even death.

The major characteristics of these three important zoonotic coronaviruses are described in Table 23.1.

Disease in Humans Caused by Other Coronaviruses

Most of the human CoVs (HCoV-229E, HCoV-OC43, HCoV-HKU1, HCoV-NL63) usually cause mild symptoms of common cold and/or diarrhoea. Epidemiological studies in adults indicate that coronavirus causes about 15% of common cold cases, and most of these are self-limiting in nature [7].

Transmission

Most of the coronaviruses are transmitted through respiratory droplets during coughing or sneezing. Droplet spread can occur when an infected person sneezes or coughs, whereupon the virus-containing droplets are propelled up to 3 ft through the air. Transmission through the ocular surface is also possible. Other possible modes for spread of the virus are shaking hands with an infected

Table 23.1 Important characteristics of zoonotic coronaviruses.

Characteristics	SARS-CoV	MERS-CoV	SARS-CoV-2
Classification	β-CoV, lineage B	β-CoV, lineage C	β-CoV, lineage B
Incubation period	2–10 d	2–14 d	1–14 d
Transmission	Respiratory droplets, fomites, faecal–oral	Respiratory droplets and fomites	Respiratory droplets, fomites, faecal–oral
Case fatality	9.5%	34.4%	2–4%
Basic reproductive number (R_0)	2–4	<1	2–2.5?
Clinical symptoms	Fever, myalgia, headache, malaise, dry cough, dyspnoea, diarrhoea, respiratory distress	Fever, cough, chills, sore throat, myalgia, arthralgia, dyspnoea, pneumonia, diarrhoea, vomiting, acute renal impairment	Fever, dry cough, dyspnoea, myalgia, headache, diarrhoea
Epidemiology	2002–2003 in China and later spread to many other countries	In 2012, first reported in the Middle East, and 2015 outbreak in South Korea. The disease is endemic in the Middle East	2019–2020 in China and global pandemic thereafter
Natural host	Bat	Bat	Bat?
Intermediate host/reservoir	Palm civets (intermediate host)	Dromedary camels (reservoir)	Pangolins? (intermediate host)
Host receptor	Angiotensin-converting enzyme 2 (ACE2)	Dipeptidyl peptidase 4 (DPP4)	Angiotensin-converting enzyme 2 (ACE2)
Human-to-human transmission	Efficient	Limited	Efficient
Pandemic potential	Yes	No	Yes
Contained	Yes	No	No

person, touching contaminated object/surface, frequent touching of the nose or mouth, or coming into contact with the patient's excreta. Healthcare professionals are particularly at risk of acquiring the infection, as high transmission has been reported among healthcare professionals [4, 5].

Disease in Animals

Animal CoVs have been known since the late 1930s. Some strains of CoVs can infect livestock, birds, bats, mice, whales and many other wild animals. In the past, some outbreaks of animal CoVs have been associated with high mortality with considerable economic losses. For example, in 2016, swine acute diarrhoea syndrome CoV (an HKU2-related bat CoV) caused a large-scale outbreak of the fatal disease in pigs in southern China which resulted in the deaths of more than 24 000 piglets. This was the first documented spillover of a bat CoV that caused severe disease in livestock [1].

Diagnosis

Various diagnostic tests are available for the detection of coronaviruses infection (including COVID-19) which is mainly based on antigen detection or specific antibody detection. In general, an antigen test would detect the virus during the current phase of infection (acute phase). The positive results of coronaviruses nucleic acids obtained by real-time reverse transcription-polymerase chain reaction (RT-PCR) of respiratory or blood specimens are considered positive cases [8]. Serological testing (mainly IgG specific) would detect the previous infection as the antibody titre would rise 1–3 weeks post infection.

During handling of samples, always follow standard protocols which include hand hygiene and the use of personal protective equipment (PPE), such as laboratory coats or gowns, gloves and eye protection. The routine viral testing of samples can be handled in a Biosafety Level 2 laboratory using standard precautions. Virus isolation in cell culture and initial characterisation of viral agents recovered from cultures of zoonotic coronaviruses specimens should only be conducted in a Biosafety Level 3 laboratory [8].

Treatment

Vaccine development for CoVs remains a challenge. It is noteworthy that the world has realised the need for safe and effective vaccines to combat the ongoing COVID-19 pandemic. The COVID-19 pandemic has challenged the scientific community to race for the development and deployment of safe and effective vaccines. As of 3 November 2021, the WHO had issued an emergency use listing (EUL) for the following eight COVID-19 vaccines which have met the necessary criteria for safety and efficacy.

1) AZD1222 (Oxford/AstraZeneca)
2) Ad26.COV2.S (Janssen/Johnson and Johnson)
3) mRNA-1273 (Moderna)
4) BNT162b2 (Pfizer/BioNTech)
5) BBIBP-CorV (Vero Cells) (Sinopharm)
6) CoronaVac® (Sinovac)
7) Covishield™ (Oxford/AstraZeneca formulation) (Serum Institute of India)
8) COVAXIN® (Bharat Biotech)

At present, there is no specific antiviral therapy for CoV. Therefore, treatment regimens are mainly supportive and symptomatic. Recombinant interferon(s) with ribavirin was found to have limited effects against COVID-19 infections in some clinical trials. Plasma and antibodies obtained from convalescent patients have been proposed for the treatment of severe cases as per some of the studies [1].

Prevention and Control

There is no specific therapy for the coronaviruses and the availability of the vaccines is limited to COVID-19, so preventive measures include controlling the source of infection, early diagnosis and reporting, quarantine and isolation of suspected cases, supportive treatment and timely publishing of outbreak(s) information to avoid panic and raise awareness. For individuals, good personal hygiene, use of protective masks and avoiding crowded places will help to prevent the spread of CoVs infection in endemic regions. Some other important considerations are provided below [2, 4, 5].

- Personal and environmental hygiene should be strictly maintained.
- During epidemics, there should be strict implementation of wearing N95 masks or medical-surgical masks when accessing public places.

- Contact tracing, strict isolation of active cases and quarantine of close contacts should be implemented at the early stage of the outbreak.
- Public health professionals must be well trained to use PPE.
- Enhancement of public health surveillance and diagnostic capacities.
- Education of the public on the infectious nature of the disease and what measures to take on a personal basis to prevent spread of the infection.
- Availability and access to safe and effective vaccines across the globe.

References

1 Chen, Y., Liu, Q., and Guo, D. (2020). Emerging coronaviruses: genome structure, replication, and pathogenesis. *Journal of Medical Virology 92* (4): 418–423.

2 Su, S., Wong, G., Shi, W. et al. (2016). Epidemiology, genetic recombination, and pathogenesis of coronaviruses. *Trends in Microbiology 24* (6): 490–502.

3 Menachery, V.D., Graham, R.L., and Baric, R.S. (2017). Jumping species – a mechanism for coronavirus persistence and survival. *Current Opinion in Virology 23*: 1–7.

4 Ye, Z.W., Yuan, S., Yuen, K.S. et al. (2020). Zoonotic origins of human coronaviruses. *International Journal of Biological Sciences* 16 (10): 1686.

5 Lee, P.I. and Hsueh, P.R. (2020). Emerging threats from zoonotic coronaviruses-from SARS and MERS to 2019-nCoV. *Journal of Microbiology, Immunology and Infection* 53 (3): 365.

6 World Health Organization (2021). MERS situation update. www.emro.who.int/health-topics/mers-cov/mers-outbreaks.html (accessed 7 December 2021).

7 Greenberg, S.B. (2016). Update on human rhinovirus and coronavirus infections. *Seminars in Respiratory and Critical Care Medicine* 37: 555–571.

8 Centers for Disease Control and Prevention (2021). Information for laboratories about coronavirus (COVID-19). www.cdc.gov/coronavirus/2019-nCoV/lab/index.html (accessed 7 December 2021).

24

Viral Haemorrhagic Fevers

Viral haemorrhagic fevers (VHFs) refer to a group of illnesses caused by four distinct families of viruses: Arenaviridae, Bunyaviridae, Filoviridae and Flaviviridae. In general, the term 'VHF' is used to describe a severe multisystem syndrome in which multiple organs of the body are affected and the overall vascular system is damaged, which impairs the body's self-regulating ability. These symptoms are often accompanied by haemorrhage (bleeding). In severe cases, vascular dysregulation and vascular damage with capillary leakage can lead to shock, which is characteristic of the terminal phase of VHFs [1]. VHF viruses cause marked morbidity and mortality and are endemic disease threats in many regions of the world. They also have serious potential as biological warfare and terrorist weapons. The Centers for Disease Control and Prevention (CDC) classified most of these viruses as 'Category A Bioweapon' agents because of their ability to cause high mortality, their ease of dissemination or transmission from person to person, and potential to cause major public panic and socioeconomic disruption [2, 3].

The four families of VHFs share several characteristic features as describes below [1].

- They are all RNA viruses and their survival is dependent on the animal or insect host.
- Humans are not the natural reservoir for these viruses. Humans are infected when they come into contact with infected hosts. However, with some VHFs, after accidental transmission from the host, human-to-human transmission is possible.
- The mechanism of haemorrhage and plasma leakage in VHFs includes pathological concentrations of cytokines and other immune mediators, platelet aggregation and consumption, activation of the coagulation cascade, endothelial injury, and insufficient coagulation factors because of severe hepatic necrosis.
- The initial clinical presentation of VHFs is usually indistinct and therefore difficult to distinguish from illnesses caused by non-VHF viruses and also from one another. Once infected, these viruses are capable of causing serious illness and mortality in humans.
- The major outbreaks of some of the VHFs (e.g. Ebola, Lassa fever and Marburg viruses) have been associated with nosocomial transmission.
- With the notable exception of yellow fever and the less common Argentine haemorrhagic fevers, there are neither vaccines available for the prevention of VHFs nor standard drug therapies or treatments for most of these viruses. The antiviral drug ribavirin is somewhat effective for some of the arenaviruses and bunyaviruses.

A summary of the important VHFs and their characteristics is provided in Table 24.1.

Textbook of Zoonoses, First Edition. Jasbir Singh Bedi, Deepthi Vijay, and Pankaj Dhaka.

Table 24.1 Summary of various viral haemorrhagic fevers (VHFs). Based on [2, 4].

<table>
<tr><th>Family</th><th>Characteristics</th><th>Viruses</th></tr>
<tr><td>Arenaviruses
Family:
Arenaviridae</td><td>• The word 'arena' is derived from a Latin word that means 'sandy'. The cross-section of the RNA genome of the virus shows grainy particles that are the ribosomes acquired from their host cells.
• The viruses are generally associated with rodent-transmitted diseases in humans. Each virus usually is associated with a particular rodent host species in which it is maintained (one notable exception is the Tacaribe virus, which has been isolated from bats and mosquitoes)
Disease transmission:
• Rodent hosts are chronically infected with the virus without any obvious illness. Some arenaviruses appear to have a vertical transmission in rodents. Viruses are shed into the environment in the urine or droppings of infected hosts.
• Human infection can occur due to contact with the excretions of infected rodents. Infection can also occur as aerosol transmission by inhalation of tiny particles soiled with rodent urine or saliva.
• Some arenaviruses, such as Lassa, Machupo and Lujo viruses, are associated with secondary human-to-human and nosocomial transmission</td><td>Arenavirus is divided into two groups:
New World or Tacaribe complex: these are generally associated with the New World rats and mice (family Muridae, subfamily Sigmodontinae)
Old World or LCM/Lassa complex: these viruses are associated with the Old World rats and mice (family Muridae, subfamily Murinae)
Various diseases due to arenaviruses are listed below
<table>
<tr><th>Virus</th><th>Disease</th><th>Year</th></tr>
<tr><td>Lymphocytic choriomeningitis virus (LCMV)</td><td>Lymphocytic choriomeningitis</td><td>1933</td></tr>
<tr><td>Junin virus</td><td>Argentine haemorrhagic fever</td><td>1958</td></tr>
<tr><td>Machupo virus</td><td>Bolivian haemorrhagic fever</td><td>1963</td></tr>
<tr><td>Lassa virus</td><td>Lassa fever</td><td>1969</td></tr>
<tr><td>Guanarito virus</td><td>Venezuelan haemorrhagic fever</td><td>1989</td></tr>
<tr><td>Sabia virus</td><td>Brazilian haemorrhagic fever</td><td>1993</td></tr>
<tr><td>Chapare virus</td><td>Chapare haemorrhagic fever</td><td>2004</td></tr>
<tr><td>Lujo virus</td><td>Lujo haemorrhagic fever</td><td>2008</td></tr>
</table></td></tr>
<tr><td>Bunyaviruses
Family:
Bunyaviridae</td><td>The family Bunyaviridae consists of single-stranded enveloped RNA viruses. The family is divided into five genera of viruses: Orthobunyavirus, Phlebovirus, Nairovirus, Hantavirus and Tospovirus (Tospoviruses infect only plants). These viruses are found in and transmitted by arthropods (e.g. mosquitoes, ticks, sandflies) and rodents, and can occasionally infect humans</td><td>Some examples of bunyaviruses are:
Hantaviruses
Nairovirus (Crimean-Congo haemorrhagic fever)
Rift Valley fever virus</td></tr>
<tr><td>Filoviruses
Family:
Filoviridae</td><td>These are negative-sense non-segmented RNA viruses. Filoviruses can cause severe haemorrhagic fever in humans and non-human primates. The two important genera of this virus family are Marburg virus and Ebola virus. These filoviruses have been detected in fruit bats and insectivorous bats in Africa.</td><td>Ebola viruses
Zaire ebolavirus
Sudan ebolavirus
Taï Forest ebolavirus
Bundibugyo ebolavirus</td></tr>
</table>

(Continued)

Table 24.1 (Continued)

Family	Characteristics	Viruses
	• Marburg virus was found to be associated with a VHF outbreak in 1967, causing severe illness in people in Marburg, Germany and Belgrade, Serbia. The patients were exposed to tissues from non-human primates shipped from Uganda. • Ebola virus was first reported from the Democratic Republic of the Congo (formerly Zaire) and Sudan, where highly lethal outbreaks occurred in 1976	Reston ebolavirus Bombali ebolavirus • Of these, four (Zaire, Sudan, Taï Forest and Bundibugyo viruses) are known to cause disease in humans • Reston virus causes disease in non-human primates and pigs • Bombali virus was recently identified in bats (pathogenesis unknown) **Marburg virus:** associated with Marburg haemorrhagic fever. Fruit bats are likely reservoirs but non-human primates are considered as a common source of index patient infection. Most cases have been reported from the Democratic Republic of Congo, Kenya, Uganda, Angola and South Africa
Flaviviruses (Latin word 'flavus' means yellow) Family: Flaviviridae	Flaviviridae are a family of positive-sense, single-stranded, enveloped RNA viruses. They are found in arthropods (primarily ticks and mosquitoes) and can occasionally infect humans	*Mosquito-transmitted viruses:* **Yellow fever:** a mosquito-borne acute viral haemorrhagic disease affecting humans and non-human primates (NHPs) **Zika virus:** the disease is asymptomatic in most cases. In few cases, the virus can trigger paralysis (Guillain–Barré syndrome). In pregnant women, the infection is associated with subsequent birth defects **Dengue fever** (also known as dengue haemorrhagic fever, dengue shock syndrome and break-bone fever): caused by dengue viruses (types 1–4) which involve the vector *Aedes aegypti* and the human cycle in South-East Asia, Africa, Pacific and Americas *Tick transmissible viruses:* **Omsk haemorrhagic fever**: mainly found in Siberia **Kyasanur forest disease (**KFD**) or monkey fever**: KFD was first described in 1957 in the Kyasanur forest of Mysore, India. The disease remains a public health concern along with the belts of the Western Ghats of India. Hard ticks (*Hemaphysalis spinigera*) are the important reservoir of the KFD virus and once infected, remain so for life. Rodents, shrews and monkeys are common hosts for the KFD virus after being bitten by an infected tick. KFDV can cause epizootics with high fatality in primates. Ruminants such as goats, cows and sheep may become infected with KFD but play a limited role in transmission of the disease. These animals provide the blood meals for ticks and it is possible for infected animals with viraemia to infect other ticks, but the transmission of KFDV to humans from these larger animals is extremely rare. Humans are mainly infected by the bite of the ticks and present with fever and other mild symptoms, and sometimes with serious haemorrhagic and/or neurological features. No person-to-person transmission has been described **Alkhurma disease**: the virus was isolated in 1995 from patients in Saudi Arabia and is closely related to KFD

Treatment

The treatment of cases of VHF syndrome needs close supervision and critical cases require intensive care. As the pathogenesis of VHFs is not entirely understood and the availability of antiviral drugs is limited, treatment largely consists of supportive management and palliative care with particular attention paid to the maintenance of hydration, circulatory volume, blood pressure and the provision of supplemental oxygen. The care is essentially the same as the conventional care given to patients with other causes of multisystem failure. The challenge with VHF patients is to provide this support while minimising the risk of infection to other patients and medical personnel [2, 4].

Although there are no currently approved antiviral drugs for treating VHFs, some drugs are available with varying efficacy for VHFs (e.g. ribavirin is effective for some of the VHFs caused by arenaviruses and bunyaviruses). Also, passive immunisation has been attempted for treating the diseases caused by VHF viruses although the results have been largely inconsistent [4].

Prevention and Control

There are no vaccines available to prevent VHFs in humans (exceptions are for yellow fever and Argentine haemorrhagic fever). Therefore, prevention and control strategies should be disease specific and evidence based as per the available resources. Some general recommendations include the following [1, 4].

- Various strategies should be undertaken to control the number of rodents in endemic regions. Prevent rodents from entering or living in homes or workplaces. While cleaning the nests and droppings of the rodents, proper preventive measures should be taken to prevent aerosol exposure.
- For viruses spread by ticks or mosquitoes, prevention should be focused on controlling mosquitoes and ticks in the environment. Use insect repellent, proper clothing, bed nets, window screens and other insect barriers to avoid being bitten.
- If travelling to an area where there is a risk for VHF, follow precautions including:
  - wearing long sleeves and long trousers treated with permethrin
  - use of insect repellent and bed nets in high-risk areas
  - avoiding contact with livestock or rodents in areas where outbreaks are occurring.

References

1 Centers for Disease Control and Prevention (2021). Viral hemorrhagic fevers (VHFs) cdc.gov/vhf/virus-families/flaviviridae.html (accessed 7 December 2021).

2 Marty, A.M., Jahrling, P.B., and Geisbert, T.W. (2006). Viral hemorrhagic fevers. *Clinics in Laboratory Medicine 26* (2): 345–386.

3 Schnittler, H.J. and Feldmann, H. (2003). Viral hemorrhagic fever – a vascular disease? *Thrombosis and Haemostasis 89* (06): 967–972.

4 Paessler, S. and Walker, D.H. (2013). Pathogenesis of the viral hemorrhagic fevers. *Annual Review of Pathology: Mechanisms of Disease 8*: 411–440.

25

Other Zoonotic Viruses of Public Health Importance

Virus and disease	Epidemiology and transmission	Clinical signs in humans	Control measures
Eastern equine encephalomyelitis (EEE) **Western equine encephalomyelitis** (WEE) **Venezuelan equine encephalomyelitis** (VEE) Family: Togaviridae	**EEE:** In North America, passerine birds act as reservoir hosts and ornithophilic mosquitoes (e.g. *Culiseta melanura*) as enzootic vectors. Rodents/marsupials may serve as principal enzootic reservoirs in South America *Equines:* Outbreaks in horses are common and often accompanied by high case fatality rates. About 80–90% of infected horses develop acute and lethal diseases **WEE:** Maintained in an enzootic cycle between passerine birds (reservoirs) and its mosquito vector (*Culex tarsalis*) in western USA *Equines*: For horses, WEE is less virulent than EEE. The case fatality rate in horses is 20–30% but can reach up to 50% in some epidemics	These are mosquito-borne pathogens that can cause non-specific illnesses and encephalitis in equids and humans in the Americas **EEE:** The mosquito *Culiseta melanura* is not considered to be an important vector of EEEV to humans because it feeds almost exclusively on birds. Transmission to humans requires mosquito species capable of creating a 'bridge' between infected birds and uninfected mammals such as some *Aedes*, *Coquillettidia* and *Culex* spp. Human infections are usually asymptomatic, but some cases can progress to severe encephalitis accompanied by a high fatality rate or incapacitating sequelae. The disease is generally more severe in the elderly and infants. Approximately 30% of people with EEE may die and the survivors can have neurological sequelae	• Vaccination of equines in high-risk regions • Quarantine and movement controls of all animals • Proper biosecurity of equine farms • Implementation of mosquito control measures

Textbook of Zoonoses, First Edition. Jasbir Singh Bedi, Deepthi Vijay, and Pankaj Dhaka.

Virus and disease	Epidemiology and transmission	Clinical signs in humans	Control measures
	VEE: The transmission cycle is maintained among rodents and other vertebrates (e.g. cotton rats, bats and opossums) as reservoirs and mosquitoes of subgenus *Culex* (*Melanoconion*) as vectors. Approximately 150 animal species may be infected under natural conditions *Equines*: Horses are most severely affected by VEE infection and half of the infected cases develop encephalitis	**WEE:** Most of the human cases of WEE are asymptomatic. Infants and children are highly susceptible to WEE infection and are most likely to develop severe encephalitis. The case fatality rate in humans is about 3–4% **VEE:** Of the three equine encephalitis alphaviruses, VEE virus is the most important zoonotic pathogen. In humans, infected patients manifest flu-like clinical signs (e.g. fever, severe headache, myalgia, etc.). Most clinical cases are self-limiting illnesses with recovery after a week. Some symptomatic cases can progress to neurological disease with symptoms including convulsions, drowsiness and disorientation, sometimes followed by incapacitating sequelae (e.g. paralysis, epilepsy, tremor). The disease is more severe in children compared to adults. The case fatality rate is approximately 20% but can reach up to 35% in children under 5 years of age	
Foot and mouth disease (FMD) Family: Picornaviridae Genus: *Aphthovirus* Seven serotypes: O, A, C, SAT1, SAT2, SAT3, Asia1	The disease affects cloven-hoofed animals and is one of the most contagious animal diseases. In animals, the disease presents with acute fever, followed by the development of blisters mainly in the mouth and on the feet	The occurrence of FMD in humans is rarely reported. Mostly, the symptoms are mild and self-limiting, including tingling blisters on hands, accompanied by fever, sore throat and blisters on the feet and in the mouth	At-risk groups (e.g. veterinarians, farm workers, etc.) should use personal protective equipment (PPE) while handling infected animals
Hendra virus (HeV) Family: Paramyxoviridae Genus: *Henipavirus*	The disease was first discovered in horses during 1994 in Hendra, Brisbane, Australia. Fruit bats have been identified as the natural host of the virus. Horses may be infected after exposure to the virus from the contaminated urine of flying foxes. Infected horses develop haemorrhagic fever and respiratory distress with a high case fatality rate	Most Hendra outbreaks in horses and humans are confined to the north-eastern coast of Australia. The transmission of Hendra virus to humans can occur after exposure to body fluids and tissues or excretions of infected horses. In humans, the infection can lead to respiratory illness with severe flu-like signs and symptoms. In severe cases, the illness may progress to encephalitis	Avoiding contact with infected horses is important to prevent the infection. Always use appropriate PPE while handling suspected animals

(*Continued*)

Virus and disease	Epidemiology and transmission	Clinical signs in humans	Control measures
Herpes B virus (*Cercopithecine herpesvirus 1*) Family: Herpesviridae (DNA viruses) Disease: Herpes B virus infection (monkey herpes infection, *Herpesvirus simiae* infection, simian B disease)	Macaque monkeys (Old World monkeys) are considered as natural hosts of the herpes B virus. The virus causes asymptomatic infection in Asian macaques (*Macaca mulatta* and *M. fascicularis*). The clinical picture in the natural hosts is comparable to human herpesvirus 1 infection in humans with mild mucocutaneous lesions upon primary infection, followed by latency in sensory ganglia and virus reactivation. The virus shedding mainly occurs through bodily fluids, like saliva or other contaminated excretions, upon primary infection or reactivation	Herpes B virus presents a serious zoonotic threat to humans. The main route of transmission in humans is exposure to saliva from infected animals by bites and scratches; however, in a few cases, needle-stick injuries and even air-borne infections were also reported. Therefore, animal handlers are more prone to infection with this virus. Transmission is also possible in laboratory conditions during the processing of central nervous tissue or other internal organs of infected monkeys. Clinical signs in humans include the formation of small vesicles under the skin and hyperaesthesia around the scratch or bite. In the majority of cases without appropriate antiviral treatment, patients develop encephalitis resulting in severe neurological disorders combined with a high mortality rate of up to 80%	There are no vaccines for protection against herpes B virus. Stay away from macaque monkeys to avoid getting bitten or scratched. Laboratory workers and veterinarians should use PPE while handling the tissues of monkeys
La Crosse encephalitis virus (LACV) Family: Bunyaviridae Disease: La Crosse encephalitis (California encephalitis)	LACV is maintained in a cycle between *Aedes triseriatus* (the eastern tree-hole mosquito) and vertebrate hosts (especially small mammals such as chipmunks and squirrels) in deciduous forest habitats	Humans can be infected with LACV from the bite of an infected mosquito. Most cases occur in the upper Midwestern United States. Most cases remain asymptomatic. However, some cases can develop the severe neuroinvasive form of the disease which involves encephalitis and seizures, coma and paralysis. This form occurs most often in children less than 16 years of age	The most effective way to prevent infection is to avoid mosquito bites

Virus and disease	Epidemiology and transmission	Clinical signs in humans	Control measures
Lymphocytic choriomeningitis virus (LCMV) Family: Arenaviridae Strains: WE, Armstrong and Traub Disease: Lymphocytic choriomeningitis (LCM)	The natural host of the LCMV is the house mouse (*Mus musculus*). Rodents are mainly asymptomatic and can spread LCMV through bite wounds or aerosols. Food contaminated with mouse excretions is also an important source of human infection	LCM has been reported in Europe, the Americas, Australia and Japan. Infection without symptoms or mild febrile illnesses is a common clinical manifestation. However, the LCMV is commonly recognised as the causative agent for neurological signs in severe cases. The second phase of illness may occur with the symptoms of meningitis, encephalitis or meningoencephalitis. LCMV has also been known to cause acute hydrocephalus, which often requires surgical shunting to relieve intracranial pressure. Serious pregnancy-related infection has been associated with congenital hydrocephalus, chorioretinitis and mental retardation	Rodent control and public awareness (especially for pregnant women and at-risk groups) are the important control measures
Monkeypox virus Family: Poxviridae Genus: *Orthopoxvirus* Disease: Monkeypox	Monkeypox occurs primarily in tropical rainforest areas of Central and West Africa and is occasionally exported to other regions. For the first time, the disease was observed in the Western hemisphere during 2003. The natural reservoir of monkeypox has not yet been identified, though rodents are considered to be most likely. Non-human primates exhibit self-limiting rash and fever with mortality in young animals	Monkeypox virus is mostly transmitted to people from rodents and non-human primates. Animal-to-human transmission may occur by bite or scratch, bush meat preparation, direct contact with body fluids of an infected animal, or indirect contact with contaminated materials. Human-to-human transmission is thought to occur primarily through large respiratory droplets or contact with body fluids. The clinical presentation of monkeypox resembles that of smallpox, although with less clinical severity. In severe cases, the complications include secondary infections, bronchopneumonia, sepsis, encephalitis and infection of the cornea with ensuing loss of vision	Avoid contact with animals that could harbour the virus (including dead animals in monkeypox endemic areas). Isolate infected patients from others who could be at risk of infection

(*Continued*)

Virus and disease	Epidemiology and transmission	Clinical signs in humans	Control measures
Powassan virus (POWV) Family: Flaviviridae Disease: Powassan virus disease	Powassan is primarily transmitted through ticks (mainly by *Ixodes* sp.). The ticks become infected when they feed on groundhogs, squirrels, mice or other rodents that carry the virus in their blood	Infected ticks can spread the Powassan virus to humans and other animals through the bite. Human disease is rare and mostly asymptomatic. In some cases, a non-specific influenza-like infection can be noticed, which rarely may be followed by meningitis and encephalitis in immunocompromised persons	Tick control is the best way to prevent the infection
St Louis encephalitis virus (SLEV) Family: Flaviviridae Disease: St Louis encephalitis (SLE)	SLEV is maintained in a mosquito–bird–mosquito cycle with periodic amplification by peridomestic birds and *Culex* spp. mosquitoes. Wild birds are the primary vertebrate hosts and sustain inapparent infection. Humans and domestic animals can acquire infection but are considered as dead-end hosts	Outbreaks of SLEV are mainly reported in the United States. Most people infected with SLEV have no apparent illness. In some cases, the initial symptoms include fever, headache, nausea, vomiting and tiredness. The severe neuroinvasive form of the disease occurs in elderly people. In rare cases, long-term disability or death can result	The effective way to prevent the infection is to prevent mosquito bites

26

Food-borne Viral Zoonoses

Unlike bacteria, viruses are strict intracellular parasites and cannot replicate in contaminated food or water. Therefore, the load of viral contamination in food does not increase during processing, transport or storage of food and in fact may decrease with time. Generally, virus-contaminated food products will have normal appearance, smell and taste, so it is difficult to detection viral contamination in foods.

Globally, food-borne enteric viruses are associated with a huge burden of illnesses. Various groups of viruses can be transmitted through the food-borne route and cause infection ranging from mild diarrhoea to severe outcomes like flaccid paralysis, rare events of myocarditis, respiratory disease or haemorrhagic fever. However, the most frequently reported outcomes are gastroenteritis and hepatitis. The food-borne viruses associated with human illnesses under respective disease categories are presented in Table 26.1.

Virus Characteristics and Transmission

Most of the food- or water-borne viruses are non-enveloped and relatively resistant to heat, disinfection and pH changes. They can survive for a prolonged duration on inanimate surfaces, on the hands of food handlers and in dried faecal suspensions. Many of the enteric viruses are host specific, however, host range variants have been reported in different animal species. For example, norovirus (NoV) has been reported from a large proportion of calf herds and in pigs [1]. However, the zoonotic potential of these viruses is still under consideration as these animal viruses are quite similar to the human NoV and, as with other RNA viruses, are also capable of mutating and expanding their host range [2].

Viral infection through contaminated foods depends on the viral stability, amount of virus shedding by an infected individual, method of food processing, infective dose needed, and susceptibility and immune status of the host. For most enteric viruses, the infective dose is less compared to bacterial food-borne pathogens, and large numbers of viral particles are shed in the stools from infected cases (e.g. for rotavirus, up to 10^{11} particles/g stool) [3, 4].

The common foods frequently associated with food-borne disease outbreaks include seafood (e.g. bivalve molluscan shellfish), contaminated fruits, vegetables and salad items that can be eaten raw or without proper treatment. The at-risk group includes infants, pregnant women, the elderly and the immunocompromised population.

Textbook of Zoonoses, First Edition. Jasbir Singh Bedi, Deepthi Vijay, and Pankaj Dhaka.

Table 26.1 List of food-borne viruses associated with human illnesses.

Disease category	Virus name	Family	Genetic structure
Viruses associated with gastroenteritis	Human norovirus	Caliciviridae	Non-enveloped/ ssRNA
	Human sapovirus	Caliciviridae	Non-enveloped/ ssRNA
	Human astrovirus (serotypes 1–8)	Astroviridae	Non-enveloped/ ssRNA
	Human rotavirus (group A, B, C)	Reoviridae	Non-enveloped/ segmented dsRNA
	Human enteric adenovirus (types 40/41)	Adenoviridae	Non-enveloped/ dsDNA
	Human parvovirus	Parvoviridae	Non-enveloped/ ssDNA
Faeco-orally transmitted hepatitis viruses	Hepatitis A virus	Picornaviridae	Non-enveloped/ ssRNA
	Hepatitis E virus	Hepeviridae	Non-enveloped/ ssRNA
Viruses associated with neurotropic symptoms	Poliovirus: can cause fever, flaccid paralysis and meningitis	Picornaviridae	Non-enveloped/ ssRNA
	Non-polio enteroviruses (including coxsackie A and B virus, echovirus and enterovirus D68 and 71): these groups of viruses can cause meningitis, flaccid paralysis, hand-foot-and-mouth disease, myocarditis and respiratory illness	Picornaviridae	Non-enveloped/ ssRNA
	Nipah virus: associated with encephalitis and respiratory illnesses	Paramyxoviridae	Enveloped/ ssRNA
	Tick-borne encephalitis virus: associated with encephalitis and meningitis	Flaviviridae	Non-enveloped/ ssRNA

Viral Gastroenteritis

The important viruses associated with viral gastroenteritis are described below.

Noroviruses

One of the important causes of viral gastroenteritis is NoV (previously known as Norwalk-like viruses and also known as 'winter vomiting bug'). The first detection of this virus occurred in Norwalk town in the United States in 1972. NoV are genetically and antigenically highly diverse agents distributed into seven genogroups (GI to GVII) with altogether more than 30 genotypes circulating worldwide [5]. The genotypes belonging to the GI, GII and GIV genogroups are infectious to humans. Despite numerous attempts, NoVs have never been isolated in cell or tissue culture, and diagnosis mainly relies on the visualisation of virus particles by electron microscopy. The infectious dose for NoV infections can be as low as 10–100 virus particles [6]. The characteristic features of viral gastroenteritis (also known as 'non-bacterial gastroenteritis' or 'winter vomiting disease') are acute onset of symptoms after an incubation period of 24–36 hours. The illness is generally considered as mild and self-limiting, with symptoms lasting for 2–3 days. The predominant clinical signs include vomiting and diarrhoea. The infection is associated with a high attack rate (average 45%) which causes a high number of secondary cases [7]. Noroviruses are transmitted by direct person-to-person contact or indirectly via contaminated food or environment through the faecal–oral route. Crop or vegetable irrigation with sewage-contaminated water has been associated with large outbreaks of NoV gastroenteritis that are linked to the consumption of raw/improperly cooked fruits, vegetables and salads [8]. Infected food handlers are an important source of virus transmission. Individuals suffering from viral gastroenteritis may shed large numbers of viruses in their faeces, in some cases more than 10^{10} NoV genome copies per gram of stool [9]. In addition, the characteristic projectile vomiting also causes dissemination of viruses over a wide area as aerosol droplets. It has been estimated that as many as 3×10^7 virus particles are released in a single episode of vomition [10].

Until recently, the NoVs were considered to be pathogens with humans as the sole host. However, the close genetic relationship of NoV and sapoviruses found in animals and humans has raised the question of the zoonotic potential of these agents [2].

Rotavirus

Since their discovery in 1973, rotaviruses have frequently been associated with common diarrhoeal disease infecting children under 5 years of age, mostly in regions where hygiene and sanitary conditions are inadequate. Rotavirus is classified into seven main groups (A–G) and two subgroups. However, only groups A, B and C are capable of causing disease in humans, and most cases are associated with group A rotavirus serotype G2 [11]. The infection can develop by consumption of sewage-contaminated tap water or using sewage water for irrigation of vegetables and fruits, consumption of contaminated shellfish and meat, and contamination of food by infected or carrier individuals. The clinical manifestation is acute gastroenteritis that usually begins with sudden vomiting with fever and is followed by watery diarrhoea that lasts for a few days [11].

Astrovirus

The astroviruses (Latin *astron*, star) form a morphologically distinct group of viruses, and are named from the five- or six-point star-shaped structure observed by electron microscopy on the surface of virus particles. Astroviruses have mainly been associated with illness in young children, often under 1 year of age, which causes acute viral gastroenteritis. Similar to other enteroviruses, the main transmission route is faecal–oral, and infection takes place through the consumption of contaminated shellfish, tap water and food washed with contaminated water.

Faeco-orally Transmitted Hepatitis Viruses

The viruses which cause hepatitis can be divided into enteric transmitted viruses (hepatitis A virus [HAV] and hepatitis E virus [HEV]), and parenterally transmitted hepatitis viruses (i.e. hepatitis B, C, D, G). A summary of the enterically transmitted viruses HAV and HEV is provided below.

HAV

Hepatitis A virus exists as a single serotype with six genotypes (I–VI). The human strains are distributed into three genotypes (I, II, III) [12]. The virus is quite resistant to acid, heat, freezing, drying, chemicals or disinfectants commonly used for water disinfection (such as chlorine and ozone, γ and ultraviolet rays) [13]. HAV is extremely stable in the environment, with only a 100-fold reduction in infectivity over 4 weeks at room temperature, and 3–10 months in water [14].

Among the risky foods, bivalve molluscan shellfish are infamous as a source of food-borne viral infections due to their filter-feeding mechanism. They can concentrate HAV up to 100-fold from large volumes of water, allowing accumulation of virus from faecally contaminated water [15]. On rare occasions, HAV infection can be transmitted by transfusion of blood or blood products collected from donors during the viraemic phase of infection.

Infection with HAV can cause asymptomatic or symptomatic infection after a median incubation period of 30 days (range 15–50 days) [14]. The virus shedding starts 10–14 days before the onset of symptoms, thereby providing a clear window for spread of the virus. The faecal shedding of HAV reaches the maximum (i.e. 10^{11} virus particles/g) just before the onset of symptoms, which poses the maximum risk of faecal–oral transmission [16]. Infected food handlers may shed the virus for longer periods and therefore may remain infectious even after full recovery.

The illness is generally self-limiting, but can last up to several months and infrequently causes fulminant disease [17]. Among children younger than 6 years of age, most HAV infections are asymptomatic and rarely develop jaundice. Among older children and adults, infection is usually symptomatic and jaundice occurs in the majority of cases.

The clinical course of HAV infection can be divided into four stages [18].

1) **Viraemic phase:** The symptoms do not exist during this phase.
2) **Pre-icteric phase:** Patients display symptoms such as nausea, vomiting and fatigue.
3) **Icteric phase:** Characterised by dark urine with hepatomegaly, pale faeces, jaundice and pain in the top right side of the abdomen.
4) **Recovery phase:** During this phase, symptoms improve and liver enzymes return to normal.

Infection with HAV induces a life-long immunity, so in endemic regions where most children are infected during early life, severe infections among adults are rare. In contrast, in non-endemic regions, the disease occurs mostly in adulthood, mainly due to consumption of contaminated food and water while travelling to endemic regions or having risky sexual practices, hence the likelihood of a severe form of illness is high. It should be noted that due to the presence of a single serotype, highly effective inactivated vaccines exist for the HAV.

HEV

Hepatitis E virus is an emerging cause of enteric viral hepatitis infection worldwide [19]. The virus is endemic over a wide geographic area, primarily in countries with inadequate sanitation (e.g. South-East Asia, the Indian subcontinent, Africa). The primary source for the infection is faecally contaminated water. However, human cases of HEV have been reported in regions where pig HEV is endemic, suggesting that zoonotic transmission of HEV cannot be ruled out. Sporadic cases of HEV have been linked to the consumption of raw or undercooked animal meats such as pig livers, wild boar, sausages and deer meat [20]. In addition, application of animal manure and runoffs can contaminate irrigation and drinking water with concomitant contamination of fresh produce or shellfish [21]. In most cases, HEV infections are asymptomatic. In symptomatic cases, the virus may cause mild to fulminant acute hepatitis (case fatality rates are generally under 0.5% but may reach up to 25% in pregnant women). Chronic hepatitis is commonly reported in immunocompromised patients [22]. In severe cases, HEV has been associated with a range of extrahepatic manifestations including aplastic anaemia, acute thyroiditis and glomerulonephritis as well as neurological disorders such as Guillain–Barré syndrome and encephalitis [23].

Diagnosis of Food-borne Viruses

The burden of viral food-borne infections is grossly underestimated due to the limited availability of diagnostics for routine surveillance in many parts of the globe.

Infection with gastroenteritis viruses is usually diagnosed by detection of the pathogen in stool samples from clinical cases. Many of these enteric viruses either cannot be cultured in the laboratory or can only be cultured with difficulty, requiring expertise. Historically, these viruses were diagnosed by scanning stool suspensions under the electron microscope. This procedure remains the gold standard assay but is considered insensitive and labour intensive.

The recently developed genome-based molecular detection methods are widely used, in which the fragments of viral RNA are amplified directly from stool samples by reverse transcription-polymerase chain reaction (RT-PCR). However, these novel sensitive molecular diagnostic tools for these viruses are not routinely available in food microbiology laboratories of resource-limited nations where the burden of these illnesses is high. Moreover, virus detection in food or water is troublesome, because many food-borne viruses do not easily grow in cell culture, so they must be detected directly in food extracts, with the associated problems of standardisation, inhibition of enzymes used in the RT-PCR, false-positive results, etc. Other diagnostics, such as enzyme-linked immunosorbent assays (ELISA), have routinely been used for detection of many food-borne viruses (e.g. group A rotavirus, adenovirus, astrovirus, NoV, HAV, HEV) in clinical specimens.

The evolving next-generation sequencing (NGS) methods have the potential for early identification of food-borne organisms and the resulting data can be integrated into risk assessment studies.

Prevention and Control

Most food-borne viruses are relatively more resistant to heat, disinfection and pH changes than are most vegetative bacteria. Therefore, the emphasis should be strongly on the prevention of contamination of food before or during processing by adopting good hygiene practices. Some important points to be considered are as follows.

- Personal hygiene is important to prevent food-borne viral infections, which includes frequent handwashing before taking or preparing meals.
- Raise awareness among food handlers about the transmission of enteric and hepatic food-borne viruses, with special emphasis on the risk of 'silent' transmission by asymptomatically infected persons and carrier cases shedding the virus following the resolution of clinical symptoms.
- Food items (e.g. fruits and vegetables) must not be grown or washed in faecal-contaminated water or sewage.
- Shellfish remains an important food source for the transmission of many of these viruses. Quality control of the growing waters can prevent the contamination of shellfish.

- Care must be taken to prevent zoonotic transmission of viral food-borne infections. Some of the infections can be transmitted through the ingestion of animal food products infected with these viruses (e.g. HEV after consumption of pork).
- Implementation of hazard analysis and critical control point (HACCP) systems to identify risks and knowledge gaps in food chains and processing units.
- Highly effective inactivated hepatitis A vaccines are available, which need to be administered to food handlers in endemic regions.
- Capacity building and routine surveillance activities are required in outbreak-prone regions to assess the true burden of these food-borne viral infections so that evidence-based prevention and control strategies can be formulated and implemented.

References

1 van Der Poel, W.H., Vinjé, J., Van der Heide, R. et al. (2000). Norwalk-like calicivirus genes in farm animals. *Emerging Infectious Diseases 6* (1): 36.

2 Bank-Wolf, B.R., König, M., and Thiel, H.J. (2010). Zoonotic aspects of infections with noroviruses and sapoviruses. *Veterinary Microbiology 140* (3–4): 204–212.

3 Sattar, S.A., Ijaz, M.K., Johnson-Lussenburg, C.M., and Springthorpe, V.S. (1984). Effect of relative humidity on the airborne survival of rotavirus SA11. *Applied and Environmental Microbiology 47*: 879–881.

4 Koopmans, M. and Duizer, E. (2004). Foodborne viruses: an emerging problem. *International Journal of Food Microbiology 90* (1): 23–41.

5 Patel, M.M., Hall, A.J., Vinjé, J., and Parashar, U.D. (2009). Noroviruses: a comprehensive review. *Journal of Clinical Virology 44* (1): 1–8.

6 Caul, E.O. (1994). Small round structured viruses: airborne transmission and hospital control. *Lancet 343* (8908): 1241–1243.

7 Hedberg, C.W. and Osterholm, M.T. (1993). Outbreaks of food-borne and waterborne viral gastroenteritis. *Clinical Microbiology Reviews 6* (3): 199–210.

8 Bernard, H., Faber, M., Wilking, H. et al. (2014). Large multistate outbreak of norovirus gastroenteritis associated with frozen strawberries, Germany, 2012. *Eurosurveillance* 19 (8): 20719.

9 Teunis, P.F.M., Sukhrie, F.H.A., Vennema, H. et al. (2015). Shedding of norovirus in symptomatic and asymptomatic infections. *Epidemiology & Infection 143* (8): 1710–1717.

10 Hall, A.J., Wikswo, M.E., Pringle, K. et al. (2014). Vital signs: foodborne norovirus outbreaks – United States, 2009–2012. *Morbidity and Mortality Weekly Report 63* (22): 491.

11 Mattison, C.P., Vinjé, J., Parashar, U.D., and Hall, A.J. (2021). Rotaviruses, astroviruses, and sapoviruses as foodborne infections. In: *Foodborne Infections and Intoxications* (ed. J.G. Morris Jr. and D. Vugia), 327–344. St Louis, MO: Elsevier.

12 Lemon, S.M., Jansen, R.W., and Brown, E.A. (1992). Genetic, antigenic and biological differences between strains of hepatitis A virus. *Vaccine* 10 (Suppl. 1): 40–44.

13 Bintsis, T. (2017). Foodborne pathogens. *AIMS Microbiology 3* (3): 529.

14 Koopmans, M., von Bonsdorff, C.H., Vinjé, J. et al. (2002). Foodborne viruses. *FEMS Microbiology Reviews 26* (2): 187–205.

15 Le Guyader, F., Miossec, L., Haugarreau, L. et al. (1998). RT-PCR evaluation of viral contamination in five shellfish beds over a 21-month period. *Water Science and Technology 38* (12): 45–50.

16 Pintó, R.M., Bosch, A., and Kaplan, G. (2014). Hepatitis A: immune response and virus evolution. In: *Liver Immunology* (ed. M. Gershwin, J. Vierling and M. Manns), 173–189. Cham: Springer.

17 Bosch, A., Pintó, R.M., and Guix, S. (2016). Foodborne viruses. *Current Opinion in Food Science 8*: 110–119.

18 Jaykus, L.A. and Escudero-Abarca, B. (2010). Human pathogenic viruses in food. In: *Pathogens and Toxins in Foods: Challenges and Interventions* (ed. V. Juneja and J. Sofos), 218–232. Washington, DC: ASM Press.

19 Lapa, D., Capobianchi, M.R., and Garbuglia, A.R. (2015). Epidemiology of hepatitis E virus in European countries. *International Journal of Molecular Sciences 16* (10): 25711–25743.

20 Sooryanarain, H., Heffron, C.L., Hill, D.E. et al. (2020). Hepatitis E virus in pigs from slaughterhouses, United States, 2017–2019. *Emerging Infectious Diseases 26* (2): 354.

21 Gao, S., Li, D., Zha, E. et al. (2015). Surveillance of hepatitis E virus contamination in shellfish in China. *International Journal of Environmental Research and Public Health 12* (2): 2026–2036.

22 EFSA Panel on Biological Hazards (BIOHAZ), Ricci, A., Allende, A. et al. (2017). Public health risks associated with hepatitis E virus (HEV) as a food-borne pathogen. *EFSA Journal 15* (7): e04886.

23 Dalton, H.R., Kamar, N., van Eijk, J.J. et al. (2016). Hepatitis E virus and neurological injury. *Nature Reviews Neurology 12* (2): 77–85.

Section 3

Parasitic Zoonoses

Introduction

The word 'parasite' (Greek – *parasitos*: *para* = besides, *sitos* = food) means a person that eats at the table of another. In parasitology, a parasite is an organism that takes benefit from another organism (the host), without providing something in return and usually causing some degree of damage to the host. Incidentally, parasites constitute a diverse group of organisms that may affect a wide range of animal hosts, including amphibians, birds, fishes, mammals and reptiles, as well as humans [1].

Parasites are responsible for many important zoonotic diseases. Thus, 'parasitic zoonoses' involve those parasites that can be naturally transmitted to humans from vertebrate animals. In many of the resource-limited regions of the world, these zoonotic parasites pose a significant burden on human and animal health. Their impact on health varies with the species of parasite involved, their abundance in the host and the host's ability to resist the infection (i.e. immune status of the host). Many of the parasitic zoonoses have been designated as neglected tropical diseases (NTDs) by the World Health Organization (WHO). These NTDs predominantly affect poor rural communities which derive income from livestock production and are deprived of basic hygiene and sanitation facilities. Some examples of parasitic zoonoses listed under NTDs are [2]:

- Chagas disease
- echinococcosis
- food-borne trematodiases
- human African trypanosomiasis
- leishmaniasis
- schistosomiasis
- soil-transmitted helminthiases
- taeniasis/cysticercosis.

Important Terms and Classifications

Hosts

A person or animal infected by a parasite is referred to as a host. Almost all zoonotic parasites have one or more host species in which the adult parasites or their equivalent stage reproduce sexually. These are known as the definitive host(s) of the parasite. Examples include the following.

- The sexual phase of the life cycle of *Toxoplasma gondii* occurs in a mammalian host (i.e. members of the family Felidae).

Textbook of Zoonoses, First Edition. Jasbir Singh Bedi, Deepthi Vijay, and Pankaj Dhaka.

- The sexual phase of *Plasmodium knowlesi*, a parasite of macaques that is a causal agent of human malaria, occurs in the mosquito vectors.
- Only one zoonotic helminth, the intestinal nematode *Strongyloides stercoralis*, reproduces sexually away from the hosts, like some of the parasitic arthropods (e.g. flies and mosquitoes).

Life Cycle

A parasite's life cycle is the sequence of events by which it completes its development through a series of stages from one generation to the next. Various types of life cycles are as follows [3].

- **Direct life cycle:** Some species of parasite require only a definitive host to complete their life cycle, alternating between the host and the environment. An example is *Trichinella spiralis*.
- **Indirect life cycle**: In addition to a definitive host, some species of parasites also infect the second type of host (i.e. intermediate host), in which their immature stages undergo essential development. In intermediate hosts, some species undergo asexual reproduction, resulting in increased number of parasites. An example is *Leishmania* spp.
- **Paratenic hosts:** Some parasites might also use a third type of host, i.e. paratenic host. These hosts harbour the sexually immature parasite but are not required for completion of the life cycle. However, they are often helpful because of their position in food chains within the local ecosystem which enhances parasite transmission. Depending on the parasite species, many types of animals can act as intermediate or paratenic hosts, from molluscs and arthropods through birds and amphibians to mammals. For example, rodents are important intermediate and paratenic hosts for carnivore parasites, including the important zoonotic agents such as *Toxoplasma*, *Echinococcus* and *Toxocara*.
- Once acquired from an animal source, some parasites can transmit from person to person without further contact with animals (e.g. some species of *Giardia*). In some parasitic zoonoses, humans are considered dead-end hosts (e.g. *Trichinella* sp.) and do not usually transmit the parasite to other human or animals.

Based on the zoonotic transmission cycle, the parasitic zoonoses can be classified as follows.

1) **Cyclozoonoses**: These require more than one vertebrate species, but no invertebrate host is required to complete the developmental cycle of the agent. This can be divided as follows.
   a) *Obligatory cyclozoonoses*: This means that transmission between animals and humans is required for the completion of their life cycles, for example *Taenia saginata*. The human acts as the definitive host, and cattle act as intermediate host for the parasite.
   b) *Non-obligatory cyclozoonoses*: In this transmission cycle, the parasites survive well in the animal population without any compulsory involvement of the human host; however, they can occasionally infect people, for example *P. knowlesi* in which the parasite is maintained in macaques but sometimes infects people.
2) **Pherozoonoses** (also called **metazoonoses**): These are zoonoses that require both vertebrates and invertebrates for completion of the infectious cycle of the parasite. In pherozoonoses, the infectious agent multiplies (propagative or cyclopropagative transmission) or merely develops (developmental transmission) in the invertebrate; there is always an extrinsic incubation period in the invertebrate host before transmission to a vertebrate host, for example vector-borne metazoonoses (e.g. *Leishmania*, *P. knowlesi*, *Trypanosoma brucei*, *Schistosoma*, etc.).
3) **Saprozoonoses**: These involve a vertebrate host and an inanimate developmental site or reservoir. The inanimate reservoir in the transmission cycle can be organic matter, food, soil or

plants. For example, *Ancylostoma braziliense* can cause cutaneous larva migrans (also known as 'creeping eruption'); humans may be infected by free-living hookworm larvae when walking barefoot in close contact with contaminated soil.

Based on the aetiological agent, parasitic zoonoses can be classified as follows.

1) **Trematode zoonoses**: The aetiological agent is a trematode (fluke), e.g. clonorchiasis, schistosomiasis, paragonimiasis, etc.
2) **Cestode zoonoses**: The aetiological agent is a cestode (tapeworm), e.g. echinococcosis, taeniasis, cysticercosis, etc.
3) **Nematode zoonoses**: The aetiological agent is a nematode (roundworm), e.g. cutaneous larva migrans, angiostrongylosis, trichinellosis, etc.
4) **Protozoonoses**: The aetiological agent is a protozoan, e.g. giardiasis, amoebiaisis, toxoplasmosis, etc.
5) **Arthropod zoonoses**: The aetiological agent is an arthropod, e.g. zoonotic scabies, tungiasis, myiasis, etc.

Transmission Routes of Parasitic Infections

Depending on the parasite involved, the human can acquire parasitic zoonoses from animals by several routes, including:

- Contact with an infected arthropod vector (e.g. *Leishmania donovani*)
- Ingestion of food or water contaminated with the parasite (e.g. *Cryptosporidium parvum* and *Giardia lamblia*)
- Ingestion of contaminated food of an infected animal (e.g. *Toxoplasma gondii*, *Trichinella spiralis* and *Taenia solium*)
- Ingestion of contaminated material from the environment containing the infective stage of the parasite's life cycle (e.g. eggs of *Toxocara canis* in soil)
- Direct contact with an infected animal (e.g. bite from fleas, scabies from mites).

Prevention and Control of Parasitic Zoonoses

Mass antiparasitic drugs administration and related parasite eradication campaigns have reduced the burden of parasitic disease in developing countries; however, many of the parasitic zoonoses continue to be a significant cause of morbidity and mortality in humans and animals worldwide. Some of the characteristics of parasitic zoonoses which make them difficult to mitigate at different levels include the following.

- The life cycle of many parasites are complex, involving animals, vectors, humans and/or transmission through the environment (e.g. food, water, soil, air).
- The resilience of some life stages in surviving adverse environmental conditions enhances their survival during unfavourable periods (e.g. environmentally resistant oocyst of *C. parvum*).
- Human encroachment into wildlife habitats allows the emergence or re-emergence of many parasitic zoonoses (e.g. outbreaks of trichinellosis).
- In rural and periurban areas, contact of domestic animals and humans with wildlife remains frequent, so there are chances of spillover of wildlife parasites to domestic animals and humans (e.g. *T. gondii*).

- In urban areas, pet animals may be involved in the transmission cycles of many parasites (e.g. echinococcosis, toxoplasmosis, etc.).
- Global climate change is associated with the introduction of parasites into new locations or new hosts, or change in the incidence or severity of disease. This can result in expansion of the horizon of the parasite, leading to emergence or resurgence of associated disease(s) (e.g. expansion of *Aedes* spp. and *Culex* spp. in Europe).
- Potential effects and consequences of changes in land use (e.g. deforestation, development of crop and pasture land) for hosts and parasites. For example, there is a positive correlation between landscape characteristics favouring the rodent population (intermediate hosts for *Echinococcus multilocularis*) and the incidence of human alveolar hydatid disease [4].
- The dispersal of infection through blood and organ donations, especially through immigrant donors from endemic regions.
- Travel to exotic locations along with changes in feeding habits, including the globalisation of exotic cuisine such as consumption of sushi, sashimi or ceviche, can lead to the emergence or re-emergence of parasitic diseases such as anisakiasis or gnathostomiasis.

The prevention and control of parasitic zoonoses require an integrated multidisciplinary approach. Reduction of parasite burden is a major objective but needs to be implemented alongside environmental and ecological modifications to reduce the risk of transmission. Therefore, the One Health framework is appropriate for studying zoonotic parasites which can provide multipronged control strategies. Interdisciplinary approaches are ideal for investigating zoonotic parasites when they take multiple hosts into account and present various evidence-based solutions for their control through inputs from relevant stakeholders such as veterinarians, entomologists, social scientists, sanitation experts, environmental experts and economists. Finally, education and behavioural changes among stakeholders are essential for the success of the control and prevention of these diseases [5, 6].

References

1 Schantz, P.M. (1991). Parasitic zoonoses in perspective. *International Journal for Parasitology 21* (2): 161–170.

2 World Health Organization. (2022). Neglecoted Tropical Diseases. www.who.int/neglected_diseases/en/ (accessed 24 January 2022).

3 Dhaliwal, B.S. and Juyal, P.D. (2013). *Parasitic Zoonoses*. New Delhi: Springer.

4 Polley, L. and Thompson, R.A. (2009). Parasite zoonoses and climate change: molecular tools for tracking shifting boundaries. *Trends in Parasitology 25* (6): 285–291.

5 Schurer, J.M., Mosites, E., Li, C. et al. (2016). Community-based surveillance of zoonotic parasites in a 'One Health' world: a systematic review. *One Health 2*: 166–174.

6 Chomel, B.B. (2008). Control and prevention of emerging parasitic zoonoses. *International Journal for Parasitology 38* (11): 1211–1217.

27
Amoebiasis

Aetiology

Amoebiasis (or amoebic dysentery) is caused by *Entamoeba histolytica*, a pathogenic intestinal protozoan that is mainly transmitted through contaminated water and food.

Transmission Factors

The three major pathways that contribute to the spread of *E. histolytica* are person to person transmission; water- and food-borne transmission; and vector- or vehicle-borne transmission. The important points to be considered are as follows.

- The disease is common in people who live in tropical areas with poor hygiene and sanitary conditions. Human-to-human and faeco-oral transmission are the major sources of human infections. Transmission occurs after ingestion of amoebic cyst from faecal contaminated food or water or sometimes via oro-anal sexual practices.
- Low infectious dose (i.e. less than 100 organisms), chlorine resistance and environmental stability of the cysts are important factors that pose the threat of easy dissemination of the cysts through contaminated food and water supplies [1]. The cysts may remain viable for one month at 4 °C in both sewage and natural surface water [2].
- Besides humans, some cases of *E. histolytica* infection among non-human primates, cats and dogs have been reported. However, it is not easily transmitted from animals to humans, as the parasite rarely encysts in the intestinal lumen of animals, which is an important factor in the transmission of this parasite.

Disease in Humans

Entamoeba histolytica is an invasive enteric protozoan. Infection typically begins with the ingestion of mature, quadrinucleated cysts found in faecal contaminated food or water. In susceptible hosts, the ingestion of 10–20 *E. histolytica* cyst cells can initiate the infection. The single infective cyst cell will divide into eight motile trophozoites, and under ideal conditions trophozoites quickly attain the maturity. Mature trophozoites adhere easily and cause damage to tissue structures mediated by galactose or N-acetyl-D-galactosamine (GalNAc) and N-acetyl-D-glucosamine (GlcNAc) polymers [3]. This allows

Textbook of Zoonoses, First Edition. Jasbir Singh Bedi, Deepthi Vijay, and Pankaj Dhaka.

the trophozoites to degrade the protective mucous barrier and subsequently penetrate the colonic epithelium which increases the risk of metastasis to distant sites. In addition, several other specific enzymes (e.g. proteinase, phospholipase, hemolysin, etc.) act as synergistic factors for cell damage. Through binary fission, the trophozoites form new cysts, and both stages are shed in faeces. Cysts can survive days to weeks in the external environment, while trophozoites are rapidly destroyed once outside the body or by gastric secretions if ingested [4].

Amoebiasis is a leading cause of severe diarrhoea worldwide. The incubation period for *E. histolytica* can be several days to several months [3]. In most cases, intestinal amoebiasis causes asymptomatic colonisation. However, in some cases the infection can progress to symptomatic intestinal disease with diarrhoea and abdominal pain. In advanced infections, patients can experience diarrhoea with blood, mucus and pus. Subsequent complications include amoebic colitis, fulminant colitis (toxic megacolon), intestinal perforation, amoebic appendicitis, haemorrhage, amoeboma (i.e. tumour-like mass of granulation tissue arising from amoebiasis) and perianal cutaneous amoebiasis. The amoebic liver abscess is the extraintestinal manifestation which can progress to pleuropulmonary amoebiasis and can take the form of pneumonitis or lung abscess.

Diagnosis

Direct visualisation of the colon by colonoscopy can be performed to diagnose amoebiasis, particularly when non-specific gastrointestinal symptoms make diagnosis difficult. It is also useful to exclude other diseases, particularly neoplasms. The most common findings are 'flask-like' ulcerations or erosions that are typically present in the cecum, followed by the rectum, ascending colon, sigmoid colon and, rarely, the transverse and descending colon.

The important diagnostics include microscopy, antigen detection, molecular tests and serology. The identification of *E. histolytica* specific nucleic acids by polymerase chain reaction (PCR) is quick, accurate, and sensitive in diagnosing both intestinal and extraintestinal disease. The stool and serum antigen detection assays are sensitive and specific and can potentially diagnose early infection. Antigen detection can be done using enzyme-linked immunosorbent assay (ELISA), radioimmunoassay or immunofluorescence. These assays use monoclonal antibodies to bind to epitopes found on *E. histolytica* which are not present on other non-pathogenic strains.

Treatment

The effective therapy for amoebic colitis is the use of nitroimidazoles, in particular metronidazole and tinidazole.

Prevention and Control

There is no vaccine available to prevent amoebiasis. Preventive efforts should be focused on hand hygiene, food and water safety, and avoidance of faeco-oral exposure. Household contacts of patients with amoebiasis should be screened to contain further cases. Fruits and vegetables that are eaten raw and not washed properly can be an important vehicle for the entry of various parasites. Parasitic cysts are resistant to water chlorination and detergents but proper washing with detergent in running water can dissolve the attached parasites on fruits and vegetables. The cysts can also be damaged with 5% acetic acid or low heating for 15 minutes.

References

1 Shirley, D.A.T., Farr, L., Watanabe, K., and Moonah, S. (2018). A review of the global burden, new diagnostics, and current therapeutics for amebiasis. In: *Open Forum Infectious Diseases*, vol. 5, ofy161.

2 Shirley, D.A., Hung, C.C., and Moonah, S. (2019). *Entamoeba histolytica* (Amebiasis). In: *Hunter's Tropical Medicine and Emerging Infectious Diseases* (ed. E.T. Ryan), 699–706. Canada, Elsevier.

3 Cornick, S. and Chadee, K. (2017). *Entamoeba histolytica*: host parasite interactions at the colonic epithelium. *Tissue Barriers 5* (1): e1283386.

4 Haque, R., Huston, C.D., Hughes, M. et al. (2003). Amebiasis. *New England Journal of Medicine 348* (16): 1565–1573.

28

Balantidiasis

Balantidiasis is a zoonotic disease and is often associated with swine, which is considered the primary reservoir host. *Balantidium* is the only ciliated protozoon known to infect humans. Sometimes, the parasite is referred to as *Neobalantidium coli* or *Balantioides coli* as per the recent classifications based on molecular analyses [1].

Transmission

Humans acquire the infection mainly from pigs through the faeco-oral route. Human infections occur more frequently in areas where pigs are intensively raised without adequate sanitary conditions. Outbreaks are commonly reported in regions where water sources may be contaminated with porcine or human faeces. Subtropical or tropical climatic conditions with high temperature and humidity favour the survival of cysts [2]. However, rodents and non-human primates can also be potential reservoirs for the parasite.

Disease in Humans

Most cases are asymptomatic in humans. In some cases, clinical manifestations may be acute or chronic with abdominal symptoms. Balantidiasis can mimic intestinal amoebiasis. The acute form of the disease is marked by rapid onset of diarrhoea or dysentery. However, the symptoms may be severe or fatal in immunocompromised persons where extraintestinal infection, although rare, can occur secondary to intestinal infection. Peritonitis and liver abscesses have been recorded following intestinal perforation or rupture of fulminant colonic ulcers [1].

Diagnosis

Freshly collected diarrhoeic stool samples are likely to contain actively swimming trophic ciliates. Due to its large size, the parasite can readily be recognised in wet-mount slide preparations. However, stool samples for examination should be collected over several days because excretion of parasites can be erratic [2].

Textbook of Zoonoses, First Edition. Jasbir Singh Bedi, Deepthi Vijay, and Pankaj Dhaka.

Treatment

Tetracyclines and metronidazole are the treatment of choice for human *Balantidium* infection.

Prevention and Control

Important strategies to protect humans from balantidiasis include the following.

- Use of clean, uncontaminated water for drinking and other purposes (normal chlorination is not effective against cysts of *Balantidium*).
- Pigs should not be allowed to roam around water sources. Also, pigs should not have access to areas where crops are being raised.
- Spreading of sludge from sewage processing as fertiliser can lead to contamination of produce or water sources with cysts of *Balantidium*.

References

1 Centers for Disease Control and Prevention. (2019). Balantidiasis. www.cdc.gov/dpdx/balantidiasis/index.html (accessed 24 January 2022).

2 Schuster, F.L. and Ramirez-Avila, L. (2008). Current world status of *Balantidium coli*. *Clinical Microbiology Reviews 21* (4): 626–638.

29

Cryptosporidiosis

The protozoan parasite *Cryptosporidium* is a well-recognised zoonotic pathogen which causes diarrhoeal disease in humans and animals. Globally, *Cryptosporidium* spp. ranks among the predominant aetiological agents of food-borne diseases. Currently, there are more than 40 recognised species of *Cryptosporidium*. Among these species, *C. parvum* is considered the most important zoonotic species for human infection. The parasite was included in the World Health Organisation's Neglected Diseases Initiative in 2004. The transmission of the parasite is linked with poor socio-economic status and inadequate hygiene and sanitation practices [1].

Life Cycle

Cryptosporidium has a complex life cycle involving both sexual and asexual replication. Some of the important points in the life cycle of *Cryptosporidium* spp. are as follows [2].

- All the species of *Cryptosporidium* are obligate intracellular parasites. The only stage found outside the host is the oocyst. The prepatent period (i.e. the time from ingestion of infective oocysts to excretion of oocysts following completion of the life cycle) can be completed in as few as 3–5 days or can take as long as 2 weeks.
- There are two types of oocysts. The 'thin wall oocysts' reinfect the gastrointestinal tract, whereas the 'thick wall oocysts' excrete into the environment through faeces.
- After ingestion by a suitable host, the oocysts excyst and release four motile sporozoites that invade and parasitise epithelial cells, primarily in the gastrointestinal tract and rarely in extraintestinal tissues. Subsequent developmental stages are intracellular but extracytoplasmic, usually found at the microvillar surface of the host's epithelial cells.
- This can cause loss of absorptive epithelium through apoptosis and villus atrophy which may result in malabsorption, and the release of inflammatory cell mediators can stimulate electrolyte secretion that leads to diarrhoea [3].

Oocyst Survival in the Environment

Cryptosporidium oocysts are microscopic spore-like body (4–6 μm in diameter) consisting of four crescent-shaped sporozoites. The oocysts have a tough waxy wall composed of lipids and glycoproteins that enables the parasite to survive a wide range of conditions, including the temperature range of −22 to 60 °C [2]. This wall protects the parasite against many commonly available

Textbook of Zoonoses, First Edition. Jasbir Singh Bedi, Deepthi Vijay, and Pankaj Dhaka.

disinfectants, which makes *Cryptosporidium* hard to control on the farm, in drinking water, swimming pools and fresh produce. It has been observed that the oocysts held in sterile water at 15 °C remained infectious for mice for 7 months [4].

Disease Transmission

Cryptosporidium spp. are highly successful parasites in transmission due to their broad host range, high oocyst excretion rates from infected hosts, water-borne and food-borne transmission route and low infectious dose required to initiate infection. Studies have demonstrated a significant risk of *Cryptosporidium* spp. infection from as low as a single oocyst among susceptible hosts [5]. Infection occurs through ingestion of the oocyst stage of the parasite from faecal contaminated food and water. Therefore, the prevalence of cryptosporidiosis is higher in regions where people do not have adequate hygiene facilities to avoid food and drinking water contamination by infectious oocysts.

The two major transmission routes of this parasite are as follows [2].

- **Direct transmission**: Direct transmission occurs through the faecal–oral route between animal to animal, animal to human (zoonosis), human to animal (reverse zoonosis) and human to human. Human-to-human transmissions are usually observed in swimming pools, water parks and hospitals and via contact with contaminated human faeces during sexual activities.
- **Indirect transmission:** This mainly occurs through consumption of contaminated water (water-borne transmission) or food (food-borne transmission).

Cattle are considered an important source of zoonotic cryptosporidiosis in humans. Contact with infected calves have been implicated in many outbreaks. Cryptosporidiosis cases are higher in areas where manure contaminated with *Cryptosporidium* oocysts is applied to land, allowing oocysts to contaminate the soil and water sources [6]. A schematic diagram depicting the possible zoonotic transmission of *Cryptosporidium* parasites is presented in Figure 29.1.

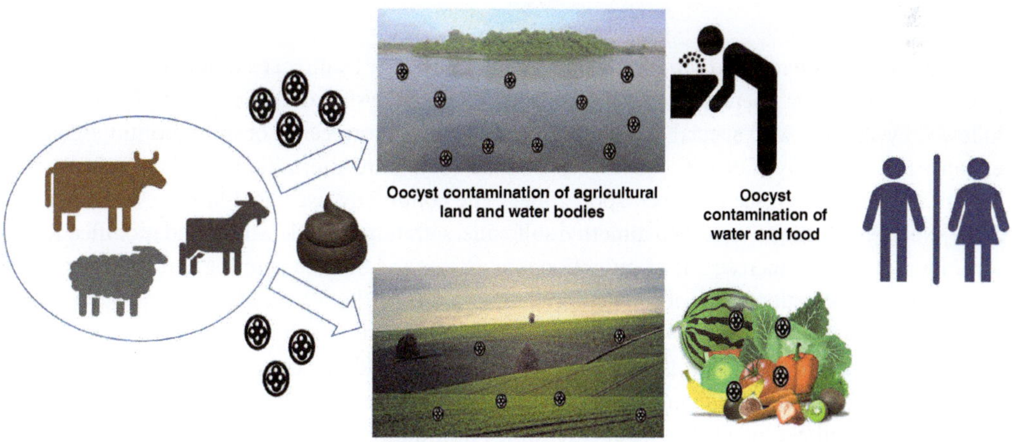

Figure 29.1 Transmission of *Cryptosporidium* spp. parasites from faecal oocysts of livestock to humans through contaminated food and environment.

Disease in Animals

Cryptosporidiosis affects a large number of animal species, including livestock (e.g. cattle, sheep, goats, pigs, rabbits, horses, donkeys, camels, poultry) and various wildlife species across the globe. Farm cattle are the frequently documented host species regarding distribution and prevalence of *C. parvum* infection. The highest prevalence of *C. parvum* has been identified in pre-weaned calves and the parasite remains an important cause for neonatal diarrhoea.

Clinical signs in infected calves include yellow watery faeces, reluctance to feed and dehydration, and in severe cases the animal may die of infection. During acute infection, or following clinical recovery, the infected calf can shed a high number of infectious oocysts in faeces. Past studies have reported that a single infected calf can shed around 100 million infectious oocysts in faeces, which is a massive source of environmental contamination and poses a risk for other vulnerable hosts, including humans [7].

Disease in Humans

Most infection in healthy individuals remains asymptomatic. The gastrointestinal symptoms among immunocompetent persons are diarrhoea (usually voluminous and watery), nausea, vomiting, fever and abdominal discomfort that usually resolve within 2 weeks. The rapid multiplication of the parasite in gut cells causes tissue damage and destruction of the intestinal epithelial cells with stunting of the villi, which result in reduction of the absorptive surface of the gut, leading to malnutrition, dehydration and diarrhoea.

Among immunocompromised individuals, such as those with human immunodeficiency virus infection/acquired immunodeficiency syndrome (HIV/AIDS), infants and the elderly, individuals undergoing cancer chemotherapy, and other conditions that compromise the immune system including malnutrition, the disease can pose a life-threatening diarrhoeal condition and the patient can experience chronic, long-term infection, often lasting several months. In severe cases, life cycle stages can affect lungs, liver, gallbladder, pancreas and other extraintestinal sites.

Diagnosis

The diagnosis of *Cryptosporidium* infection is traditionally done by direct examination of faecal samples for the oocyst by microscopic methods. Detection of oocysts can be performed by wet mount followed by staining with special dye such as acid-fast dye, fluorescence or immunofluorescence to enhance the sensitivity of detection. Acid-fast stained oocysts are intermittently red with size around 4–6 μm and contain crescent-shaped sporozoites. The commonly used acid-fast dyes are modified Ziehl–Neelsen technique, modified dimethyl sulfoxide, safranin-methylene blue and modified Koster technique. However, microscopic examination is laborious and time-consuming and lacks sensitivity and specificity. Detection limits of conventional microscopy methods have been reported to be as low as 50 000–500 000 oocysts per gram of human faeces, which can result in non-detection of oocysts among individuals with low levels of infection or sporadic shedding of oocysts [8].

Immunology-based techniques have been developed for rapid detection of the infection which include direct fluorescent antibody, enzyme-linked immunosorbent assay (ELISA), indirect ELISA and dipstick-like tests. Although immunological techniques increase laboratory efficiency due to their high sensitivity, many oocyst antigens are conserved within the genus of *Cryptosporidium* and appear in several species. Therefore, reliable differentiation of numerous species of *Cryptosporidium* using antibodies is difficult. For this reason, DNA-based molecular detection methods are widely used to identify and characterise *Cryptosporidium* sp. which include polymerase chain reaction (PCR) assay, partial gene sequencing, restriction fragment length polymorphism (RFLP), real-time PCR assays, etc. [9].

Treatment

The infection among immunocompetent individuals is self-limiting. The mild clinical symptoms including watery diarrhoea, vomiting, nausea, stomach cramps and dehydration, can be managed with supportive treatments. However, antiprotozoal therapy is necessary in serious cases. There is no consistently effective and approved drug for cryptosporidiosis for either animals or humans. However, nitazoxanide (a nitrothiazole benzamide with a wide spectrum of activity against bacteria, protozoa and helminths) has shown efficacy in clinical trials with human subjects and is the only anticryptosporidial agent which has been approved by the US Food and Drug Administration (FDA) [2, 10].

Prevention and Control

Cryptosporidiosis is a zoonosis that needs to be tackled by collaborative interdisciplinary efforts adopting the One Health approach [2]. Vaccine development for the parasite in animals and humans is mainly hampered by an incomplete understanding of the host immune response to *Cryptosporidium*. Hence, close co-operation between veterinarians, physicians, environmental managers and public health operators is essential to properly control this disease. Some of the important prevention and control measures are listed below.

In Humans

The most common route for *Cryptosporidium* spp. infection among susceptible hosts is through the faeco-oral route of transmission. Strategies for the prevention of transmission of *Cryptosporidium* spp. in humans include [2, 10]:

- Practice of good personal hygiene including handwashing before preparing and consuming food, after using the toilet and after contact with diarrhoeic patients and handling animals
- Raw food must be washed, heated, cooked or boiled before consumption
- Patients who have diarrhoea symptoms should avoid using public swimming pools, water parks or rivers in order to prevent transmission to others.

It should be noted that chlorine, which is effective against many micro-organisms, is not very effective against the oocysts of *Cryptosporidium*, even at high concentrations. Therefore, in drinking water, the destruction of *Cryptosporidium* oocysts can be managed by heating (*Cryptosporidium* oocysts are inactivated within a few seconds at 62 °C) or use of chemical disinfection such as hydrogen peroxide or sterilisation processes through steam, ethylene oxide, ozone (O_3) and ultraviolet light (UV light).

Mass education and awareness programmes about the routes of disease transmission and applied prevention measures can help in reduction of disease incidence in endemic regions.

In Animals

There is no effective vaccine for cryptosporidiosis in livestock so prevention and control of disease remain the key and include the following factors.

- Supporting the resilience of young animals in the first few weeks of life. Ensure that newborn animals receive adequate colostrum in the first few hours of life.
- Young animals should be housed in clean, dry, warm pens with raised feeding and water troughs to minimise exposure to *Cryptosporidium* parasites as environmental contamination.
- It is advisable to house calves in similar age groups, as younger calves are more susceptible to disease, and may be vulnerable to infection if they are moved into an environment contaminated by older calves.
- Deep, clean straw bedding will also help in minimising contact with contaminated faeces.
- Regular steam cleaning of calf pens can be helpful in destruction of oocysts, as they are inactivated at temperatures above 60 °C.
- Disinfection with recommended products can help to reduce build-up of contaminated faeces on the farm. Disinfectants containing hydrogen peroxide are considered effective in destroying oocysts.
- Fencing of livestock away from streams and water courses can help to reduce the transmission of *Cryptosporidium* oocysts from livestock faecal matter into water courses.

Environmental Control

As manure is applied to land, oocysts can be transported via run-off into surface waters and may be a source of infection to both animals and humans. The effective management of manure and slurry on farms is crucial to reduce viability of *Cryptosporidium* oocysts, which will reduce the risk of wider environmental contamination and in particular water catchments. Such on-farm management practices include proper composting of manure (as heating over 60 °C will inactivate the oocysts), slurry storage (as ammonia and low pH will help to inactivate oocysts), and treatment with mesophilic and thermophilic anaerobic digestion to reduce oocyst viability.

References

1 Savioli, L., Smith, H., and Thompson, A. (2006). *Giardia* and *Cryptosporidium* join the 'neglected diseases initiative'. *Trends in Parasitology 22* (5): 203–208.
2 Innes, E.A., Chalmers, R.M., Wells, B., and Pawlowic, M.C. (2020). A One Health approach to tackle cryptosporidiosis. *Trends in Parasitology 36* (3): 290–303.
3 Gookin, J.L., Nordone, S.K., and Argenzio, R.A. (2002). Host responses to *Cryptosporidium* infection. *Journal of Veterinary Internal Medicine 16* (1): 12–21.
4 Jenkins, M., Trout, J., Higgins, J. et al. (2002). Comparison of tests for viable and infectious *Cryptosporidium parvum* oocysts. *Parasitology Research 89* (1): 1–5.
5 Messner, M.J. and Berger, P. (2016). *Cryptosporidium* infection risk: results of new dose-response modeling. *Risk Analysis 36* (10): 1969–1982.
6 Lake, I.R., Harrison, F.C., Chalmers, R.M. et al. (2007). Case–control study of environmental and social factors influencing cryptosporidiosis. *European Journal of Epidemiology 22* (11): 805.

7 Nydam, D.V., Wade, S.E., Schaaf, S.L., and Mohammed, H.O. (2001). Number of *Cryptosporidium parvum* oocysts or *Giardia* spp cysts shed by dairy calves after natural infection. *American Journal of Veterinary Research 62* (10): 1612–1615.

8 Weber, R., Bryan, R.T., Bishop, H.S. et al. (1991). Threshold of detection of *Cryptosporidium* oocysts in human stool specimens: evidence for low sensitivity of current diagnostic methods. *Journal of Clinical Microbiology 29* (7): 1323–1327.

9 Pumipuntu, N. and Piratae, S. (2018). Cryptosporidiosis: a zoonotic disease concern. *Veterinary World 11* (5): 681.

10 Fayer, R. (2004). *Cryptosporidium*: a water-borne zoonotic parasite. *Veterinary Parasitology 126*: 37–56.

30

Cutaneous Larva Migrans

Cutaneous larva migrans (CLM) (also known as creeping eruption) is caused by penetration of larvae of the hookworm species of dogs or cats into the skin of humans. Zoonotic hookworm species include *Ancylostoma braziliense*, *Ancylostoma caninum*, *Ancylostoma ceylanicum* and *Uncinaria stenocephala*. Other than hookworms of dogs and cats, a cattle hookworm (*Bunostomum phlebotomum*) is also capable of causing short-lived CLM in humans [1]. Infection occurs after contact with soil contaminated by animal faeces. CLM is a self-limiting disease; as humans are an incidental host, the larvae cannot reach their programmed destination and migrate in the epidermis for up to several weeks, resulting in severe inflammation.

Epidemiology and Transmission

Cutaneous larva migrans is endemic in resource-poor communities of the developing world where inadequate hygiene remains a major concern. It is also reported sporadically in developed countries and in tourists who have visited the tropical countries [1].

Transmission Cycles

The hookworms are generally present in the intestine of domestic dogs and cats, which shed their eggs via faeces and contaminate soil. Under favourable conditions of moisture, warmth and shade, the larvae hatch in 1–2 days. The rhabditiform larvae grow in the faeces or soil and after 5–10 days they become filariform (third-stage) larvae (L3) that are infective for humans and animals. These infective larvae can survive 3–4 weeks in favourable environmental conditions [1]. Humans are infected by contact of unprotected skin with these larvae, especially when walking barefoot or sitting on contaminated soil or sand [2]. The hookworm larva (filariform L3 larva) burrows through intact skin but remains confined to the upper dermis.

On contact with the definitive animal hosts (e.g. dogs for *A. caninum*), the larvae penetrate their skin and migrate to the small intestine, from which they are carried through the blood vessels to the heart and then to the lungs and pharynx, and are swallowed to the small intestine. The larvae reside and mature into adults in the lumen of the small intestine, and then suck blood when attached to the intestinal wall. Some larvae become arrested in the tissues and serve as a source of infection for pups via transmammary and possibly transplacental routes.

Textbook of Zoonoses, First Edition. Jasbir Singh Bedi, Deepthi Vijay, and Pankaj Dhaka.

Disease in Animals

The clinical signs of ancylostomosis in dogs and cats are associated with the blood-sucking nature of worms, characterised by anaemia, pale membranes, weight loss, stool with blood, weakness, poor growth in puppies and stunted growth in young animals [3].

Disease in Humans

The clinical features of CLM vary from non-specific dermatitis to typical 'creeping eruption' with varying levels of pruritus. An erythematous itchy papule is usually observed at the site of larval penetration. Later, there is formation of raised red linear serpentine (serpiginous) or bizarre tracks in the skin where the larvae could grow for weeks to months, and these tracks may move in the skin by following the larvae's movements. The symptoms of intense pruritus and pain can last several weeks before the larvae die and disease is usually self-limiting. Secondary bacterial infection caused by scratching is common.

Diagnosis and Treatment

Mostly, the clinical diagnosis is confirmed by the presence of a linear serpiginous track moving forward in the skin, associated with itching and a history of exposure [4]. Itching is typically very intense and can prevent patients from sleeping. Treatment is based on oral antiparasitic drugs (e.g. albendazole or ivermectin) or the topical application of thiabendazole in affected regions [5].

Prevention and Control

To control hookworm-related CLM at the community level, regular treatment of dogs and cats with anthelmintic drugs is necessary. Prompt disposal of animal faeces prevents eggs from hatching and contaminating soil, which makes it important for control of this parasitic infection.

At an individual level, care should be taken to avoid the skin coming into contact with possibly contaminated soil. Wearing shoes and taking other protective measures to avoid skin contact with sand or soil will prevent infection with zoonotic hookworms. Travellers to endemic areas, especially at beaches, should be advised to wear shoes and use protective mats or other suitable coverings.

References

1 Centers for Disease Control and Prevention. (2020). Zoonotic hookworm. www.cdc.gov/parasites/zoonotichookworm/health_professionals/ (accessed 24 January 2022).

2 Shinkar, R.M., Stocks, R., and Thomas, E. (2005). Cutaneous larva migrans, creeping eruption, sand worm. *Archives of Disease in Childhood 90* (10): 998–998.

3 Sharma, R., Singh, B.B., and Gill, J.P.S. (2015). Larva migrans in India: veterinary and public health perspectives. *Journal of Parasitic Diseases 39* (4): 604–612.
4 Karthikeyan, K. and Thappa, D.M. (2002). Cutaneous larva migrans. *Indian Journal of Dermatology, Venereology and Leprology 68* (5): 252.
5 Despommier, D.D. and Hotez, P.J. (2012). Tissue nematodes. In: *Principles and Practice of Pediatric Infectious Diseases* (ed. S.S. Long), 1334–1341. St Louis, MO: Elsevier.

31

Diphyllobothriasis

Diphyllobothriasis is a cestode zoonosis caused by *Diphyllobothrium* spp. The infection is acquired by humans after ingestion of plerocercoid larvae of *Diphyllobothrium* spp. which can be present in raw, undercooked, pickled or untreated smoked fish [1]. Four recognised species, *Diphyllobothrium latum*, *D. pacificum*, *D. klebanovskii* and *D. nihonkaiense*, are associated with human cases of diphyllobothriasis [2]. However, *D. latum*, also known as 'broad fish tapeworm', is usually considered the most common agent of human diphyllobothriasis. The infection of *D. latum* in humans is common in regions with cold-water lakes, such as Europe and North America. The growing popularity of raw fish dishes such as Japanese sushi and sashimi can be an important risk factor for human infection [1].

Transmission Cycle

All species associated with human infections with diphyllobothriid cestodes have marine or aquatic life cycles, and transmission occurs via ingestion of undercooked or raw fish. The life cycle of *D. latum* requires two intermediate hosts. Many of the fish-eating mammals, including humans, and birds act as definitive hosts for the parasite which can excrete the eggs through faeces. The egg passed in faeces hatch into a small ciliated coracidium in water, which swims freely until ingested by a suitable crustacean (first intermediate host) where development of the second larval stage (the procercoid) is completed. Procercoid larvae are released from the crustacean upon predation by the second intermediate host (usually a small fish) and migrate into the deeper tissues where they develop into plerocercoid larvae (spargana), which is the infectious stage for the definitive host. As the humans usually do not eat these small fish species in raw form, the second intermediate host probably does not represent an important source of human infection. However, these small second intermediate hosts can be eaten by larger predator species (such as perch, pike, burbot, whitefish, salmon and trout) that then serve as paratenic hosts, which harbour the infective plerocercoid stages within their tissue. Thus, humans (and other definitive host species) mainly acquire the parasite through the consumption of raw or undercooked fish [1].

Clinical Signs in Humans

Most cases of human diphyllobothriasis remain asymptomatic. However, in severe cases, symptoms such as transient abdominal discomfort, diarrhoea, anorexia, nausea, vomiting, vertigo, weakness and weight loss can be observed. Occasionally, infection can cause acute abdominal pain

Textbook of Zoonoses, First Edition. Jasbir Singh Bedi, Deepthi Vijay, and Pankaj Dhaka.

and intestinal obstruction. In rare cases, inflammation of the bile duct system (cholangitis) or the gallbladder (cholecystitis) may be caused by migrating proglottids. Prolonged or heavy *D. latum* infection is associated with megaloblastic anaemia due to parasite-mediated dissociation of the vitamin B12–intrinsic factor complex within the gut lumen, which causes unavailability of vitamin B12 to the host [1, 2].

Diagnosis

Diagnosis is generally carried out by coprological detection of the parasite stages (proglottids or eggs) from patients' faeces. Identification of an operculated egg with a small knob in the antioperculum side is the reliable diagnostic method for diphyllobothriasis. However, this approach is not always appropriate for species-specific identification, as there is close morphological similarity among the different species of fish tapeworms. Therefore, modern molecular tools such as polymerase chain reaction (PCR) can be used in epidemiological studies for accurate species-specific diagnosis during outbreaks.

Treatment

Praziquantel is reported to be highly effective against intestinal tapeworms. The supplementation of vitamin B12 may be needed to correct megaloblastic anaemia, if present.

Prevention and Control

Fish should only be consumed if thoroughly cooked, properly brine-cured or frozen at −10 °C for 24–48 hours. Control of the faecal contamination of water bodies can help in breaking the life cycle of parasite. Health education campaigns with objectives to change human eating behaviour and improvement in health-seeking attitudes are warranted.

References

1 Centers for Disease Control and Prevention. (2020). Parasites - *Diphyllobothrium* Infection. www.cdc.gov/parasites/diphyllobothrium/biology.html (accessed 24 January 2022).
2 Chou, H.F., Yen, C.M., Liang, W.C., and Jong, Y.J. (2006). Diphyllobothriasis latum: the first child case report in Taiwan. *Kaohsiung Journal of Medical Sciences 22* (7): 346–351.

32
Echinococcosis

Echinococcosis is a parasitic zoonosis of great public health significance which is caused by larval stages of cestodes of the genus *Echinococcus* (family Taeniidae) in intermediate hosts, such as ungulates and rodents, and can accidentally infect humans.

Epidemiology and Transmission

Out of the six species in the genus *Echinococcus*, four are of major public health concern: *Echinococcus granulosus* (causes cystic echinococcosis), *E. multilocularis* (alveolar echinococcosis), *E. vogeli* (polycystic echinococcosis) and *E. oligarthrus* (unicystic echinococcosis) [1].

Cystic echinococcosis, also known as hydatid disease or hydatidosis, occurs worldwide, including tropical and subtropical regions, whereas alveolar echinococcosis is widely distributed in the temperate northern hemisphere [2]. Polycystic echinococcosis and unicystic echinococcosis are confined to Latin America and are therefore collectively termed 'neo-tropical echinococcosis' [3]. The human disease burden is highly variable in the different endemic areas, mainly depending upon human behavioural risk factors, diversity and ecology of animal hosts, and genetic diversity within *Echinococcus* species which differ in their zoonotic potential and pathogenicity [4].

Hosts

Various herbivorous and omnivorous animals such as goats, swine, cattle, camels and yaks act as intermediate hosts of *E. granulosus*. Carnivores can be infected through the consumption of viscera of intermediate hosts containing the parasite larvae. Infected carnivores act as definitive hosts for the parasite where the larva matures to the adult tapeworm (3–6 mm long) in the intestine. Alveolar echinococcosis is typically maintained in a wild animal cycle with canids, particularly foxes and wolves, as the definitive hosts and rodents as the intermediate hosts [4]. Although the infection is more common in dogs, cats can become infected with alveolar echinococcosis by eating infected rodents (e.g. mice and squirrels) [2]. For *E. vogeli*, bush dogs and domestic dogs act as definitive hosts, whereas wild felids act as definitive hosts for *E. oligarthrus*. Small rodents act as intermediate hosts for both *E. vogeli* and *E. oligarthrus* [3].

The intermediate hosts become infected by ingesting parasite eggs from contaminated food and water, and the eggs then develop into larval stages in the viscera. The eggs are adapted to survive in the environment for as long as a year in cool moist conditions but are susceptible to desiccation [5].

Textbook of Zoonoses, First Edition. Jasbir Singh Bedi, Deepthi Vijay, and Pankaj Dhaka.

Humans can be accidentally infected through ingestion of parasite eggs from contaminated food, water or soil, or after direct contact with animal hosts.

Transmission Cycles

The most widespread transmission cycle for *E. granulosus* exists between dogs and sheep (Figure 32.1). The disease is endemic in pastoral communities where dogs are used to care for sheep flocks. The dogs can be infected when they are fed offal or scavenge infected sheep carcasses containing cysts. The infected dogs contaminate pasture with their faeces and sheep can be reinfected as they graze on these pastures. There exist many similar cycles in nature between dogs and horses, dogs and camels, etc., and also in wildlife between wolves and moose/deer [5]. *E. multilocularis* is mainly transmitted within the predator–prey relationship between foxes and small mammals, mostly rodents such as voles. Sometimes cattle, sheep and pigs can be exposed to infection but develop small non-viable lesions of *E. multilocularis,* and therefore are not considered to be involved in transmission [5].

Pathogenesis

After ingestion of *Echinococcus* spp. eggs by an intermediate host (e.g. sheep, goats, pigs, etc.) or humans (as accidental host), the egg hatches in the small intestine and releases oncosphere larvae which can penetrate the lamina propria of the intestine. After penetration, the larvae are passively transported through blood or lymphatics to the liver, lungs or other internal organs where they develop into hydatid cysts (metacestode larvae). The metacestode is a fluid-filled, spherical, unilocular or multilocular cyst, depending on the species, having an inner germinal layer and an outer laminated layer surrounded by a fibrous capsule derived from the host. The small vesicles (called brood capsules) bud internally from the germinal layer and develop asexually into pre-adult worms called protoscolices [6]. The cysts grow slowly and can be up to many litres in volume and contain thousands of protoscolices. Accidental rupture of the cysts can be followed by the massive

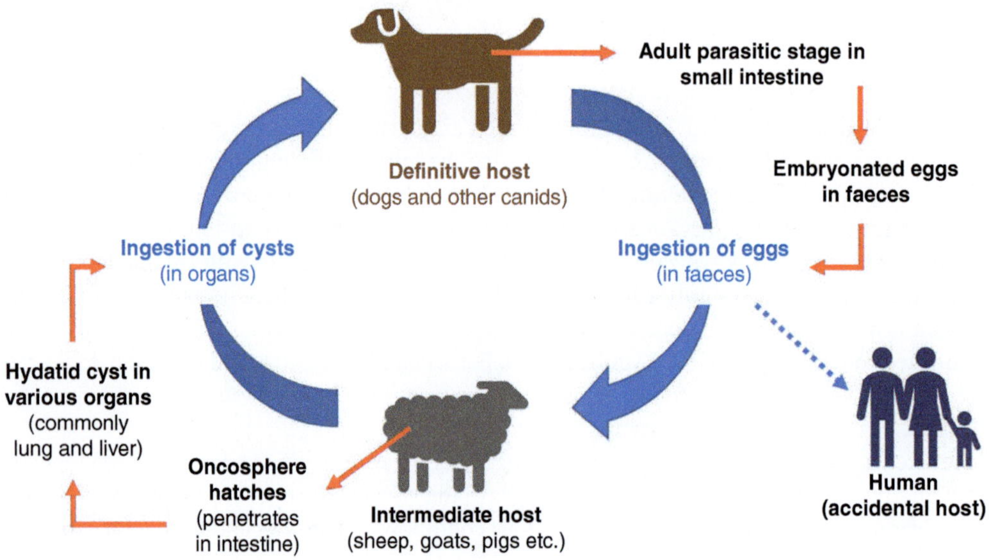

Figure 32.1 Transmission cycle of *Echinococcus granulosus.*

release of cyst fluid and haematogenous dissemination of protoscolices. This can result in anaphylactic reactions and multiple secondary echinococcosis (as protoscolices can develop into secondary cysts within the same intermediate host).

Disease in Animals

Tapeworms in the small intestine of the definitive host cause few ill effects. In intermediate hosts, the hydatid cysts gradually displace or induce fibrosis in normal tissue, and result in disease manifestation. In infected livestock, the cysts act like tumours that can disrupt the function of the affected organ and lead to slow body growth, decrease in the production of milk, meat and wool, reduced birth rate, and economic losses due to condemnation of organs during postmortem examination [5]. However, due to the slow growth of the cysts, many infected animals are slaughtered before the cysts ever cause clinical signs.

Disease in Humans

The clinical signs in humans depend on the location and growth of the hydatid cysts (metacestode larvae). The asymptomatic incubation period of the disease can last many years until the cysts grow to an extent that triggers clinical signs. The symptoms in humans depend on where in the body the cyst develops, and the size and numbers of cysts or metacestode mass. The clinically important forms of human echinococcosis are described below [2].

1) **Cystic echinococcosis** is caused due to infection with *E. granulosus*. Cystic echinococcosis is clinically related to the presence of one or more well-delineated spherical primary cysts, most frequently formed in the liver, but other organs such as the lungs, kidney, spleen, brain, heart and bone may also be affected. Clinical signs include weight loss, abdominal pain, general malaise and hepatic failure [7]. If the cyst is located in the lungs, clinical signs include chronic cough, chest pain and shortness of breath. Other signs depend on the location of the hydatid cysts and the pressure exerted on the surrounding tissues. The disease can be severe, occasionally fatal, and the treatment is lengthy and expensive.
2) **Alveolar echinococcosis** is caused by infection with *E. multilocularis*. The infection manifests primarily in the liver, showing a tumour-like malignant growth which, left untreated, can be fatal [7].
3) **Neotropical echinococcosis**: polycystic echinococcosis is caused by infection with *E. vogeli* and unicystic echinococcosis is caused by *E. oligarthrus*.

The cysts found in those with alveolar and polycystic echinococcosis are similar to those found in those with cystic echinococcosis; however, the alveolar and polycystic echinococcosis cysts usually have multiple compartments and display infiltrative growth as opposed to expansive growth in cystic echinococcosis [8].

Diagnosis

In definitive hosts, diagnosis is usually carried out by demonstration of adult worms in the intestine at postmortem or in the mucus after arecoline purgation, or finding the proglottids (tapeworm segments) in faeces. Genus-specific antigen detection tests in faeces such as coproantigen enzyme-linked immunosorbent assay (ELISA) can be used [5]. For molecular diagnosis, eggs can be sampled from soil (or faeces) for specific amplification of DNA to detect the presence of *Echinococcus* spp.

In intermediate hosts, diagnosis depends on the postmortem detection of the cysts, particularly in the liver and lungs. Serological testing for cystic echinococcosis in cattle, sheep and pigs can be carried out during epidemiological studies, but the sensitivity and specificity of these tests should be checked.

In humans, ultrasonography imaging is the technique of choice for the diagnosis of both cystic and alveolar echinococcosis. This technique is usually complemented or validated by computed tomography (CT) and/or magnetic resonance imaging (MRI) scans. Serological tests such as ELISA and indirect haemagglutination test (IHA) are widely used for screening of cases, whereas the immunoblotting (IB) test is used for confirmatory purposes [2].

Treatment

The treatment of echinococcosis is often expensive and complicated, and may necessitate extensive surgical intervention and/or prolonged drug therapy. The four main treatment options for cystic echinococcosis are as follows.

- Percutaneous treatment of hydatid cysts with PAIR (Puncture, Aspiration, Injection, Reaspiration) technique. This involves percutaneous treatment of cysts, where a scolicidal agent is injected into the cyst cavity aiming to evacuate the cyst contents and inactivate the protoscolices and germinal layer of the endocyst.
- Surgical intervention is one of the most common methods used to remove cysts from the body. However, the release of cyst fluid and dissemination of protoscolices due to cyst rupture or spillage during surgery or percutaneous interventions can result in allergic reactions. Moreover, the protoscolices can develop into secondary echinococcosis, which can lead to the genesis of multiple secondary cysts.
- Anti-infective drug treatments include chemotherapy with benzimidazole compounds.
- If the cyst does not affect organ functions or cause symptoms, then a 'watch and wait' approach can safely be taken, leaving the cysts untreated. Cyst transition from an early active stage into an inactive cyst is possible over a period of time [2].
- For alveolar echinococcosis, early diagnosis and surgical interventions followed by anti-infective prophylaxis with albendazole remain the key elements [5].

Prevention and Control

Without adequate control measures, infection rates can be very high in livestock and dogs, with associated significant incidence in humans. Control measures aim at interruption of the life cycle of the parasite. Some of the important control measures for cystic and alveolar echinococcosis are described below.

Cystic Echinococcosis

Surveillance of cystic echinococcosis in animals is difficult because the infection is asymptomatic in livestock and dogs. The cycle of *E. granulosus* in wildlife is not easy to control, but by discouraging scavenging and implementing hygiene, the infection of domestic animals and subsequent spread to humans can be reduced [9]. Some of the prevention and control measures include the following.

- Preventing access of dogs to livestock carcasses or slaughter wastes from farms, households, abattoirs, etc.
- Periodic deworming of dogs with praziquantel to kill the adult stages of tapeworm.
- Detecting cysts during meat inspection, thereby targeting infected farms or communities.
- *Echinococcus granulosus* recombinant antigen (EG95) offers encouraging prospects for disease prevention. Vaccination of sheep (or other livestock) can be carried out to protect against development of the larval stage of *E. granulosus*. The vaccine is currently being produced commercially and is registered in China and Argentina [2].
- Public education campaigns should be carried out. Washing hands with soap and warm water after handling dogs and before handling food is crucial for preventing the disease in humans.

Alveolar Echinococcosis

The control of *E. multilocularis* is complex because of the wildlife cycle between foxes and rodents. Reduction in parasite transmission has been observed by the use of praziquantel baits for foxes and regular deworming of domestic carnivores that have access to wild rodents [5].

References

1 Moro, P. and Schantz, P.M. (2009). Echinococcosis: a review. *International Journal of Infectious Diseases 13* (2): 125–133.

2 World Health Organization. (2021). Echinococcosis Fact Sheet. www.who.int/news-room/fact-sheets/detail/echinococcosis (accessed 24 January 2022)

3 Stojkovic, M., Gottstein, B., and Junghanss, T. (2014). Echinococcosis. In: *Manson's Tropical Infectious Diseases* (ed. J. Farrar, P. Hotez, T. Junghanns, et al.), 795–819. Philadelphia, PA: WB Saunders.

4 Deplazes, P., Rinaldi, L., Rojas, C.A. et al. (2017). Global distribution of alveolar and cystic echinococcosis. In: *Advances in Parasitology*, vol. 95 (ed. D. Rollinson and R. Stothard), 315–493. New York: Academic Press.

5 World Animal Health Organisation (2020). Echinococcosis. www.oie.int/en/disease/echinococcosis/ (accessed 24 January 2022)

6 Almulhim, A.M. and John, S. (2019). *Echinococcus Granulosus (Hydatid Cysts, Echinococcosis)*. Treasure Island, FL: StatPearls Publishing.

7 Torgerson, P.R., Schweiger, A., Deplazes, P. et al. (2008). Alveolar echinococcosis: from a deadly disease to a well-controlled infection. Relative survival and economic analysis in Switzerland over the last 35 years. *Journal of Hepatology 49* (1): 72–77.

8 Tappe, D., Stich, A., and Frosch, M. (2008). Emergence of polycystic neotropical echinococcosis. *Emerging Infectious Diseases 14* (2): 292.

9 Centers for Disease Control and Prevention. (2012). Echinococcosis. www.cdc.gov/parasites/echinococcosis/disease.html (accessed 24 January 2022)

33

Giardiasis

Aetiology

Giardiasis is an intestinal infection caused by the flagellated protozoan parasite *Giardia duodenalis* (synonyms *Giardia lamblia* and *Giardia intestinalis*). Giardiasis is associated with water-borne and food-borne diarrhoea, day-care centre outbreaks and traveller's diarrhoea. The disease is also known by other names including lambliasis, beaver fever, runner's diarrhoea and backpacker disease. Outbreaks are common in tropical countries where unhygienic environmental conditions prevail. *Giardia* is also a very common enteric parasite of domestic animals, including livestock, dogs, cats and wildlife. The parasite has a significant zoonotic potential [1].

Transmission Factors

Giardia is commonly transmitted through the ingestion of infective cysts shed in human or animal faeces. Ingestion is mostly indirect through faecal contaminated water, food or fomites. Out of the identified eight genetic groups (or assemblages) of *G. duodenalis* (A–H), assemblages A and B are considered zoonotic, which can infect humans, domestic animals, rodents and livestock [1]. Other assemblages can also infect many species of animals and humans.

The life cycle of *Giardia* is direct; the infective cyst is encysted when released through the faeces of the host and is immediately infectious. The cysts remain infectious for months in cool, damp areas, and rapidly accumulate in the environment. In addition, the cysts are more resistant to chlorine disinfection than most microbes, thus many *Giardia* outbreaks have been linked to contaminated drinking water and swimming pools [2].

Pathogenesis

After ingestion of the infective cysts in the host, the actively multiplying trophozoite form of the protozoan hatches from the cyst and attaches to the small intestine, where it induces epithelial inflammation, villous flattening and diarrhoea due to malabsorption. In the large intestine, the trophozoites differentiate to form new cysts, which are shed in the faeces and contaminate the environment. Cysts present in faeces can remain viable in a variety of environments, particularly in water and at lower temperatures. The viability of the cysts ranges from 28 to 84 days in lake or river water [3].

Textbook of Zoonoses, First Edition. Jasbir Singh Bedi, Deepthi Vijay, and Pankaj Dhaka.

Disease in Humans

Giardia infections can be asymptomatic and generally cause self-limited clinical illness. Clinical symptoms include diarrhoea, flatulence, abdominal pain, bloating, weight loss and malabsorption [2]. Giardiasis can have deleterious effects on the growth and development of children and can have serious consequences among immunocompromised patients.

Diagnosis

Giardiasis is usually diagnosed by the laboratory analysis of stool samples for identification of trophozoites or cysts, either by traditional microscopy or by stool antigen detection assays. The modern sensitive molecular methods (e.g. polymerase chain reaction) are increasingly being used for epidemiological studies and outbreak investigations.

Treatment

Tinidazole and metronidazole are considered equally effective as first-line treatment.

Prevention and Control

The faeco-oral route is the most common pathway for giardia infection. The infectious cysts of *Giardia* can survive for months in the environment and can cause cross-contamination of water resources. Therefore, strict hygiene and sanitation are considered as the key measures to break the parasite chain. The prevention of secondary transmission is mainly through antiparasitic treatment of cases and stringent personal hygiene measures for the prevention of person-to-person spread.

References

1 Feng, Y. and Xiao, L. (2011). Zoonotic potential and molecular epidemiology of *Giardia* species and giardiasis. *Clinical Microbiology Reviews 24* (1): 110–140.
2 Minetti, C., Chalmers, R.M., Beeching, N.J. et al. (2016). Giardiasis. *BMJ 355*: i5369.
3 Olson, M.E., Goh, J., Phillips, M. et al. (1999). *Giardia* cyst and *Cryptosporidium* oocyst survival in water, soil, and cattle feces. *Journal of Environmental Quality 28* (6): 1991–1996.

34

Leishmaniasis

Leishmaniasis is caused by a protozoan parasite of *Leishmania* spp. which infects animals, humans and sandflies [1]. Leishmaniasis is prevalent in tropical and subtropical regions and southern Europe. It has been classified as a neglected tropical disease (NTD) by the World Health Organization [2] and is considered among the top parasitic diseases causing outbreaks with potential mortality [2]. Over 90 sandfly species are known to transmit *Leishmania* parasites, mainly *Lutzomyia* in the Americas and *Phlebotomus* elsewhere [1].

Epidemiology

Classically, leishmaniasis can be divided into two major syndromes as per the geographical distribution: Old World leishmaniasis and New World leishmaniasis [2–4].

- Old World leishmaniasis includes two clinical presentations: cutaneous leishmaniasis and visceral leishmaniasis. In the Old World (Eastern hemisphere), leishmaniasis is found in some parts of Asia, the Middle East, Africa (particularly in the tropical region and North Africa) and southern Europe. It is not found in Australia or the Pacific Islands.
- New World leishmaniasis mainly consists of cutaneous leishmaniasis and mucocutaneous leishmaniasis. In the New World (Western hemisphere), leishmaniasis is found in some parts of Mexico, Central America and South America. It is not found in Chile or Uruguay.

The clinical forms of disease and associated organisms are listed below [1]/BMJ publishing.

Disease	Old World organisms	New World organisms
Visceral leishmaniasis	*L. donovani* (India, Kenya) *L. infantum* (southern Europe and North Africa) *L. tropica*	*L. chagasi* *L. amazonensis*
Cutaneous leishmaniasis	*L. tropica* *L. major* *L. aethiopica* *L. infantum* *L. donovani*	*L. mexicana* species complex *L. major*-like organisms *L. chagasi*

Textbook of Zoonoses, First Edition. Jasbir Singh Bedi, Deepthi Vijay, and Pankaj Dhaka.

Mucosal leishmaniasis	*Viannia* subgenus *L. (V) braziliensis* *L. (V) panamensis* *L. (V) guyanensis* *L. amazonensis*

Transmission

Around 70 animal species, including humans, are the natural reservoir hosts of *Leishmania* spp. [2]. The epidemiology of leishmaniasis depends on the characteristics of the parasite species, sand fly species, local ecological characteristics, current and past exposure of human population, and human behaviour.

The transmission of *Leishmania* parasites occurs through the bites of infected female phlebotomine sand flies. Sand flies become infected by sucking blood from an infected animal or person and the sand fly ingests the organism as an amastigote into its digestive tract. The amastigote develops into a promastigote in the digestive tract and is then injected into a susceptible host during the next feeding of the fly. The promastigote then infects macrophages of the host and develops into amastigotes. The life cycle of *Leishmania* spp. in sand fly and natural hosts is presented in Figure 34.1.

Sand flies are usually active at twilight, evening and night-time hours. Being weak fliers, they tend to remain close to their breeding area, not too high above the ground. Although sand flies are less active during the hottest time of the day, they may bite if they are disturbed (e.g. if a person brushes up against the trunk of a tree or some other site where sand flies are resting) [3]. Most of

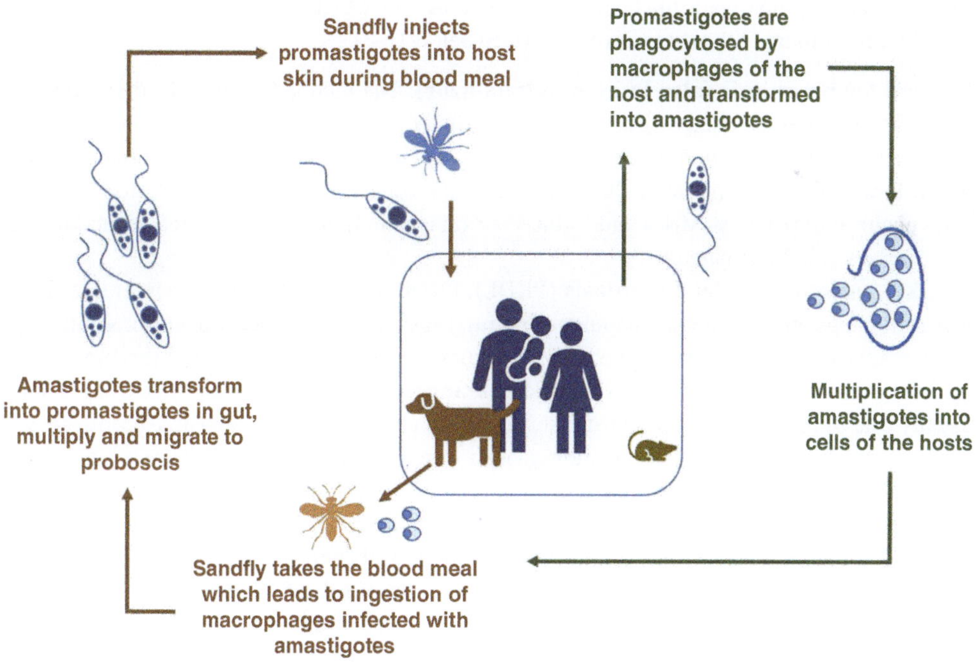

Figure 34.1 The life cycle of *Leishmania* spp. in sand fly and natural hosts.

the time, people do not observe the presence of sand flies as they are small (about a quarter the size of mosquitoes), they do not make any noise, and their bites might be painless.

Some species of *Leishmania* parasites may spread via contaminated needles or blood transfusions. Congenital transmission from pregnant woman to baby has also been reported [2]. High-risk groups include travellers, ecotourists, soldiers, ornithologists and field epidemiologists [3]. The major risk factors for leishmaniasis include the following [1, 2].

- **Socioeconomic conditions**: Poor housing and sanitary conditions such as lack of waste management or open sewerage may increase sand fly breeding and resting sites, as well as their access to humans. Human behaviour, such as sleeping outside or on the ground, may increase the risk of sand fly bite.
- **Population mobility**: Epidemics of both cutaneous and visceral leishmaniasis are often associated with migration and movement of non-immune people into areas with existing transmission cycles. Occupational exposure and widespread deforestation are important factors for the emergence of leishmaniasis.
- **Climate change**: Climate change may be responsible for the extension of leishmaniasis to previously non-endemic regions. Changes in temperature, rainfall and humidity can have strong effects on vector density and reservoir hosts by altering their distribution and influencing their survival and population size. Moreover, drought, famine and flood can lead to massive displacement and migration of people to areas with high risk of transmission of *Leishmania*, and poor nutrition could compromise their immunity.

Clinical Signs

Some people have asymptomatic infection. However, those who develop clinical evidence of infection may exhibit one or more of the three forms described below [1–3].

1) **Visceral leishmaniasis (also known as kala-azar)**: The incubation period varies from 3 to 8 months. It is characterised by irregular bouts of fever, weight loss, hepatosplenomegaly (usually spleen much larger than liver) and anaemia. Skin pigmentation may be a clinical feature, which is why the other name of the disease is 'kala azar', which means 'black disease'. Most cases occur in Brazil, East Africa and India. Visceral leishmaniasis is considered as fatal in over 95% of cases, if left untreated.

   Post-kala-azar dermal leishmaniasis (PKDL)**:** PKDL is usually a sequel of visceral leishmaniasis that appears as a macular, papular or nodular rash usually on face, upper arms and trunk but can appear on other parts of the body. It occurs mainly in East Africa and the Indian subcontinent, where 5–10% of patients with kala-azar are reported to develop PKDL [2]. This is usually due to infection by *L. donovani* sensu stricto cluster and may appear 1 month to 1 or more years after kala-azar has apparently been cured. People with PKDL are considered a potential source of *Leishmania* infection [1].
2) **Cutaneous leishmaniasis:** This is the most common form of leishmaniasis and causes skin lesions, mainly ulcers (like a volcano, with raised edge and central crater) on exposed parts of the body. These lesions can cause life-long scars with serious disability or stigma. The incubation period lasts from 2 weeks to several months, and in some cases up to 3 years have been reported. About 95% of the cases occur in the Americas, Mediterranean basin, Middle East and Central Asia.

3) **Mucocutaneous leishmaniasis (also known as espundia):** The incubation period is 1–3 months, but mucocutaneous leishmaniasis may occur years after healing of the initial cutaneous ulcer. This form of disease can cause partial or total destruction of mucous membranes of nose, mouth and throat. The severe form can cause difficulty in eating and an increased risk of secondary infection which results in significant mortality. Over 90% of mucocutaneous leishmaniasis cases occur in Bolivia, Brazil, Ethiopia and Peru.

Diagnosis

For visceral leishmaniasis, diagnosis is made by combining clinical signs with parasitological or serological tests. In cutaneous and mucocutaneous leishmaniasis, serological tests have limited value and clinical manifestations along with parasitological tests confirm the diagnosis [2]. Tissue specimens from bone marrow (for visceral leishmaniasis) or skin sores (for cutaneous leishmaniasis) can be examined for the parasite under microscope or by using serological and molecular tests [3]. Sometimes the parasite can be cultured from microscopy-negative tissue samples on special media such as Novy, McNeal, Nicolle (NNN) medium or can be inoculated into experimental animals such as hamsters [1].

Treatment

There is no effective vaccine for leishmaniasis [1]. Often, the skin sores of cutaneous leishmaniasis heal on their own, but this can take months or even years and can leave ugly scars. The cutaneous form may further develop to the mucocutaneous form of leishmaniasis that might spread from the skin and cause sores in the mucous membranes of the nose, mouth or throat. Ensuring adequate treatment of the cutaneous infection may help in prevention of mucosal leishmaniasis [2]. All patients diagnosed with visceral leishmaniasis require prompt and complete treatment. If not treated, severe cases of visceral leishmaniasis typically are fatal [2].

Leishmaniasis is a treatable and curable disease but the medicines will not get rid of the parasite from the body; thus, there is a risk of relapse in cases of immunosuppression. The treatment of leishmaniasis depends on several factors including type of disease, concomitant pathologies, parasite species and geographic location.

Prevention and Control

Prevention and control of leishmaniasis requires a combination of intervention strategies. The key strategies for prevention are listed below [2–4].

- Vector control programmes can help to reduce or interrupt transmission of the parasite by decreasing the number of sand flies. Control methods include insecticide spray, use of insecticide-treated nets, environmental management and personal protection in endemic regions.
- In areas where sand flies are mostly endophilic (rest mostly indoors after feeding), spraying houses with insecticide is effective in reducing the likelihood of contracting cutaneous leishmaniasis. During outdoor activities, minimise the area of exposed (uncovered) skin and apply appropriate insect repellent.

- Effective disease surveillance is important to monitor and act effectively during epidemics.
- Early diagnosis and treatment reduce the prevalence of the disease and prevent disabilities and death. They also help to reduce transmission and to monitor the burden of disease. In regions where anthroponotic transmission prevails (e.g. India), the successful treatment of patients, especially those with PKDL (who may act as long-term reservoirs), has been effective in controlling transmission of the parasite.
- The control of animal reservoir hosts is complex and should be tailored as per local ecology. In places where the dog is a reservoir for the disease, insecticide treatment of dogs and use of dog collars can be effective.
- Education of the community with effective behavioural change interventions must be carried out in endemic regions.

References

1 Piscopo, T.V. and Mallia Azzopardi, C. (2007). Leishmaniasis. *Postgraduate Medical Journal 83* (976): 649–657.
2 World Health Orgnaization. (2022). Leishmaniasis. www.who.int/news-room/fact-sheets/detail/leishmaniasis (accessed 24 January 2022).
3 Centers for Disease Control and Prevention. (2020). www.cdc.gov/parasites/leishmaniasis/gen_info/faqs.html (accessed 24 January 2022).
4 Kobets, T., Grekov, I., and Lipoldova, M. (2012). Leishmaniasis: prevention, parasite detection and treatment. *Current Medicinal Chemistry 19* (10): 1443–1474.

35

Sarcocystosis

Sarcocystis species are coccidian parasites of warm-blooded and poikilothermic animals, including humans. *Sarcocystis* spp. usually have a two-host cycle which includes herbivores or omnivorous mammals as intermediate hosts, and carnivorous animals and humans as definitive hosts. Of all the *Sarcocystis* species, *S. hominis* and *S. suihominis* are of zoonotic importance, where humans and non-human primates act as definitive hosts and cattle and pigs are intermediate hosts, respectively [1, 2].

Transmission Cycle

Sarcocystis species are ubiquitous and are found worldwide. Two important species known to infect humans as definitive hosts are *S. hominis* from beef and *S. suihominis* from pork. The definitive host (e.g. humans) becomes infected by ingesting the tissues of herbivores with the encysted stage (i.e. sarcocyst) of the parasite containing hundreds of bradyzoites. The oocysts sporulate *in situ* within 1 week after ingestion of bradyzoites and release two sporocysts, each sporocyst containing four sporozoites. The herbivore hosts acquire infection by ingesting feed and water contaminated with *Sarcocystis* sporocysts. After ingestion of sporocysts, sporozoites are liberated and initiate a complex asexual cycle [1]. A brief overview of the life cycle of *Sarcocystis* spp. is illustrated in Figure 35.1.

The ingestion of meat containing mature sarcocysts is the predominant source of intestinal sarcocystosis in humans. The extraintestinal infection in humans can occur due to non-human *Sarcocystis* spp. such as *S. nesbitti* (a species with a reptilian definitive host), after the accidental ingestion of oocysts via contaminated food or water containing sporocysts excreted by infected carnivores. In such cases, humans serve as an accidental and aberrant intermediate host, replacing the intermediate hosts found in nature [1].

Clinical Signs

The infection is mostly asymptomatic in cattle and pigs. In humans, *Sarcocystis* spp. are mainly associated with intestinal infection due to ingestion of oocysts and sporocysts. As a definitive host, humans can experience nausea, vomiting, acute and severe enteritis, or chronic enteritis, but many infections appear to be mild or asymptomatic. In some cases, humans can serve as an accidental

Textbook of Zoonoses, First Edition. Jasbir Singh Bedi, Deepthi Vijay, and Pankaj Dhaka.

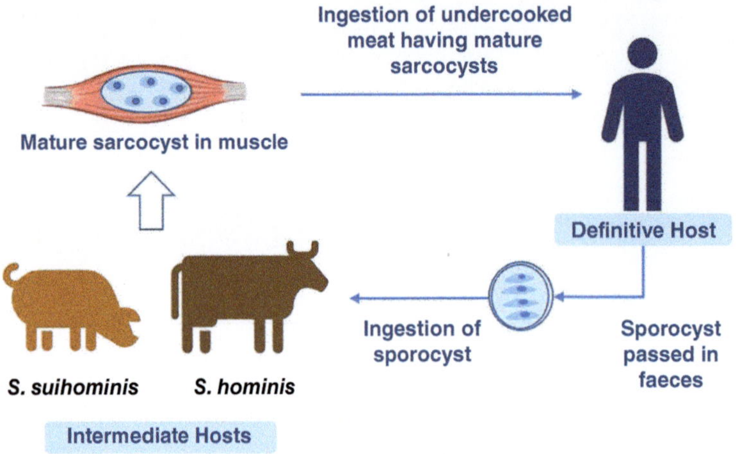

Figure 35.1 Life cycle of *Sarcocystis* spp. in intermediate and definitive hosts.

and aberrant intermediate host by ingestion of sporocysts, which can cause an extraintestinal form of the disease and lead to the development of sarcocysts in myocytes of skeletal, cardiac and smooth muscle [1, 2].

Diagnosis

The presumptive diagnosis of intestinal sarcocystosis includes enteritis and a history of consumption of undercooked meat. Confirmation requires the identification of oocysts and or sporocysts in the stool. Most cases have been diagnosed by use of incidental biopsy specimens, with no associated clinical symptoms, or during autopsies. Serological diagnosis using enzyme-linked immunosorbent assays (ELISAs), immunofluorescence assays (IFAs), etc. for detection of antibodies against *Sarcocystis* using bradyzoite antigen is limited to specialised laboratories. Molecular tests can be employed to determine the species-level identification of the parasite [1].

Treatment

Treatment remains mostly symptomatic which includes albendazole for suppressing chronic symptoms of muscular sarcocystis, and the use of metronidazole and co-trimoxazole for eosinophilic myositis. Corticosteroids can be used to reduce the inflammation associated with myositis.

Prevention and Control

To prevent intestinal sarcocystosis, meat must be thoroughly cooked or frozen to kill the bradyzoites in the sarcocysts. Clean drinking water can reduce exposure to sporocysts, but contact with contaminated recreational water and soil is also a potential risk factor for infection. It should be noted that the chemical disinfection with chlorine is not effective in killing sporocysts of *Sarcocystis*, so boiling and other appropriate methods of water disinfection should be employed in endemic regions [1]. Strict postmortem meat inspection can be helpful in detection of contaminated carcasses and thus reduce infection in humans. To prevent infection of food animals, human faeces containing sporocysts must not be permitted to contaminate water, bedding and feed.

Sanitation is the key to control the environmental contamination of sporocysts, where the contamination can be reduced or eliminated by the proper use of toilets and hand washing.

References

1 Fayer, R., Esposito, D.H., and Dubey, J.P. (2015). Human infections with *Sarcocystis* species. *Clinical Microbiology Reviews 28* (2): 295–311.

2 Dubey, J.P. (2015). Foodborne and waterborne zoonotic sarcocystosis. *Food and Waterborne Parasitology* 1 (1): 2–11.

36

Schistosomiasis

Human schistosomiasis (also known as bilharzia) is a parasitic disease caused by trematode flukes of the genus *Schistosoma*. Schistosomiasis is considered as one of the most prevalent human parasitic infections, especially in resource-limited regions. The transmission cycle of the parasite involves specific freshwater snails as intermediate hosts and human contact with infested water. The main disease-causing species are *Schistosoma haematobium*, *S. mansoni* and *S. japonicum*.

Epidemiology

Schistosomiasis is prevalent in tropical and subtropical areas, predominantly among resource-restricted communities having inadequate access to safe drinking water and sanitation. It is estimated that at least 90% of those requiring treatment for schistosomiasis reside in Africa [1]. The main species of schistosomes that infect human beings, along with their geographical distribution, are described below (Based on[1]).

Disease condition	Species	Geographical distribution	Clinical symptoms
Intestinal schistosomiasis	*Schistosoma mansoni*	Africa, Middle East, Caribbean, Brazil, Venezuela, and Suriname	Abdominal pain, diarrhoea and blood in the stool. In advanced cases, liver and spleen enlargement is common, and frequently associated with the accumulation of fluid in the peritoneal cavity
	Schistosoma japonicum	China, Indonesia, the Philippines	
	Schistosoma mekongi	Cambodia and the Lao People's Democratic Republic	
Urogenital schistosomiasis	*Schistosoma haematobium*	Africa, Middle East, Corsica (France)	The classic sign of urogenital schistosomiasis is haematuria. In advanced cases, fibrosis of the bladder and ureter along with kidney damage is usually observed. Bladder cancer is another possible complication in the later stages of the infection

Textbook of Zoonoses, First Edition. Jasbir Singh Bedi, Deepthi Vijay, and Pankaj Dhaka.

Transmission Cycle

In the human body, the larvae develop into adult schistosomes. The adult male and female worms live within the veins of their human host, where they mate and produce fertilised eggs. Some of the eggs are shed into the environment through faeces or urine to continue the parasite's life cycle, while others may be trapped in body tissues and may cause immune reactions and progressive damage to organs. The eggs that reach fresh water will hatch, releasing free-living ciliated miracidia that then infect a suitable snail host (intermediate host). In the snail, the parasite undergoes asexual replication, eventually shedding thousands of cercariae (the form infectious for human beings) into the water. People become infected when cercariae penetrate the skin during contact with infested water [1].

The important risk factors of the infection to humans include agricultural, domestic, occupational and recreational activities, which expose humans to infested water. The lack of hygiene and activities like swimming or fishing in infested water increase the risk of infection in endemic regions [1].

Clinical Signs

The eggs of *Schistosome* spp. are mainly responsible for the induction of clinical signs in human schistosomiasis. During infection, many eggs are not excreted and lodge in various organs such as the intestine or liver (for *S. mansoni*, *S. japonicum* and *S. mekongi*) or the bladder and urogenital system (for *S. haematobium*). The eggs induce a granulomatous host immune response in the infested organs, where the process of granuloma formation induces chronic inflammation that leads to the disease manifestation of schistosomiasis.

These two important clinical forms of human schistosomiasis are described below [2].

- **Intestinal schistosomiasis**: The acute form of intestinal schistosomiasis is sometimes referred to as *Katayama syndrome*. It commonly occurs among travellers or immigrants who visit schistosome endemic regions and are exposed to schistosome antigens for the first time as an adult. The clinical signs manifest weeks to months after the infection as a consequence of worm maturation, egg production and the release of egg antigen, and associated host granulomatous and immune complex responses. Typical clinical signs include a sudden onset of fever, malaise, myalgia, headache, eosinophilia, fatigue and abdominal pain. Gradually, the granulomatous immune response to eggs is downregulated, leading to progression to the chronic intestinal form of the disease. The chronic form exhibits non-specific intermittent abdominal pain, diarrhoea and rectal bleeding.
  The frequency of symptoms often relates to the intensity of infection. Some people with intestinal schistosomiasis poorly immune-regulate their response to parasite egg antigens and consequently develop extensive fibrosis and subsequent hepatosplenic disease with periportal fibrosis. Clinical features include upper abdominal discomfort with palpable nodular hepatomegaly, often with splenomegaly. The time from initial infection to advanced fibrosis can range from 5 to 15 years [2].
- **Urogenital schistosomiasis**: This form of infection is mainly associated with *S. haematobium*. The clinically important symptom is haematuria, which often presents with high urinary frequency, burning micturition and suprapubic discomfort. In endemic regions with low awareness about the disease, haematuria is so widespread that it is considered a natural sign of puberty for boys, and is confused with menses in girls. The severe form of urogenital schistosomiasis results from poor immune regulation of antischistosome egg responses, leading to chronic fibrosis of the urinary tract resulting in obstructive uropathy which can cause hydronephrosis. The

concomitant bacterial superinfection and renal dysfunction can have lethal consequences among the infected individuals. Cases of squamous cell carcinoma of the bladder are also strongly associated with *S. haematobium* infection [2].

In females, the genital schistosomiasis caused by *S. haematobium* strongly affects reproductive health as the eggs migrate to the genital tract, causing inflammatory lesions in the ovaries, fallopian tubes, cervix, vagina and vulva. In addition, urogenital schistosomiasis is also considered to be a risk factor for human immunodeficiency virus (HIV) infection, especially in women. Among women with genital schistosomiasis, inflammation, friability and neovascularisation of the genital epithelial tissue can lead to a compromised physical barrier to HIV exposure through sexual activity.

The socioeconomic and health effects of schistosomiasis are significant. In children, schistosomiasis can cause anaemia, stunting and impaired development, and also affects cognitive function. Chronic schistosomiasis may cause high disability, which in some cases can result in death. Mortality rates associated with schistosomiasis are difficult to estimate because of hidden pathologies such as liver damage, kidney failure, bladder cancer and ectopic pregnancies due to female genital schistosomiasis. The ectopic deposition of *Schistosoma* eggs can lead to unexpected morbidities and may involve the migration of parasites or eggs to the central nervous system, with symptoms of spinal compression or encephalopathy.

Cerebral schistosomiasis occurs most commonly during *S. japonicum* infections, and the clinical presentation includes meningoencephalitis with pyrexia, headache, vomiting, blurred vision and altered sensorium or Jacksonian epilepsy [2].

Diagnosis

Schistosomiasis can be diagnosed through the detection of parasite eggs in stool or urine specimens. Antibody and/or antigen detection in blood or urine samples are also indications of infection [1]. For urogenital schistosomiasis, filtration using nylon, paper or polycarbonate filters is the standard diagnostic technique. Children with *S. haematobium* almost always have microscopic blood in their urine which can be detected by chemical reagent strips. The eggs of intestinal schistosomiasis can be detected in faecal specimens through a technique using methylene blue-stained cellophane soaked in glycerin or glass slides, known as the Kato–Katz technique. In *S. mansoni* transmission areas, the CCA (circulating cathodic antigen) test can also be used. For people living in non-endemic or low-transmission areas, serological and immunological tests may be useful in assessing exposure to infection and indicating the need for a thorough examination, treatment and follow-up [1].

Treatment

Praziquantel is the drug of choice for schistosomiasis. It is effective against all *Schistosoma* species [2].

Prevention and Control

Schistosomiasis control should focus on reducing disease through periodic large-scale population treatment with praziquantel. As per World Health Organization guidelines, the targeted groups for treatment are as follows [1].

- School-aged children in endemic areas.
- Adults are considered to be at risk in endemic areas, and people with occupations involving contact with infested water (e.g. fishermen, farmers, irrigation workers and women performing washing activities).
- Entire communities living in highly endemic areas.

An integrated approach including access to potable water, adequate sanitation, the prevention of sewage contamination of fresh water and snail control is important in reducing transmission in endemic regions.

References

1 World Health Organization. Schistosomiasis. (2022). www.who.int/news-room/fact-sheets/detail/schistosomiasis (accessed 24 January 2022).

2 Gryseels, B., Polman, K., Clerinx, J., and Kestens, L. (2006). Human schistosomiasis. *Lancet* 368 (9541): 1106–1118.

37

Taeniasis/Cysticercosis Complex

Taeniasis/cysticercosis complex is a zoonotic infection in which humans are the obligate definitive hosts for the three cestode species: *Taenia saginata*, *Taenia solium* and *Taenia asiatica*; however, the intermediate hosts can vary with the parasitic species. The parasites belong to the family Taeniidae (subclass Eucestoda, order Cyclophyllidea) and have flat ribbon-like bodies, with an anterior scolex and a posterior tape (known as strobila) made up of multiple segments (known as proglottids) which attach to the small intestine of humans. The larval stage or metacestode (also known as cysticerci) is found in the intermediate hosts, which in the case of *T. solium* (pork tapeworm) and *T. asiatica* (Asian tapeworm) are pigs, and for *T. saginata* (beef tapeworm) is cattle. The intestinal infection in humans with the adult stage of the cestode is referred to as 'taeniasis', which usually does not cause any serious symptoms. Cysticercosis is caused by the larval stage or metacestode (cysticerci) of *T. solium* in humans, where the tapeworm larvae can lodge in the muscles, skin, eyes and central nervous system, which may result in serious health effects.

Epidemiology and Transmission

The World Health Organization (WHO) and Food and Agriculture Organization (FAO) have classified the taeniasis/cysticercosis complex as a neglected zoonotic disease, and ranked *T. solium* as the most important food-borne parasite in terms of public health and related socioeconomic impact [1].

Human taeniasis is caused by ingestion of the metacestode larval stage, the cysticerci of *T. saginata* in beef (*Cysticercus bovis*) or *T. solium* (*Cysticercus cellulosae*), or *T. asiatica* in pork, resulting in sexual reproduction of the adult tapeworm in the human intestine. Cysticercosis is only acquired from the faecal–oral route by ingestion of *T. solium* eggs, and not through the ingestion of cysticerci in undercooked pork which is associated with intestinal taeniasis.

The zoonotic *Taenia* species (with the exception of *T. asiatica*) have a worldwide distribution, and the largest disease burden is observed in remote and rural areas where people traditionally raise pigs and cattle without adequate farm biosecurity measures [2]. *T. asiatica* appears to be restricted to Asian countries. *T. solium* occurs mostly in developing countries such as regions of Asia, Africa and Latin America [2]. The distribution of each of the species depends on the community's cultural characteristics which may involve the consumption of undercooked meat or organs of intermediate hosts infected with viable metacestodes [3]. Cysticercosis mainly affects impoverished segments of society, where poor sanitary practices prevail. Therefore, cysticercosis is often designated as a 'biological marker' for the social and economic development of the community.

Textbook of Zoonoses, First Edition. Jasbir Singh Bedi, Deepthi Vijay, and Pankaj Dhaka.

Host Range

Since humans are the only definitive hosts for *T. solium*, *T. saginata* and *T. asiatica*, these species are also referred to as 'human taenia'. The metacestodes of these species develop in the intermediate hosts and exhibit different tissue tropism. Swine serve as intermediate hosts for *T. solium* and *T. asiatica*. The metacestode stages of *T. solium* are usually found in the muscle and brain of pigs, whereas metacestode stages of *T. asiatica* are found in the visceral organs such as the liver of pigs. Domestic cattle are the common intermediate hosts for *T. saginata* where the cysticerci are mainly observed in the muscles of the host. In addition, domestic yaks, buffaloes and reindeer are also important intermediate hosts for *T. saginata* in certain geographical regions [4].

Transmission Cycles

Humans can become infected with *T. saginata* or *T. solium* when they consume inadequately cooked contaminated beef (measly beef) or pork (measly pork) respectively, contaminated with cysticerci. In the human intestine, the cysticercus develops over 2 months into an adult tapeworm, which can survive for years [5]. Humans can also host the intermediate forms of the *T. solium* mainly by:

- ingestion of *T. solium* eggs present in food and water contaminated by faeces from a person harbouring the adult worm
- through autoinfection, when ova are carried from faeces to the mouth via the hands of infected persons
- through reverse peristalsis bringing ova back to the stomach or duodenum where they hatch.

These accidental ingestions of *T. solium* eggs can cause cysticercosis, where the extraintestinal development of larvae occurs in muscles, eyes and central nervous system of infected individuals.

The eggs released by definite hosts in their stool can contaminate the ground, where the eggs can survive for 8 months or more in warm and humid climates [6]. These eggs can be swallowed by intermediate hosts such as cattle grazing on fields contaminated with human excreta either through fertilisation with 'night soil' or from poor sanitation. In areas where pigs have access to infected human waste, foraging pigs can ingest the eggs or proglottids. Once ingested by the intermediate host, the eggs hatch to release the larval oncospheres, which attach to and penetrate the wall of the gut. The larvae enter the bloodstream and migrate to the tissues, where they develop into cysticerci in the intermediate host over a few weeks. A cysticercus can survive for several years in the animal host [5].

The transmission cycle of taeniasis/cysticercosis complex in humans and pigs is shown in Figure 37.1.

Pathogenesis

The pathogenic mechanisms of cysticercosis vary according to the location of the parasites, their volume and the inflammatory response of the patient, which in turn relates to the evolutionary stage of the parasites. Adult tapeworms reach length of several metres in the human intestine and these worms shed eggs and/or gravid proglottids intermittently into the faeces. Human cysticercosis occurs due to the ingestion of eggs from a tapeworm carrier. The eggs hatch in the upper intestine, releasing oncospheres (invasive larvae) that penetrate the intestinal mucosa using their hooklets and excretory proteases, which later can enter the bloodstream and migrate to the tissues, where they mature into cysticerci. The cysticerci may lodge in skeletal and cardiac muscles, subcutaneous tissue and even in lung tissue. In most of these locations, they cause few

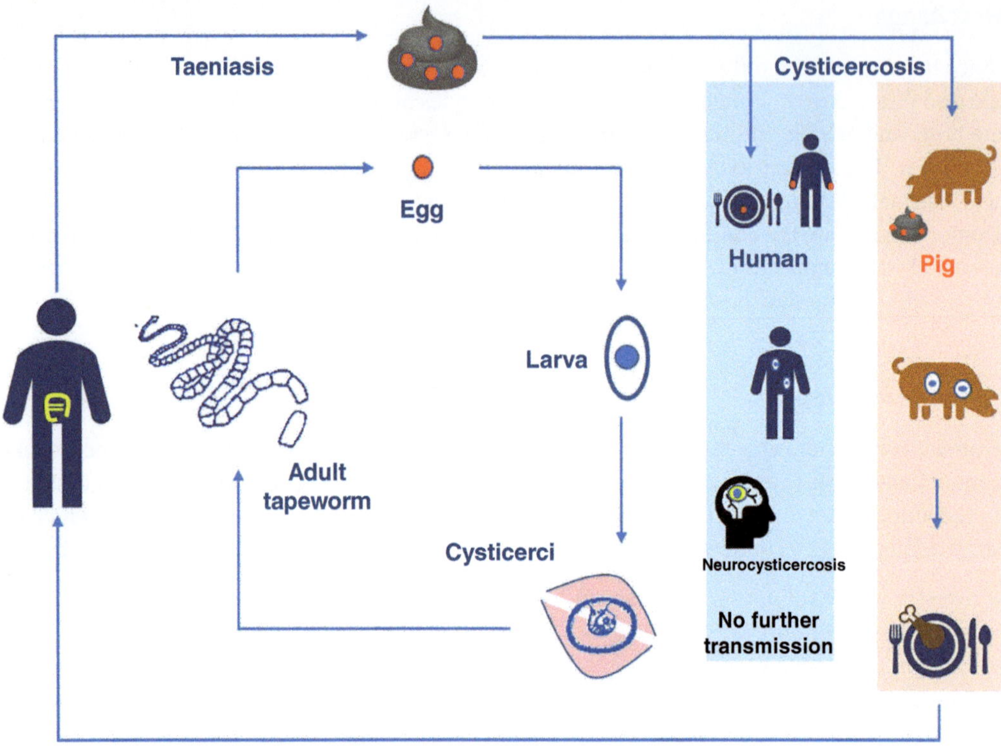

Figure 37.1 Transmission cycle of taeniasis/cysticercosis complex in humans and pigs.

symptoms and spontaneously degenerate, which may lead to the formation of calcified granulomas. However, in some cases, cysticerci can be found in the brain, meninges or spinal cord, which can result in serious health effects [7]. The inflammatory reactions have an evident role in triggering seizures and other symptoms in neurocysticercosis [8].

Disease in Animals

Cysticercosis in bovines and pigs is usually not associated with apparent clinical signs. However, heavy infections in cattle may cause myocarditis and heart failure associated with developing cysts in the heart. Pigs with neurocysticercosis can develop clinical signs such as excessive salivation, blinking and tearing, and may also suffer from tonic muscle contractions and seizures [9]. Bovine and porcine cysticercosis is associated with economic losses due to the requirement for special handling (i.e. condemnation, freezing, export restrictions) of the infected carcasses.

Disease in Humans

The intestinal infection in humans with the adult stage of the cestode is referred to as 'taeniasis' and the 'cysticercosis' is caused by the larval stage or metacestode (cysticerci) of *T. solium* in humans. Brief descriptions of these forms are provided below.

Taeniasis

Despite being a long tapeworm measuring several metres, intestinal taeniasis is usually asymptomatic. Some infected individuals may exhibit clinical signs of abdominal pain, intermittent diarrhoea or constipation, loss of appetite and weight, and generalised allergic manifestations, including urticaria, anal pruritus and eosinophilia. Patients with *T. saginata* taeniasis often experience more symptoms than those with *T. solium* because the *T. saginata* tapeworm is larger (up to 10 m) than *T. solium* (usually 3 m) [5].

Cysticercosis

The incubation period is variable and infected people may remain asymptomatic for many years. The clinical manifestation depends on the affected organs and the number of cysts in the body. The important clinical manifestations as per the location of cysts are described below.

- **Cysts in the muscles**: In general, the cyst in muscles does not cause any apparent clinical manifestation beyond detectable masses and local mass effect due to its size. However, these lumps may occasionally become tender and painful.
- **Cysts in the eyes**: Although rare, cysts may float in the eye and cause blurry or disturbed vision. Cysts in the orbital space, particularly those compromising oculomotor muscles, may cause deviations in gaze. Cysts in the anterior chamber or those floating freely in the vitreous may block visual fields, and subretinal or retinal cysticerci can affect visual acuity.
- **Neurocysticercosis (cysts in the brain and/or spinal cord)**: Neurocysticercosis is associated with an array of clinical manifestations varying from asymptomatic infections to aggressive, lethal effects which are mainly dependent on where and how many cysts are located in the brain. Symptoms may include severe headache, blindness, convulsions, epileptic seizures, difficulty with balance, cerebral hypertension and excess fluid deposition around the brain (hydrocephalus) [5]. Neurocysticercosis is a frequent cause of epilepsy worldwide and is estimated to cause 30% of all epilepsy cases in endemic regions where people and pigs co-exist [10].

Diagnosis

Commonly used diagnostic techniques for taeniasis and cysticercosis are as follows.

Taeniasis

Taenia human infections can be diagnosed through the morphology of eggs and gravid proglottids, and by using immunological or molecular techniques as explained below.

- **Microscopic examination**: Intestinal infections in humans can be diagnosed by the detection of eggs or gravid segments in faeces. Tapeworm eggs can be detected in the stools after 2–3 months of infection. The gravid segments of *T. saginata* are more active than those of *T. solium*, and they have more lateral branches of the uterus. However, morphological examination of gravid proglottids based on internal structures (i.e. the number of uterine branches) relies heavily on them being intact; therefore, it does not always allow accurate species identification.
- **Immunoserological tests**: These include immunodiagnostic assays such as enzyme-linked immunosorbent assay (ELISA) for coproantigen detection (i.e. adult parasite antigens in human stool). However, this does not support the differentiation of *T. saginata* from *T. solium*. Other

immunodiagnostic approaches include the detection of antibodies against purified antigens in the blood serum of infected individuals.
- **Molecular tools**: The use of molecular methods such as PCR allows differentiation between *Taenia* species by detecting the presence of species-specific DNA in human stool samples. Many of the PCR-based assays display adequate sensitivity and specificity.

Cysticercosis

For animal cysticercosis, the diagnosis is mainly based on postmortem surveys in pigs and cattle, using tongue or meat inspection, which remains the gold standard test. However, seroprevalence studies using serological tests such as ELISA can be carried out to determine the status of specific antibodies. For cysticercosis in humans, various diagnostic and imaging techniques can be used as described below.

- **Immunodiagnostic tests**: These diagnostics include antibody and antigen detection methods in blood, serum or cerebrospinal fluid (CSF). The most reliable assay for the detection of antibodies specific for *T. solium* in serum is enzyme-linked immune-electrotransfer blot (EITB) assay, which uses an enriched fraction of glycoproteins from *T. solium* of porcine origin [11].
- **Tissue biopsy**: In certain cases, tissue biopsy is used in diagnosis of the infection, but this invasive procedure lacks specificity.
- **Modern medical imaging techniques (magnetic resonance imaging** [MRI]**, computed axial tomography** [CT] **scans, and X-rays)**: MRI or CT scans may detect cysticerci in soft tissues such as the brain, while X-rays generally detect calcified cysticerci in the body.

Treatment

In animals, there is no specific treatment available. However, oxfendazole has been reported to be effective against porcine cysticercosis. The veterinarian can provide a long course of suitable anthelmintics to address clinical signs or offer corticosteroids as a supportive therapy.

In humans, the treatment of taeniasis includes a single oral dose of praziquantel (5–10 mg/kg) or niclosamide followed by a laxative after 2 hours [10]. Cases of cysticercosis are generally treated with antiparasitic drugs in combination with anti-inflammatory drugs, since the destruction of cysts may lead to an inflammatory response. Praziquantel plus prednisolone (prednisone), albendazole or niclosamide can be curative. Treatment of active disease may include surgery to treat cysts in certain locations, when patients are not responsive to drug treatment, or to reduce brain swelling [10].

Prevention and Control

A multisectorial approach, including public health, animal health and environmental aspects, is crucial for the prevention and control of taeniasis/cysticercosis. The high fecundity and extended longevity of adult parasites exacerbate the challenge of breaking the cycle of transmission. In addition, the resistance of the eggs to environmental conditions poses a challenge in controlling the parasite. The spread of taeniasis/cysticercosis is facilitated by poor hygiene and sanitation practices, lack of knowledge and awareness, and the consumption of raw or undercooked beef. Prevention and control approaches include measures targeting the final host and intermediate host [12].

Control measures targeting humans as the final host include the following.

- Community health education and awareness, including hygiene and food safety.
- Improved sanitary practices, such as restricting open defaecation and safe disposal of human faeces.
- Proper hygiene habits such as washing hands with soap after using the toilet, changing babies' nappies and before handling food.
- Wash and peel all raw vegetables and fruits before eating and use good food and water safety practices when travelling in endemic regions.
- Chemoprophylaxis by mass drug administration or treatment of individual cases is important to break the chain in endemic regions.
- Effective meat inspection at abattoirs, with special attention paid to the muscles and organs (heart, masseters, diaphragm, liver, tongue) having high chances of cyst infestations, is crucial to control the transmission of *Taenia* spp.
- Proper cooking of meat to a core temperature of at least 60 °C or freezing at −10 °C or less for at least 10 days can destroy the parasite.

Control measures targeting the intermediate host include the following.

- Pigs can be vaccinated with TSOL18 vaccine along with anthelmintic treatment using oxfendazole [10]. Vaccination prevents pigs from being infected, whereas oxfendazole cures pigs that are already infected at the time of vaccination. For cattle, none of the vaccine candidates have reached the commercial stage.
- Establishment of biosecurity measures in pig husbandry to avoid the free-roaming of pigs and feeding on human faeces.
- Preventing the use of untreated sewage effluent to irrigate or fertilise land to be used by pigs for forage.

References

1 Symeonidou, I., Arsenopoulos, K., Tzilves, D. et al. (2018). Human taeniasis/cysticercosis: a potentially emerging parasitic disease in Europe. *Annals of Gastroenterology* 31 (4): 406.

2 Ito, A., Li, T., Wandra, T. et al. (2019). Taeniasis and cysticercosis in Asia: a review with emphasis on molecular approaches and local lifestyles. *Acta Tropica* 198: 105075.

3 Ale, A., Victor, B., Praet, N. et al. (2014). Epidemiology and genetic diversity of *Taenia asiatica*: a systematic review. *Parasites & Vectors* 7 (1): 45.

4 Saratsis, A., Sotiraki, S., Braae, U.C. et al. (2019). Epidemiology of *Taenia saginata* taeniosis/cysticercosis: a systematic review of the distribution in the Middle East and North Africa. *Parasites & Vectors* 12 (1): 113.

5 Centers for Disease Control and Prevention. (2020). Cysticercosis. www.cdc.gov/parasites/cysticercosis (accessed 24 January 2022).

6 Bobes, R.J., Fragoso, G., Fleury, A. et al. (2014). Evolution, molecular epidemiology and perspectives on the research of taeniid parasites with special emphasis on *Taenia solium*. *Infection, Genetics and Evolution* 23: 150–160.

7 Guerrant, R.L., Walker, D.H., and Weller, P.F. (2011). *Tropical Infectious Diseases: Principles, Pathogens and Practice*. Philadelphia: Elsevier Health Sciences.

8 Gonzales, I., Rivera, J.T., Garcia, H.H., and Cysticercosis Working Group in Peru (2016). Pathogenesis of *Taenia solium* taeniasis and cysticercosis. *Parasite Immunology* 38: 136–146.

9 Trevisan, C., Mkupasi, E.M., Ngowi, H.A. et al. (2016). Severe seizures in pigs naturally infected with *Taenia solium* in Tanzania. *Veterinary Parasitology* 220: 67–71.

10 World Health Organization. (2022). Taeniasis/cysticercosis fact sheet. www.who.int/news-room/fact-sheets/detail/taeniasis-cysticercosis (accessed 24 January 2022).

11 Deckers, N. and Dorny, P. (2010). Immunodiagnosis of *Taenia solium* taeniosis/cysticercosis. *Trends in Parasitology* 26 (3): 137–144.

12 De Coster, T., Van Damme, I., Baauw, J., and Gabriël, S. (2018). Recent advancements in the control of *Taenia solium*: a systematic review. *Food and Waterborne Parasitology* 13: e00030.

38

Toxoplasmosis

Toxoplasma gondii is an obligate intracellular protozoan parasite (phylum Apicomplexa, subclass Coccidia), which infects almost all mammals and birds. The parasite was first described in the common gundi (*Ctenodactylus gundi*), a rodent from North Africa, by Nicolle and Manceaux in 1908. However, it took several decades until its entire life cycle was conclusively understood in the late 1960s [1], with the demonstration of cats as definitive hosts responsible for oocysts shedding through faeces and thereby infecting intermediate hosts. Due to its ubiquitous distribution and high prevalence, *T. gondii* remains one of the most important zoonotic agents of high medical and veterinary importance [2].

Life Cycle

Toxoplasma gondii is a tissue-cyst forming coccidium cycling in a prey–predator system that alternates between definitive (sexual reproduction) and intermediate (asexual replication) hosts [3]. It is unique among this group because it can be transmitted not only between intermediate and definitive hosts (sexual cycle) but also between intermediate hosts via carnivorism (asexual cycle) or even between definitive hosts. In general, there are three infective stages of *T. gondii*.

- The sporozoite of an oocyst: an environmental stage.
- Tachyzoite: a rapidly dividing invasive stage of the parasite.
- Bradyzoite: a slowly dividing stage in tissue cysts.

It is important to understand the stages of the life cycle of *T. gondii* to identify the transmission and clinical relevance of the parasite. The important stages in the life cycle of *T. gondii* are as follows [2, 3].

1) **Oocysts**: Oocysts are the product of the parasite's sexual cycle in the intestine of its definitive host, i.e. Felidae (cat family). Unsporulated oocysts are excreted in cat faeces and following sporulation in the environment, the sporozoites become infective.
   Environmental resistance of oocysts: The oocysts can remain viable for long periods in water and can resist freezing and moderately high water temperatures. The survival of sporulated oocysts in the environment is favoured by humidity, and under optimal conditions, the sporulated oocysts may remain infective for more than 1 year [2].
2) **Tachyzoites**: On oral uptake of sporulated oocysts by new hosts, the sporozoites transform to the invasive tachyzoite stage. Tachyzoites actively penetrate all nucleated cells and replicate rapidly in an intracytoplasmic vacuole. Due to repeated intravacuolar replication, host cells

Textbook of Zoonoses, First Edition. Jasbir Singh Bedi, Deepthi Vijay, and Pankaj Dhaka.

disrupt and tachyzoites invade neighbouring cells which causes tissue destruction and is responsible for the clinical manifestations of the disease.
Relevance of tachyzoites in human transmission: Tachyzoites are the delicate stage of the parasite, and are destroyed by gastric secretions and are unable to survive outside their host. Therefore, contamination by this route is rare except in the case of congenital infection due to transplacental transmission from an infected mother to the foetus. Tachyzoites can also be rarely transmitted by blood/bone marrow transfusions or via laboratory accidents.
3) **Bradyzoites**: After the onset of efficient immune response by the host, the tachyzoites are not eradicated but convert into bradyzoites within cells. Bradyzoites are slowly replicating intracellular stages that form persisting cysts. These tissue cysts, which can be found in the retina, brain, skeletal and heart muscles, are infective for other intermediate and definitive hosts via consumption of muscle or brain tissue.

Transmission Route

The only known definitive hosts for *T. gondii* are domestic cats and other members of the family Felidae. The global seroprevalence for *T. gondii* in domestic cats is around 30–40% and the seropositivity rates in wild felids are also high [4]. Infected animals usually shed the oocysts for 1–2 weeks but in large numbers. Remarkably, a single cat can pass more than 100 million non-sporulated oocysts [2]. The oocysts take 1–5 days to sporulate in the environment and become infective. Intermediate hosts (including birds and rodents) become infected after ingesting soil, water or plant material contaminated with oocysts. The oocysts develop into cysts in muscular and neural tissue. Cats can become infected after eating intermediate hosts harbouring tissue cysts or by ingestion of sporulated oocysts. Food animals and wild game may also be infected with tissue cysts after ingestion of sporulated oocysts from a contaminated environment. Since humans are dead-end hosts in the life cycle of the parasite, the natural cycle comprising domestic animals and wildlife is crucial for the survival of *T. gondii* and to cause human infection [2].
Humans can be infected by any of several routes as described below and illustrated in Figure 38.1.

- Consumption of undercooked meat harbouring tissue cysts is considered the predominant route for human infection [5]. In addition, the consumption of raw milk has been associated with toxoplasmosis in humans [2].
- Consuming food or water contaminated with cat faeces can cause infection in humans. Only cooking (≥60 °C), but not freezing or disinfection, reliably destroys the sporulated oocysts from contaminated vegetables and other foods. In water, the oocysts can remain infective for a long time and are not reliably destroyed by freezing and moderate temperature, chemical and physical treatments, including chlorination and ozone treatment of the water [6].
- Contaminated environmental samples, such as soil or a litter box, can transmit the oocysts to humans.
- Transplacental transmission from mother to foetus, and rarely the transmission of oocysts/cysts through blood transfusion or organ transplantation, have been reported to be associated with *T. gondii* infection.

Disease in Animals

Toxoplasma gondii infection is generally inapparent, or with mild symptoms, in most animal species. However, some species show high susceptibility which leads to clinical manifestation and associated mortality. Marsupials and New World monkeys, which have evolved separately from cats, are

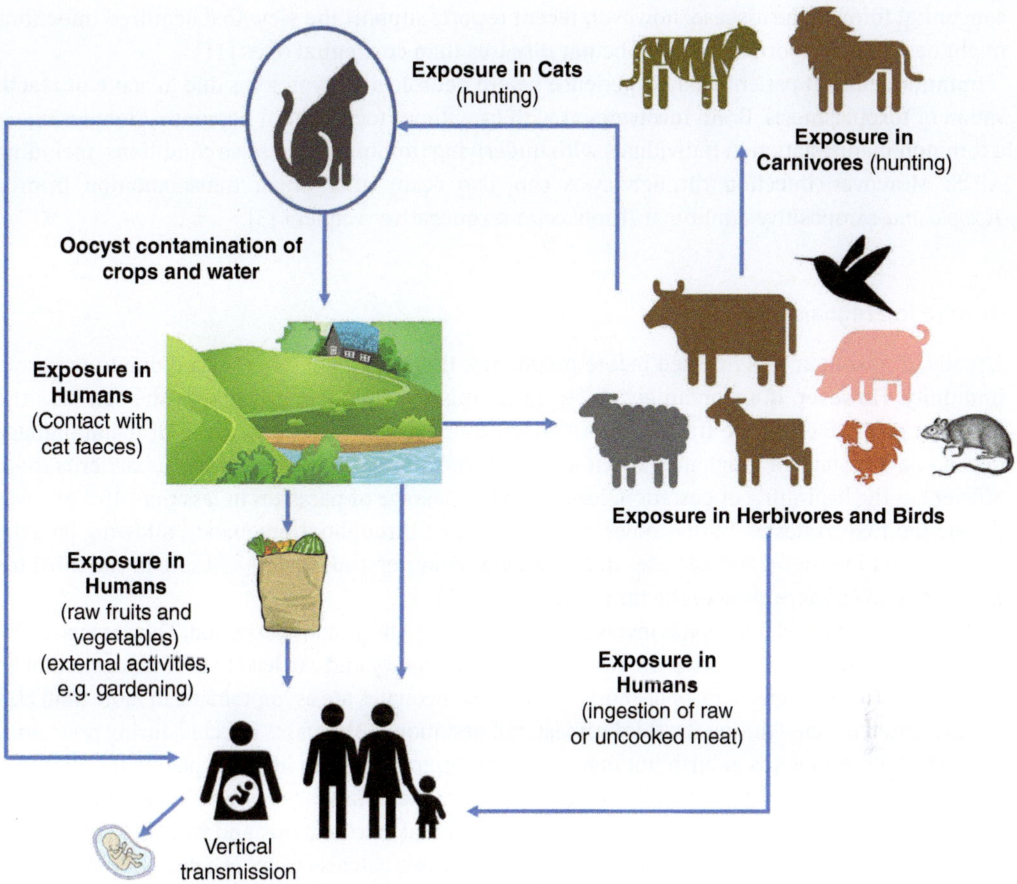

Figure 38.1 Transmission pathways of *Toxoplasma gondii* in humans.

among the most vulnerable species [7]. *T. gondii* infection can be present at a high level in many wild birds without any clinical impact, but the outcome can be clinically severe in pigeons and canaries. The ingestion of infected birds is considered an important source of infection for cats [8].

In small ruminants, mainly sheep, clinical toxoplasmosis causes abortion and neonatal mortality. Abortion is usually associated with primary infection during pregnancy in non-immune animals and is most commonly observed in young animals. Following the primary exposure, a long-lasting immunity develops and animals are unlikely to abort again due to *T. gondii* infection [9].

Disease in Humans

In epidemiological studies, the seroprevalence of toxoplasmosis varies greatly (10–80%) between different regions of the globe [10]. Immunocompetent individuals often do not develop any symptoms of infection with *T. gondii*. When illness occurs, it is usually mild with 'flu-like' symptoms that last for weeks to months. Some patients may develop lymphadenopathy, especially of cervical and occipital lymph nodes. However, the parasite can stay in the body in an inactive state and can be reactivated if the person becomes immunosuppressed. Severe disease outcomes, including myocarditis, pneumonia, encephalitis and hepatitis, are very rare among immunocompetent patients [2, 3]. Ocular toxoplasmosis was considered to be the result of recurrence of the congenital form of the disease; however, recent reports support the view that acquired infections might be a more important cause of ocular diseases than congenital ones [11].

Immunodeficient patients may experience severe neurological symptoms due to acute or reactivation of toxoplasmosis. Brain involvement with or without focal central nervous system lesions is a common manifestation in individuals with underlying immunosuppressive conditions, including AIDS. Moreover, infection through cysts can also occur after organ transplantation from a *Toxoplasma*-seropositive donor to a *Toxoplasma*-seronegative recipient [3].

Disease in Pregnant Women

Usually, if a woman gets infected before pregnancy, the foetus will be protected due to maternal immunity. However, if a woman gets infected during or just before pregnancy, she can pass the infection to the foetus. The frequency of vertical transmission and the severity of foetal damage depend on the stage of pregnancy when maternal infection occurs. The placental barrier is more efficient at the beginning of gestation, leading to the passage of parasites in less than 10% of cases during the first trimester, but becomes more permeable throughout pregnancy, allowing parasite transmission in around 30% of cases in the second trimester and 60–70% of cases in the third trimester and even more close to the time of delivery [12].

The severity of foetal infection is inversely correlated with the gestational period. The damage to the foetus is often more severe during the early period of pregnancy and can lead to miscarriage, stillbirth or a child born with signs of toxoplasmosis. In contrast, neonates are asymptomatic in more than 80% of cases when infected during the third trimester of gestation [13]. Infants infected during pregnancy often show no symptoms at birth but may develop symptoms later in life with potential vision loss, mental disability and seizures. Involvement of the central nervous system is a hallmark of congenital toxoplasmosis. The presence of chorioretinitis, intracranial calcifications and hydrocephalus is the classic triad of congenital toxoplasmosis [14]. Toxoplasmosis can also cause eye disease and is one of the most frequent causes of uveitis [3]. Eye lesions from congenital infection are often not identified at birth but occur in 20–80% of infected persons by adulthood. The eye disease can reactivate months or years later, each time causing more damage to the retina and even leading to blindness [2].

Diagnosis

The diagnosis of *T. gondii* infection in animals and humans can be established by conventional microscopic methods, bioassays for isolation of the organism, serological tests and nucleic acid detection assays. Some of the important diagnostic methods are described below [12].

- **Microscopic diagnosis**: The detection of *T. gondii* in faecal, water, environmental and tissue samples has traditionally relied on microscopic examination. However, identification using light microscopy is less sensitive and specific. The oocysts in faecal, water and environmental samples can be enriched by filtration or centrifugation for proper detection, and tissue cysts can be stained to distinguish the parasites from host cells.
- **Bioassay**: Isolation using laboratory animals is generally considered as the standard method for detection of *T. gondii* infection. Mice and cats are the commonly used laboratory animals to conduct the bioassay of *T. gondii*. Excretions, body fluids, lymph nodes, muscle and brain tissues of suspected cases can be used for isolation of the parasite.

- **Serological tests**: *T. gondii* infection usually exhibits no or non-specific clinical symptoms in most animals and humans, so the diagnosis mainly relies on serological testing for the antibodies against the parasite. A variety of serological tests, such as dye test (DT), modified agglutination test (MAT), enzyme-linked immunosorbent assays (ELISA), immunosorbent agglutination assay (ISAGA), indirect fluorescent antibody test (IFAT) and indirect haemagglutination assays (IHA), have been developed to detect different antibody classes against the *T. gondii* infection.
  Sabin–Feldman dye test: The dye test was developed by Sabin and Feldman in 1948, and is considered as the gold standard for the detection of anti-*T. gondii* antibodies in humans. The test is both specific and sensitive in humans, but may be unreliable in cattle and avian species. The Sabin–Feldman dye test is based on the observation that when living organisms (e.g. from the peritoneal exudate of mice) are incubated with normal serum, they become swollen and stain deep blue if methylene blue is added to the suspension. However, when the parasites are exposed to antibody-containing serum, due to the lysis of the organisms they appear thin and distorted without retaining the dye stain. The titer reported is that dilution of serum at which half of the organisms are not killed (stained) and the other half are killed (unstained).
- **Molecular tools**: Conventional and real-time PCR can detect target nucleic acids even at low concentrations. For epidemiological studies, it is important to identify genotypes of *T. gondii* infection, and novel molecular technologies, like microsatellite analysis, multi-locus sequence typing, restriction fragment length polymorphism (RFLP), etc., are commonly used for genotyping purposes.

Treatment

In Animals

At present, a single vaccine (S48 strain live vaccine, Toxovax™) is licensed for use in sheep to protect against abortion due to *T. gondii* infection. However, it is a live vaccine which may raise safety concerns and the short shelf-life can cause issues in production and distribution [2].

Toxoplasma gondii rarely causes clinical symptoms in cats and there is currently no vaccine available for felines. Therefore, early diagnosis and treatment is the effective strategy. Clindamycin is considered the drug of choice for treating clinical toxoplasmosis in dogs and cats. However, the available drugs usually suppress the replication of *T. gondii* but are not completely effective in killing the parasite.

In Humans

There is no available vaccine for toxoplasmosis in humans. Most healthy people do not exhibit any symptoms and recover without treatment. Clinical cases can be treated with a combination of drugs such as pyrimethamine and sulfadiazine. Special care should be taken with infection during pregnancy, where the mother and foetus should be closely monitored during the pregnancy and after delivery of the baby. Often, the parasites can remain within tissue cells as bradyzoites, and their location makes it difficult for the medication to eliminate them. Therefore, persons with compromised immune systems, such as AIDS patients, might need medication for the rest of their lives or for as long as they are immunosuppressed [2, 3].

Prevention and Control

Intervention strategies against toxoplasmosis should be focused on the susceptibility of the population for the infection, public health education and high biosecurity measures at animal farms and agricultural production sites [2–4]. Some of the important risk factors along with appropriate prevention strategies for toxoplasmosis are described below.

Risk factors	Preventive measures
Contact with cat(s)	• Wash hands carefully after stroking a cat • Change litter frequently (since it takes 1–5 days for oocysts to become infective) and wash the tray with hot water (>60 °C) • Wear gloves when changing cat litter • Wash hands with soap and water after cleaning out a cat's litter box and discard the litter properly • Avoid litter contamination in the kitchen and home environment
Food	• Cook food well. Tissue cysts are killed immediately at 67 °C • During freezing, the killing of tissue cysts takes at least 3 days at less than −12 °C, depending on the thickness of the piece of meat. The cysts can survive in refrigerated meat for up to 3 weeks • Avoid microwave cooking for meat, as the internal temperature might not be high enough to kill the parasite • Avoid raw vegetables and salads at restaurants, and wash vegetables, fruits and herbs thoroughly • Avoid raw shellfish • Avoid raw goat milk • Wash hands, knives, any containers and table thoroughly after meat manipulation or cutting
Water	• Oocysts can survive for long periods in water and resist freezing, chlorination and ozone treatment. Therefore, use boiled water or safe water for drinking in endemic regions • Avoid ingestion of water during recreational activities in lakes or rivers
Gardening or outdoor activities	• Wear gloves and use other personal protective equipment for gardening • Wash hands thoroughly after any outdoor activities having contact with soil
Farm-level measures in animals	• It is necessary to implement efficient measures at farm level to exclude the transmission of *T. gondii* through water, fodder or other routes into livestock animals • Poor rodent control can be an important risk factor for toxoplasmosis in farm animals. Rodents are potential intermediate hosts for the parasite and their presence could either increase the risk of farm cats shedding *T. gondii* oocysts or these rodents could serve as a direct source of infection for farm animals

References

1 Frenkel, J.K. (1970). Pursuing toxoplasma. *Journal of Infectious Diseases* 122 (6): 553–559.

2 Robert-Gangneux, F. and Dardé, M.L. (2012). Epidemiology of and diagnostic strategies for toxoplasmosis. *Clinical Microbiology Reviews* 25 (2): 264–296.

3 Schlüter, D., Däubener, W., Schares, G. et al. (2014). Animals are key to human toxoplasmosis. *International Journal of Medical Microbiology* 304 (7): 917–929.

4 Elmore, S.A., Jones, J.L., Conrad, P.A. et al. (2010). *Toxoplasma gondii*: epidemiology, feline clinical aspects, and prevention. *Trends in Parasitology* 26 (4): 190–196.

5 Cook, A.J.C., Holliman, R., Gilbert, R.E. et al. (2000). Sources of toxoplasma infection in pregnant women: European multicentre case-control study commentary: congenital toxoplasmosis – further thought for food. *BMJ* 321 (7254): 142–147.

6 Dumètre, A., Le Bras, C., Baffet, M. et al. (2008). Effects of ozone and ultraviolet radiation treatments on the infectivity of *Toxoplasma gondii* oocysts. *Veterinary Parasitology* 153 (3–4): 209–213.

7 Tenter, A.M., Heckeroth, A.R., and Weiss, L.M. (2000). *Toxoplasma gondii*: from animals to humans. *International Journal for Parasitology* 30 (12–13): 1217–1258.

8 Al-Kappany, Y.M., Rajendran, C., Ferreira, L.R. et al. (2010). High prevalence of toxoplasmosis in cats from Egypt: isolation of viable *Toxoplasma gondii*, tissue distribution, and isolate designation. *Journal of Parasitology* 96 (6): 1115–1118.

9 Smith, M.C. and Sherman, D.M. (2009). *Goat Medicine*. Hoboken: Wiley.

10 Dubey, J.P. and Jones, J.L. (2008). *Toxoplasma gondii* infection in humans and animals in the United States. *International Journal for Parasitology* 38 (11): 1257–1278.

11 Park, Y.H. and Nam, H.W. (2013). Clinical features and treatment of ocular toxoplasmosis. *Korean Journal of Parasitology* 51 (4): 393.

12 Dunn, D., Wallon, M., Peyron, F. et al. (1999). Mother-to-child transmission of toxoplasmosis: risk estimates for clinical counselling. *Lancet* 353 (9167): 1829–1833.

13 Montoya, J.G. (2002). Laboratory diagnosis of *Toxoplasma gondii* infection and toxoplasmosis. *Journal of Infectious Diseases* 185 (Supplement_1): S73–S82.

14 Jones, J.L., Lopez, A., and Wilson, M. (2003). Congenital toxoplasmosis. *American Family Physician* 67 (10): 2131–2138.

39

Trichinellosis

Trichinellosis (also called trichinosis) is a zoonotic disease that is responsible for huge economic losses in the piggery sector. The disease is caused by nematodes of *Trichinella* spp. which are considered as one of the most widespread parasites infecting humans and animals. In 1835, James Paget, a medical student in London, first detected the larvae of the parasite as coiled worms in the muscle tissue of a human cadaver; however, the association of pork consumption and trichinellosis was established later in 1860 [1].

Aetiology

A total of eight species of *Trichinella* have been documented as responsible for infection in wild and domestic animals in various regions of the world (*Trichinella spiralis*, *T. britovi*, *T. nativa*, *T. pseudospiralis*, *T. murelli*, *T. nelsoni*, *T. papuae* and *T. zimbabwensis*) [2]. The important *Trichinella* species causing public health-related issues are listed below.

- *Trichinella spiralis*: This species has a wide global distribution and is considered the most important aetiological agent causing disease in humans. The species is adapted to domestic and wild swine but can also include synanthropic rats in its life cycle. In the domestic cycle, pork scraps from *T. spiralis*-infected pigs are the main source of infection for synanthropic animals (e.g. rats, horses, stray cats and dogs).
- *Trichinella britovi*: This is the most widely distributed species within sylvatic life cycles of Europe, Asia and northern and western Africa. It can also affect domestic pig populations, mainly through extensive grazing systems or feed with scraps or carrion originating from sylvatic carnivores. The parasite can also affect human health, thereby exhibiting zoonotic potential.
- *Trichinella nativa*: This mainly affects sylvatic carnivores living in cold climate zones of Asia, northern states of North America and north-eastern Europe.

Epidemiology and Disease Transmission

Trichinella infection in humans is mainly associated with consumption of raw or undercooked meat. Overall, domestic pork remains the predominant source of *Trichinella* infection in humans, especially when pigs are raised under free-ranging or backyard production conditions without appropriate biosecurity measures. *Trichinella* is a highly prolific parasite and an infected animal

Textbook of Zoonoses, First Edition. Jasbir Singh Bedi, Deepthi Vijay, and Pankaj Dhaka.

might have up to several hundred larvae per gram of muscle. The larvae of the parasite can survive in decaying carcasses for a long time, thus facilitating transmission by scavenging.

Life Cycle of *Trichinella* spp.

The parasite is a tissue-dwelling nematode that can be acquired by the ingestion of raw or inadequately cooked meat products containing encapsulated larvae. The larvae are released after gastric digestion and mature into adult worms that can penetrate the mucosa of the host's intestine. After fertilisation, the female sheds new larvae which disseminate throughout the host to find their definitive location, i.e. the striated muscle, where they encyst. The larval migration may result in severe lesions, particularly when they migrate into the heart or brain. After invasion of striated skeletal muscle cells, the larvae induce changes that culminate in a new cell phenotype, termed a 'nurse cell', which in the case of the encapsulated *Trichinella* spp. is surrounded by a collagenous capsule. After 21 days, the larvae are fully infective and resistant to gastric juice. In muscle nurse cells, parasite larvae can survive for years (up to 40 years in humans and over 20 years in polar bears) [3, 4]. In humans, calcification of the cyst may begin within 6 months to a year, a process that eventually is followed by death of the encysted larvae [2].

Transmission Cycle

Most *Trichinella* species, except for *T. spiralis*, parasitise predominantly wild animals. Spillover from wild animals to domestic animals can occur when there is improper biosecurity management to prevent contact between domestic animals and wildlife. One of the important biological factors promoting transmission is the physiological ability of the larvae to survive in decaying carcasses/carrion for a long period. Encapsulated larvae of *T. spiralis* are infective for laboratory animals for up to 4 months in extremely rotten meat [5].

The two important transmission cycles, the domestic cycle and the sylvatic cycle, are described below. These cycles can function either independently from each other or interactively.

- **Domestic cycle**: In this cycle, domestic swine can be infected by feeding on uncooked pork scraps, carrion, garbage or infected carcasses that are not promptly removed from the farm. Transmission can also occur through synanthropic animals (e.g. rats) living near domestic swine.
- **Sylvatic cycle**: In this cycle, the pathogen circulates between wildlife hosts. The sylvatic cycle includes all *Trichinella* species, including *T. spiralis* for mammals, *T. pseudospiralis* for mammals and birds, and *T. papuae* and *T. zimbabwensis* for mammals and reptiles. Per-oral infection usually occurs through ingestion of muscle tissue from an infectious prey animal. Despite the potential broad host spectrum for *Trichinella* spp., the predominant biotic potential concerns carnivores and porcine omnivores (mainly domestic pigs, wild pigs, wild boars, bush pigs and warthogs).

Disease in Animals and Humans

In Animals

Serious clinical signs are rarely observed in swine naturally infected with *T. spiralis*. However, experimentally infected swine show signs of intense muscle pain and a decrease in weight gain, but recovery can be observed after some time.

In Humans

Most human infections with *Trichinella* have been attributed to *T. spiralis*. The degree of illness is usually related to the number of larvae ingested per gram of muscle. Serious outcome is rare in trichinellosis, which normally occurs only in massive infections and is associated with myocarditis, encephalitis and pneumonitis. The incubation period ranges from 1–2 days for the enteral phase to 2–8 weeks for the parenteral phase; however, the incubation period depends on the infectious dose and possibly the species of parasite [6]. The clinical signs seen during different phases of the infection are described below [2].

- **Intestinal or enteral phase**: This occurs within the first week after ingestion of L1 larvae in inadequately cooked meat. Mucosal irritation is common as the adult worms grow in the small intestine. Other symptoms include nausea, abdominal cramps, loss of appetite, vomiting, low-grade fever and either mild diarrhoea or constipation. Frontal headache, dizziness and weakness can also occur, especially in low-to-moderate infections. Severe diarrhoea persisting for weeks can be observed in cases with a heavy parasitic load.
- **Muscle invasion or parenteral phase**: This phase can start as early as 9–10 days after exposure and is associated with penetration of the newborn larvae into muscle cells. Symptoms include myositis, which is initiated with the immunological response and results in enlarged and oedematous muscle fibres. Myositis mainly occurs in the extraocular muscles, masseters, intercostals, muscles of the larynx, tongue, diaphragm and neck, and muscular attachments to tendons and joints. These symptoms reach a peak at about 5–6 weeks after infection and diminish when the larvae become encapsulated.
  - Early symptoms include swelling of the eyelids and facial oedema. Muscle swelling and pain on movement can develop. In some cases, respiratory symptoms, including dyspnoea resulting from involvement of respiratory muscles, and myocarditis due to larval invasion of the heart can be observed. Neurological symptoms are the result of larval migration through the central nervous system (CNS), which can lead to intracerebral haemorrhage and meningitis. Patients can exhibit dizziness, ataxia, hysteria, psychotic disturbances, seizures and eventually coma in severe CNS infections.
- **Convalescent phase**: After the second month of infection, the myalgia and itching recede. However, the larvae can remain alive in the cysts for one or more years, depending on the species, even after the cyst wall becomes calcified. The larvae can release antigens that may lead to a persistent low-to-moderate eosinophilia and stimulate specific circulating antibodies.

Diagnosis

In Animals

The diagnosis of infection in an animal is crucial to prevent the entry of the parasite into the human food chain. Important diagnostic tools for detection of *Trichinella* infection in animals include the following.

- **Direct methods**: Postmortem meat inspection for the detection of *Trichinella* larvae in muscle samples of pigs and other animals intended for human consumption is important. On microscopic examination, the encysted parasites are easily observed, and if there are degenerative changes or necrotic muscle fibres, an inflammatory reaction with many eosinophils may be present around them. However, direct detection of the larvae is greatly influenced by sample size

and the muscle type selected for sampling. Some of the sampling sites recommended by the International Commission on Trichinellosis for different domestic and wild animals subjected to meat inspection or epidemiological studies are as follows [2].
  - *Domestic swine*: Diaphragm, tongue, masseter
  - *Horse*: Tongue and masseter
  - *Wild boar:* Forearm, diaphragm, tongue
  - *Fox:* Diaphragm, forearm muscles, tongue
- **Serology**: The serological diagnosis of *Trichinella* is suitable for the surveillance and epidemiological investigations of domestic animals and wildlife. Animals can be tested for the presence of anti-*Trichinella* antibodies in the serum or meat juice. Following ingestion of *T. spiralis* larvae, anti-*Trichinella* immunoglobulin G (IgG) can be detected in animals about 2–3 weeks post infection. Enzyme-linked immunosorbent assay (ELISA) is the most commonly used method for the detection of *Trichinella* infection and its high sensitivity allows the detection of as low as 1 larva per 100 g of muscle tissue [7].
- **Molecular techniques**: The use of molecular tools, including polymerase chain reaction, is a sensitive and rapid diagnostic approach that can identify even a low number of larvae infections. These tools are also important to characterise the isolates to the species or genotype level during epidemiological studies.

In Humans

The early clinical diagnosis of trichinellosis is difficult in humans because of the lack of any specific or pathognomonic signs. This is a point of concern for patients because delay in diagnosis and treatment favours the establishment of larvae in muscle tissue and the development of a collagen capsule, which may render the larvae resistant to drugs. The diagnosis of trichinellosis in humans should be based on three main criteria as provided below [2].

- **Clinical findings**: Recognition of the signs and symptoms of trichinellosis.
- **Laboratory findings**: The clinical picture can be correlated with laboratory parameters, such as eosinophilia and elevation in muscle enzymes, antibody detection and larval detection in a muscle biopsy. These procedures can be carried out by biochemical, molecular and serological means.
- **Epidemiological investigation**: This involves the identification of the source and detection of the outbreak origin.

Treatment

In Animals

Treatment is generally impractical in animals. The prevention of ingestion of viable *Trichinella* cysts is the best way to prevent the disease in both animals and people. Any suspected outbreak of trichinellosis in animals should be reported to the animal health authorities.

In Humans

During treatment, factors such as the species involved, worm burden, duration of symptoms and host immune response need to be considered. Prompt treatment with antiparasitic drugs such as mebendazole and albendazole can help to prevent the progression of trichinellosis by killing the adult worms, and thereby preventing the further release of larvae [6]. Symptomatic treatment includes analgesics, antipyretics and corticosteroids, especially in severe infections to prevent shock-like symptoms [6]. Once the larvae are established in skeletal muscle cells (usually by 3–4 weeks post-infection), treatment may not eliminate the infection and associated symptoms.

Prevention and Control

Trichinellosis is an ubiquitous zoonotic infection with high economic consideration, so the key efforts should be focused on the control or elimination of *Trichinella* from the food chain. The main control measures should target the domestic and sylvatic cycles of the parasite as well as risky human food consumption habits [2, 6].

Control of *Trichinella* Infection in Pigs

Pigs raised on extensive grazing with minimal confinement are at the highest risk for *Trichinella* infection. These so-called 'backyard pigs' are often fed food scraps or other forms of meat-containing waste, and have ready access to rodents and wildlife. Furthermore, pigs raised in such systems are generally not sold through organised marketing channels and therefore are not subjected to reliable methods of veterinary inspection.

Proper awareness of the modes of transmission of *Trichinella* to domestic pigs can be helpful to pig farmers and producers to allow the design of farm management systems that can prevent or reduce the risk of exposure to the parasite. Commercial and backyard pig production needs to have stringent barriers to exposure to wild animals, rodents and uncooked meat scraps. Some of the important measures include architectural and environmental barriers to reduce contact with wildlife and rodents, farm hygiene including proper disposal of dead animals, proper hygienic feeding of animals, and rearing of piglets with controlled housing conditions in endemic regions.

Control of *Trichinella* Infection in Wildlife

The importance of wildlife as a reservoir host for relevant species of *Trichinella* is underscored by the fact that the parasite's biomass is greater in wildlife than in domestic animals. To reduce the prevalence of infection among wildlife, hunters can be instructed to avoid leaving the leftovers of animal carcasses in the field after skinning or removing and discarding the entrails, as this increases the probability of transmission to new hosts. Due to inadequate biosecurity measures, *Trichinella* infection can be transmitted from the sylvatic environment into domestic animals. In addition, the parasite can be transferred in a reversible path from domestic animals to wildlife when the carrion of domestic animals is not properly disposed of or the carcasses of dead free-ranging pigs are not appropriately removed from the field.

Prevention of Trichinellosis in Humans

The consumption of contaminated meat and meat products remains the important route of trichinellosis in humans. Meat from animals that might contain *Trichinella* larvae but cannot be tested by an appropriate laboratory method should be treated by a procedure that has been proven to inactivate *Trichinella* before distribution for human consumption. It is also important to spread awareness and education among consumers about the risk of consumption of raw meat and meat products from both domestic (e.g. pigs, horses, dogs) and wild (e.g. wild boars, bears, foxes, jackals, armadillos, crocodiles, etc.) animals that can be carriers of the parasites if they are not properly tested for *Trichinella* larvae upon meat inspection. Common methods that have been shown to reliably inactivate *Trichinella* larvae in meat are as follows [2].

- Cooking of meat to reach a core temperature of not less than 71 °C (159.8 °F) for at least 1 minute.
- During freezing, meat processors should ensure that meat cuts up to 15 cm in thickness are kept in frozen state at the minimum temperature of −15 °C for not less than 3 weeks, and cuts of meat up to 50 cm in thickness should be frozen solid for not less than 4 weeks. It is important to note that the species *T. nativa* is considered somewhat resistant to freezing [8].
- Irradiation at appropriate levels (i.e. 0.3 kGy) has been proven to inactivate *Trichinella*, and is thus considered an acceptable method for rendering meat safe for human consumption in those countries where irradiation of food is permitted [8].

Other commonly used methods, including cooking by microwave ovens, curing, drying or smoking, are not considered safe for reliable inactivation of *Trichinella* larvae from meat and meat products. Particular attention should be given to the putative presence of freeze-resistant *Trichinella* species or genotypes in meats.

References

1 Campbell, W.C. (1983). Historical introduction. In: *Trichinella and Trichinosis* (ed. W.C. Campbell), 1–30. New York: Plenum Press.

2 Gottstein, B., Pozio, E., and Nöckler, K. (2009). Epidemiology, diagnosis, treatment, and control of trichinellosis. *Clinical Microbiology Reviews* 22 (1): 127–145.

3 Fröscher, W., Gullotta, F., Saathoff, M., and Tackmann, W. (1988). Chronic trichinosis. *European Neurology* 28 (4): 221–226.

4 Kumar, V., Pozio, E., De Borchgrave, J. et al. (1990). Characterization of a *Trichinella* isolate from polar bear. *Annales de la Societe Belge de Medecine Tropicale* 70 (2): 131–135.

5 Madsen, H. (1974). The principles of the epidemiology of trichinelliasis with a new view on the life cycle. In: *Proceedings of the 3rd International Conference on Trichinellosis, Florida, USA*, 615–638.

6 Centers for Disease Control and Prevention. (2020). Parasites – Trichinellosis (also known as Trichinosis). www.cdc.gov/parasites/trichinellosis/ (accessed 24 January 2022).

7 Office International des Epizooties (2004). Trichinellosis. In: *Manual of Standards for Diagnostic Tests and Vaccines*, 5e, 649–659. Paris, France: Office International des Epizooties.

8 Gamble, H.R., Bessonov, A.S., Cuperlovic, K. et al. (2000). International Commission on Trichinellosis: recommendations on methods for the control of *Trichinella* in domestic and wild animals intended for human consumption. *Veterinary Parasitology* 93 (3–4): 393–408.

40

Trypanosomiasis

Trypanosomiasis is caused by the flagellate protozoan *Trypanosoma* (derived from the Greek word *trypanon* meaning 'borer' and *soma* means 'body'). The two important forms of the disease in humans are human African trypanosomiasis (HAT) and American trypanosomiasis.

Human African Trypanosomiasis

Human African trypanosomiasis (also known as sleeping sickness) is a vector-borne parasitic disease caused by an extracellular protozoan belonging to the genus *Trypanosoma* and species *brucei*. The parasite is transmitted to humans through bites of the tsetse fly (*Glossina* spp.), where both male and female flies can transmit the infection. The two subspecies of *T. brucei* which are mainly pathogenic to humans are *T. brucei gambiense* and *T. brucei rhodesiense*. The important characteristics of these species are provided below (Based on [1]).

Trypanosoma brucei gambiense	*Trypanosoma brucei rhodesiense*
Causes West African sleeping sickness and is mainly found in western and Central Africa	Causes East African sleeping sickness and is mainly found in eastern and southern Africa
Responsible for the chronic form of disease, named 'gambiense'	It is less adapted to humans and causes an acute and rapidly progressive disease, known as 'rhodesiense'
T. b. gambiense is generally not considered zoonotic. It is an anthroponotic disease with a minor role in animal reservoirs	It is considered a zoonotic disease that mainly affects animals (livestock and wildlife), where humans are accidental host

Disease Transmission and Clinical Signs

Transmission of the parasite can occur during a blood meal on a mammalian host by infected tsetse flies, which can inject metacyclic trypomastigotes into the skin tissue. The parasites enter the lymphatic system and pass into the bloodstream where they transform into trypomastigotes and are carried to other sites throughout the body.
The disease can be broadly classified into two stages.

- **Early stage**: This phase includes non-specific signs (e.g. skin lesions, chancre, pruritus and cardiac, endocrine and gastrointestinal problems). In more severe cases, it may include

Textbook of Zoonoses, First Edition. Jasbir Singh Bedi, Deepthi Vijay, and Pankaj Dhaka.

hepatosplenomegaly, weight loss and intermittent fevers lasting 1 day to 1 week. Lymphadenopathy, mainly posterior cervical but in some cases axillary, inguinal or epitrochlear, may also occur. Posterior triangle cervical lymphadenopathy (also known as Winterbottom's sign) is commonly seen in *T. b. gambiense* infections.
- **Late stage (i.e. parasitic infection of the central nervous system)**: Parasitic invasion of the central nervous system causes a variety of neuropsychiatric manifestations which may include reversal of the sleep/wake cycle with daytime somnolence, nocturnal insomnia and sudden urges to sleep, therefore the disease is also called 'African sleeping sickness'. Clinical signs include tremors, motor weakness, walking difficulties, sensory disorders, visual impairments, headache and sleep disturbances that can deteriorate into a coma [1].

Diagnosis

Diagnosis of the disease involves confirmation of the presence of the parasite in body fluids. Parasitaemia is usually higher during *T. b. rhodesiense* infection in comparison to *T. b. gambiense*. Therefore, symptomatic patients typically have detectable parasites in the blood. For diagnosing *T. b. gambiense* infection, the classic approach involves light microscopic detection of the parasite in lymph node aspirate (usually from the posterior cervical node). Serological testing for *T. b. gambiense* can be used for screening purposes. In addition, molecular tools such as polymerase chain reaction (PCR) can be employed to characterise the parasite [2].

Treatment

There is no vaccine or drug prophylaxis against African trypanosomiasis. The recommended drug for the first stage of *T. b. gambiense* infection is pentamidine. Other drugs such as suramin, melarsoprol, eflornithine and nifurtimox in combination with eflornithine can also be used to treat African trypanosomiasis.

Prevention and Control

The preventive and control measures can include:

- minimising contact with tsetse flies
- use of proper clothing to avoid the bites of tsetse flies during outdoor activities
- avoid roaming around bushes during outdoor activities. The tsetse fly is less active during the hottest part of the day but will bite if disturbed
- use of appropriate insect repellent during travel and tourism to endemic areas.

American Trypanosomiasis

American trypanosomiasis (also known as Chagas disease) is caused by the parasite *Trypanosoma cruzi*, which is mainly found in South America. The disease is named after Carlos Chagas who first described it in 1909. The disease is considered as a zoonosis and infections are found in small mammals in the sylvatic cycle that can be transmitted to humans by blood-sucking triatomine bugs. Infected humans, pet animals (e.g. cats and dogs) and wild animals (e.g. rodents, monkeys, opossums, armadillos) can serve as the reservoir of the parasite. The triatomine bugs hide in crevices in the walls and roofs of houses during the daytime. At night, these bugs come out and tend to bite people's faces, hence they are also named 'kissing bugs'. After the bite, the bugs defaecate on the person, who can be infected if *T. cruzi* parasites in the bug faeces enter the body through mucous membranes or breaks in the skin. The person in sleep may accidentally scratch or rub the bug faeces into the bite wound, eyes or mouth and become infected. The disease can also be transmitted to humans by other pathways such as blood transfusion, organ transplantation and congenital transmission [3].

Clinical Signs in Humans

The disease in humans can occur in two phases [3].

- **Acute phase**: This phase can last for the first few weeks or months. During this phase, the person may have no symptoms or can have mild symptoms (e.g. fever, fatigue, body aches, headache, rash, loss of appetite, diarrhoea, vomiting). Other specific clinical signs include mild enlargement of the liver or spleen, swollen glands or swelling at the site of the bite (also called a chagoma). Some patients may have swelling of the eyelids on the side of the face near the bite wound or where the bug excreta were accidentally rubbed into the eye, which is known as Romaña's sign. In rare instances, young children can die from severe inflammation, myocarditis or meningoencephalitis during the acute phase.
- **Chronic phase**: This phase can last for decades or even for an entire lifetime. Most people do not exhibit any symptoms, but approximately 20–30% of infected people can develop cardiac complications (e.g. enlarged heart, altered heart rate or rhythm, cardiac arrest) and/or gastrointestinal complications (e.g. mega-oesophagus or megacolon).

Diagnosis

During the acute phase of Chagas disease, there will be many parasites in the peripheral blood so the infection can be detected by microscopical examination of wet or dry blood smears or by parasitological tests such as xenodiagnoses or blood culture. Molecular tools such as PCR can provide high detection sensitivities with species-level identification. Diagnosis during the chronic phase can be based on immunological tests targeting IgG class antibodies against the parasitic antigens.

Treatment

Benznidazole and nifurtimox are considered important drugs for the treatment of Chagas disease.

Prevention and Control

Prevention and control strategies involve:

- improved housing and spraying of insecticide to eliminate the bugs
- screening of blood donations for the parasite to prevent the spread of the disease through blood transfusions
- the early detection and treatment of new cases, including congenital cases, will also help in reducing the burden of disease.

References

1 Fevre, E.M., Wissmann, B.V., Welburn, S.C., and Lutumba, P. (2008). The burden of human African trypanosomiasis. *PLoS Neglected Tropical Diseases 2* (12): e333.

2 Centers for Disease Control and Prevention. (2020). Parasites – African Trypanosomiasis (also known as Sleeping Sickness). www.cdc.gov/parasites/sleepingsickness/disease.html (accessed 24 January 2022).

3 Centers for Disease Control and Prevention. (2021). Parasites – American Trypanosomiasis (also known as Chagas disease). www.cdc.gov/parasites/chagas/prevent.html (accessed 24 January 2022).

41

Visceral Larva Migrans

Many of the nematodes of the family Ascarididae are the causative agents of zoonoses transmitted to humans via contaminated soil. Within the ascarids, *Toxocara canis*, *Toxocara cati* and *Baylisascaris procyonis* are the predominant zoonotic parasites of dogs, cats and raccoons, respectively. These are among the most widespread causes of visceral larva migrans (VLM), ocular larva migrans (OLM) and neural larva migrans (NLM) [1]. VLM is due to the aberrant migration of the larvae in human tissues with incomplete maturation which can produce clinical manifestations in the visceral organs such as lungs and liver. When invading the eye, the parasitic larvae may lead to OLM. NLM is the invasion of the brain and/or spinal cord by parasitic larvae, especially of *B. procyonis* [2]

Epidemiology

Although widely distributed, toxocariasis is a neglected parasitic zoonosis that is most commonly seen in tropical countries, where sanitary and hygienic conditions are poor [3]. Children, especially those less than 5 years old, are more vulnerable to infection due to the high risk of exposure while playing in soil [4].

Transmission Cycles

All wild and domestic canids can act as definitive hosts for *T. canis*, which is considered the most important aetiological agent for OLM and NLM in humans [5], whereas *T. cati* is found in wild and domestic felids of all ages. *B. procyonis* primarily infects raccoons and is considered the most prevalent and pathogenic of several *Baylisascaris* species with the potential to cause clinical larva migrans, especially NLM [2]. The definitive hosts may be infected congenitally or perinatally or through the ingestion of eggs where the hatched larvae penetrate the intestinal mucosa and reach the lungs via liver and bloodstream. These larvae are coughed up, swallowed and mature to egg-producing adults in the small intestine of the host.

Numerous species of mammals and birds can act as paratenic hosts for these species of worms, with livestock being the important paratenic hosts [6]. Humans are accidental hosts who become infected by ingesting infective eggs from contaminated soil, vegetables, unwashed hands and ingestion of undercooked muscles or viscera of paratenic hosts such as chicken, sheep and cattle. The larva hatches in the intestine, can penetrate through the small intestine and undergoes widespread somatic migration. The liver may become infected as larvae pass through the portal system and hepatic sinusoids, and later can disseminate to other organs.

Textbook of Zoonoses, First Edition. Jasbir Singh Bedi, Deepthi Vijay, and Pankaj Dhaka.

Disease in Animals

Toxocariasis causes serious disease in pups and kittens, but adult dogs and cats usually remain asymptomatic. The parasite causes serious blood loss, acute gastrointestinal haemorrhages, anaemia, poor growth and loss of condition in young animals. Death may also occur in severe cases.

Disease in Humans

The clinical manifestations may vary from asymptomatic to severe clinical presentations which depend on the degree of involvement of host tissue by the larvae and the site of larval migration [7]. The most important larval migration sites are the lungs, heart, liver and CNS. The infection is mostly asymptomatic or usually compartmentalised in the viscera, brain and eyes (VLM or NLM or OLM) as described below.

- In VLM, hepatomegaly, splenomegaly and myocarditis are the important clinical manifestations, usually accompanied by hypereosinophilia. The liver is the organ most commonly affected in VLM, with the formation of granulomatous lesions and hepatitis [8]. Pulmonary involvement can result in pneumonia or asthma.
- In NLM, seizures, neuropsychiatric symptoms, encephalopathy or eosinophilic meningoencephalitis are usually observed.
- In OLM, the larvae produce various ophthalmological lesions and may cause diffuse unilateral subacute neuroretinitis. Involvement is typically unilateral (affecting one eye) and associated visual impairment usually presents with uveitis, retinitis or endophthalmitis. Permanent visual damage or blindness can occur in severe cases.

Diagnosis

In definitive hosts like dogs and cats, the eggs of the parasite can be detected via faecal examination.

In humans, the diagnosis of toxocariasis should rely on clinical, radiographic and laboratory evidence of the disease. Serological tests such as enzyme-linked immunosorbent assay (ELISA) based on excretory and secretory antigens of the third stage larvae (L3) of *T. canis* are widely used for diagnosis. The persistent eosinophilia and increase in the total IgE levels and an elevation of parasite-specific immunoglobulins help to establish the diagnosis. Various imaging techniques such as ultrasonography, CT scan and MRI could also aid in diagnosis. A liver biopsy can be performed to diagnose VLM. Molecular diagnostic tests based on PCR are widely used to identify *T. canis* larvae collected from human biopsies and also for accurate species-level identification of *Toxocara* eggs isolated from faeces or soil [9].

Treatment

A variety of anthelmintic drugs can be used for the treatment of toxocariasis in definitive hosts. The key component of toxocariasis therapy is anthelmintics (e.g. albendazole, mebendazole, thiabendazole) and anti-inflammatory drugs. In humans, the administration of corticosteroids can be used to suppress the intense allergic manifestations of the infection.

Prevention and Control

In the absence of effective treatment protocols, prevention of the infection remains the best strategy [9]. Important prevention and control measures include the following.

- Control of the stray dog population is important to combat larva migrans. Environmental contamination with *Toxocara* eggs can be prevented by restricting the entry of stray dogs to public places, parks and playgrounds.
- Dogs and cats should be periodically dewormed against these zoonotic helminths.
- Owners should dispose of dog and cat faeces properly. The public must be educated regarding the potential dangers of contact with faeces of pets and raccoons.
- All fruits and vegetables should be properly washed before consumption and meat should be properly cooked.
- Good hygienic measures like washing hands after playing on the beach or with dogs or cats, or after gardening, should be advocated.
- Discourage geophagia in children and encourage them to adopt good hygienic practices.
- An awareness campaign should be carried out to educate pet owners and others. Information for travellers on how to avoid exposure to these parasites is also important.

References

1. Sharma, R., Singh, B.B., and Gill, J.P.S. (2015). Larva migrans in India: veterinary and public health perspectives. *Journal of Parasitic Diseases* 39 (4): 604–612.
2. Graeff-Teixeira, C., Morassutti, A.L., and Kazacos, K.R. (2016). Update on baylisascariasis, a highly pathogenic zoonotic infection. *Clinical Microbiology Reviews* 29 (2): 375–399.
3. Yu, T., Zhao, L.N., Fan, M.J. et al. (2012). Visceral larva migrans associated with earthworm and gecko ingestion: a case report. *Journal of Medical Case Reports* 6 (1): 210.
4. Manini, M.P., Marchioro, A.A., Colli, C.M. et al. (2012). Association between contamination of public squares and seropositivity for *Toxocara* spp. in children. *Veterinary Parasitology* 188 (1–2): 48–52.
5. Fan, C.K., Holland, C.V., Loxton, K., and Barghouth, U. (2015). Cerebral toxocariasis: silent progression to neurodegenerative disorders? *Clinical Microbiology Reviews* 28 (3): 663–686.
6. Centers for Disease Control and Prevention. (2019). Toxocariasis. www.cdc.gov/dpdx/toxocariasis/index.html (accessed 24 January 2022).
7. Santarém, V.A., Leli, F.N.C., Rubinsky-Elefant, G., and Giuffrida, R. (2011). Protective and risk factors for toxocariasis in children from two different social classes of Brazil. *Revista do Instituto de Medicina Tropical de São Paulo* 53 (2): 66–72.
8. Musso, C., Castelo, J.S., Tsanaclis, A.M., and Pereira, F.E. (2007). Prevalence of *Toxocara*-induced liver granulomas, detected by immunohistochemistry, in a series of autopsies at a Children's Reference Hospital in Vitoria, ES, Brazil. *Virchows Archiv* 450 (4): 411–417.
9. Chen, J., Liu, Q., Liu, G.H. et al. (2018). Toxocariasis: a silent threat with a progressive public health impact. *Infectious Diseases of Poverty* 7 (1): 59.

42

Other Parasitic Zoonoses of Public Health Importance

Angiostrongyliasis

Angiostrongylus cantonensis is a parasitic worm of rats (also called the rat lungworm). The adult form of the parasite is found only in rodents. Infected rats pass larvae of the parasite in their faeces that can lead to infections in snails and slugs. These larvae mature in snails and slugs but do not become adult worms. The life cycle is completed when rats eat infected snails or slugs and the larvae further mature to become adult worms [1].

Humans can be infected by eating raw or undercooked snails or slugs that are infected with the parasite. However, accidental infection by eating raw produce (such as lettuce) that contains a small snail or slug has also been reported. In addition, certain animals such as freshwater shrimp, crabs or frogs can be infected with larvae of the parasite. Therefore, it is also possible that eating undercooked or raw animals that are infected could result in human infection. Of note, fish do not spread this parasite.

Most infected people do not have any symptoms, or have only mild symptoms that do not last very long. Sometimes the infection causes a rare type of meningitis (eosinophilic meningitis). Symptoms can include headache, stiff neck, tingling or painful feelings in the skin, low-grade fever, nausea and vomiting. Even if infected, most people recover fully without treatment. Even people who develop eosinophilic meningitis usually do not need antiparasitic drugs. The important prevention measures include avoiding the consumption of raw or undercooked snails or slugs, frogs or shrimp/prawns. Use gloves while handling snails or slugs and wash the hands properly after handling them [1].

Anisakiasis

Anisakiasis (also known as herring worm disease) is a parasitic disease caused by nematodes – *Anisakis simplex* and *Pseudoterranova decipiens*. The disease is commonly found in areas, such as Japan, where eating raw fish is popular. *A. simplex* infects humans accidentally when raw or undercooked fish contaminated with larvae is consumed. These larvae are in their third developmental stage (L3) and further development is arrested until they are ingested by sea mammals such as seals and dolphins, whereupon they progress through two more developmental stages until adulthood. Once in the human gastrointestinal tract, the L3 of *A. simplex* and *P. decipiens* may progress to L4, but only in exceptional cases may the immature adult stage be reached [2].

Textbook of Zoonoses, First Edition. Jasbir Singh Bedi, Deepthi Vijay, and Pankaj Dhaka.

Inside the human body, the larvae can invade the gastrointestinal tract. Eventually, the parasite dies and produces an inflamed mass in the oesophagus, stomach and/or intestine. The gastrointestinal symptoms may be associated with mild-to-severe immunological, usually allergic-type, reactions. In addition, some patients show more generalised hypersensitivity reactions, without any associated digestive disorders.

The treatment for anisakiasis may require removal of the worm from the body by endoscopy or surgery. The best way to prevent this disease is to avoid eating raw or undercooked fish or squid [2].

Clonorchiasis

Clonorchiasis (also known as Chinese liver fluke disease) is caused by infection with *Clonorchis sinensis*. Clonorchiasis is a common infection of dogs and other fish-eating carnivores in China, the Republic of Korea and Vietnam. During the life cycle, the adult flukes inhabit the bile ducts and lay eggs that are dispersed into the environment during defaecation. When they reach fresh water, eggs develop into miracidia that are ingested by various species of aquatic snails. The miracidia further develop and reproduce asexually into cercariae (larvae). The cercariae leave the snail and swim to penetrate beneath the scales of various species of carp-like freshwater fishes where, as metacercariae, they encyst in the subcutaneous tissue. When dogs or other carnivores eat raw fish, the metacercarial cysts hatch in the intestine and the young worms migrate to the bile ducts, thus completing the cycle [3].

Humans may replace reservoir hosts in the transmission cycle when they eat raw or partially cooked fish, thus ingesting the metacercariae. In humans, acute clonorchiasis may be asymptomatic, but if the number of worms is significantly high, fever and right upper quadrant pain may occur and may be associated with intermittent colic pain caused by the worms obstructing the gallbladder. Chronic clonorchiasis, which results from protracted episodes of reinfection over time, is severe in most cases. The presence of the worms in the walls of the smaller bile ducts causes chronic inflammation, resulting in fibrosis of the ducts and destruction of the adjacent liver parenchyma. Cholangiohepatitis, or recurrent pyogenic cholangitis, is also a frequent clinical outcome. Chronic clonorchiasis is strongly associated with cholangiocarcinoma, a severe and often fatal form of bile duct cancer.

Praziquantel is recommended for the treatment of clonorchiasis. Proper cooking of fish before consumption is the best way to prevent clonorchiasis in humans [3].

Dracunculiasis (Guinea Worm Disease)

The infection is caused by the parasite *Dracunculus medinensis*. Dracunculiasis is primarily a human disease. It affects people in rural and deprived communities who depend mainly on open surface water sources such as ponds for drinking water [4].

People become infected with Guinea worms by drinking unfiltered water from ponds and other stagnant water containing copepods (tiny 'water fleas'). Alternatively, it is believed that people and animals might also become infected by eating certain aquatic animals, like fish or frogs, that might have swallowed infected copepods and might carry Guinea worm larvae but do not themselves suffer from infection [5]. In many endemic regions, due to the advocacy of hygiene and distribution of clean water supply by national and international health agencies, the disease is on the verge of eradication [4].

Clinical Signs

People mainly remain asymptomatic for about 1 year after they become infected. After that, when the worms come out of the skin, the person may develop fever, swelling and pain in the affected area. More than 90% of worms come out of the legs and feet, but worms can also appear on other body parts. In remote rural communities, in the absence of healthcare facilities, the emergence of adult female worms from the skin can be very painful and disabling. Often, the wound caused by the emerging worm develops a secondary bacterial infection. Sometimes, permanent damage occurs if a joint is infected [5].

Treatment

There is no drug to treat Guinea worm disease and no vaccine to prevent infection. Once a part of the worm begins to come out of the wound, the rest of the worm can only be pulled out a few centimetres each day by winding it around a piece of gauze or a small stick. Care must be taken not to break the worm during removal. If part of the worm is not removed, there is a risk for secondary bacterial infections and resulting complications. Anti-inflammatory medicine can help in reducing pain and swelling. Antibiotic ointment can help to prevent secondary bacterial infections [4, 5].

Prevention and Control

Important measures that can prevent the spread of the disease include the following [5].

- Use of drinking water from protected sources (such as from boreholes or protected hand-dug wells) that are free from contamination. If this is not possible, always filter drinking water to remove the copepods that carry the Guinea worm larvae.
- Cook fish and other aquatic animals (e.g. frogs) well before eating. Also, avoid feeding raw or undercooked fish or aquatic animals to dogs.
- Prevent people with blisters, swellings, wounds and visible worms emerging from their skin from entering ponds and other water sources.
- Tether dogs that have blisters, swellings, wounds and visible worms emerging from their skin to prevent them from entering ponds and other water sources.
- Awareness programmes on health education and behavioural change are important in endemic regions.

Fasciolopsiasis

Fasciolopsiasis is caused by the intestinal fluke *Fasciolopsis buski*. The disease is found in South and South-Eastern Asia where pigs and humans are the major reservoirs of infection. Humans can be infected with *Fasciolopsis* when they eat raw or undercooked aquatic plants that have the parasite encysted on them [6].

The infection mainly remains asymptomatic but in some cases, abdominal pain and diarrhoea can occur after 1–2 months of infection. In addition, heavy infections of *Fasciolopsis* flukes can cause intestinal obstruction, abdominal pain, nausea, vomiting and fever. Allergic reactions and swelling of the face and legs can also occur, and in some cases, anaemia may be present.

The infection can be treated with praziquantel. Preventive measures include proper cooking of aquatic plants before consumption. In endemic areas, prevent faecal contamination (from humans or pigs) of water where aquatic plants are grown. Do not feed raw aquatic plants to pigs [6].

Paragonimiasis

Among the more than 10 species of *Paragonimus* reported to infect humans, the most common is *Paragonimus westermani* (also known as the oriental lung fluke). *P. westermani* is distributed in South-East Asia and Japan [7]. Human infection with *P. westermani* occurs by eating inadequately cooked or pickled crab or crayfish that harbour the metacercariae stage of the parasite. The metacercariae excyst in the duodenum, and penetrate through the intestinal wall into the peritoneal cavity, then through the abdominal wall and diaphragm into the lungs, where they become encapsulated and develop into adults. The worms can also reach other organs and tissues, such as the brain and striated muscles.

The acute phase (i.e. invasion and migration) of infection may be marked by diarrhoea, abdominal pain, fever, cough, urticaria, hepatosplenomegaly, pulmonary abnormalities and eosinophilia [7]. During the chronic phase, pulmonary manifestations include cough, expectoration of discoloured sputum (rusted sputum), haemoptysis and chest radiographic abnormalities. Extrapulmonary locations of the adult worms result in more severe manifestations, especially when the brain is involved.

Prevention measures include proper cooking of seafood before consumption.

Pentastomiasis

Pentastomiasis (also known as linguatulosis or linguatuliasis) is caused by crustaceans known as pentastomids or pentastomes. The majority of human pentastomiasis is caused by two species. The first, *Armillifer armillatus*, infects humans as secondary hosts. Infection is usually asymptomatic but has characteristic postmortem and radiological features. The second, *Linguatula serrata*, can infect humans as does *Armillifer* or can cause a self-limiting nasopharyngitis, i.e. the halzoun or marrara syndrome, where humans act as a temporary definitive host.

There is no proven pharmacotherapy but ivermectin, praziquantel or mebendazole can be tried in severe cases [8]. Surgery may be needed to relieve obstructive symptoms. Prevention is by avoiding eating raw meat and boiling drinking water.

Primary Amoebic Meningoencephalitis or Amoebic Encephalitis

Naegleria fowleri (commonly referred to as the 'brain-eating amoeba') is a free-living microscopic amoeba. It can cause a rare and devastating infection of the brain called primary amoebic meningoencephalitis (PAM). The amoeba is commonly found in warm fresh water (e.g. lakes, rivers, hot springs) and soil. *N. fowleri* usually infects people when contaminated water enters the body through the nose. Once the amoeba enters the nose, it travels to the brain where it causes PAM, which is usually fatal. Infection typically occurs when people go swimming or diving in warm freshwater sites, such as lakes and rivers. *N. fowleri* can grow in pipes, water heaters and water systems, including treated public drinking water systems [9].

Personal actions to reduce the risk of *N. fowleri* infection should focus on limiting the amount of water going up the nose and lowering the chances that *N. fowleri* may be present in the water.

References

1 Centers for Disease Control and Prevention. (2020). Parasites – Angiostrongyliasis. www.cdc.gov/parasites/angiostrongylus/gen_info/faqs.html (accessed 24 January 2022).

2 Centers for Disease Control and Prevention. (2020). Parasites – Anisakiasis. www.cdc.gov/parasites/anisakiasis/faqs.html#what (accessed 24 January 2022).

3 World Health Organization. (2021). Foodborne trematode infections. https://www.who.int/news-room/fact-sheets/detail/foodborne-trematode-infections (accessed 24 January 2022).

4 World Health Organization. (2022). Dracunculiasis (guinea worm disease) – Fact Sheet. www.who.int/news-room/fact-sheets/detail/dracunculiasis-(guinea-worm-disease) (accessed 24 January 2022).

5 Centers for Disease Control and Prevention. (2021). Parasites – Guinea Worm. www.cdc.gov/parasites/guineaworm/gen_info/faqs.html (accessed 24 January 2022).

6 Centers for Disease Control and Prevention. (2014). Parasites – Fasciolopsiasis. www.cdc.gov/parasites/fasciolopsis/faqs.html (accessed 24 January 2022).

7 Centers for Disease Control and Prevention. (2020). Parasites – Paragonimiasis. www.cdc.gov/dpdx/paragonimiasis/index.html (accessed 24 January 2022).

8 Drabick, J.J. (1987). Pentastomiasis. *Reviews of Infectious Diseases* 9 (6): 1087–1094.

9 Centers for Disease Control and Prevention. (2017). Parasites – *Naegleria fowleri* – Primary Amebic Meningoencephalitis (PAM) – Amebic Encephalitis. www.cdc.gov/parasites/naegleria/index.html (accessed 24 January 2022).

Section 4

Fungal Zoonoses

Introduction

Fungi are a group of non-photosynthetic micro-organisms which live as saprophytes in soil and on dead organic matter, or as parasites of plants and animals, including humans. The fungal kingdom includes some of the most important organisms, in terms of both their ecological and economic roles. Fungi perform a variety of key roles, such as breaking down organic material, supplying the roots of plants with essential nutrients, providing humans with life-saving antibiotics, supplying the bubbles in bread, champagne and beer, providing foods such as mushrooms, truffles, morels, etc. There are approximately 1.5 million different species of fungi on Earth but only about 300 of those are known to cause disease in humans [1].

Fungal infections with zoonotic and/or sapronotic modes of transmission (the source is an abiotic substrate) are associated with considerable socioeconomic and public health impact worldwide. A number of these infections are common fungal diseases, such as dermatophytosis, aspergillosis, sporotrichosis, and histoplasmosis. Fungi are eukaryotic and so are genetically more similar to animals and humans, which makes them more challenging to treat.

Most of the fungi are free-living and can thrive in the environment for extended periods without requiring any host to complete their life cycle. Nevertheless, a pathogenic fungus has an evolutionary advantage of the use of a vertebrate vector as a part of their life cycle. The importance of fungal infections in both humans and animals has increased over recent decades. Many of these fungal infections are considered as emerging or re-emerging, associated with the outbreaks in resource-limited regions due to inadequate public health infrastructure and diagnostic facilities. Until the 1980s, most fungal infections in humans were limited to sporadic outbreaks with a low incidence, which might be attributed to the lack of diagnostics. However, the emergence of the human immunodeficiency virus (HIV) infection and other immunosuppressive disorders, which led to the generalised use of immunosuppressive drugs, has caused the flaring up of fungal infections [2]. The invasive fungal infections, i.e. systemic and subcutaneous mycoses, are major causes of morbidity and mortality in immunosuppressed hosts. In the recent past, access to molecular and other novel tools for detection of fungal infections and their epidemiological characteristics has improved their better reporting from many parts of the world.

Humans and animals are generally tolerant to fungi but fungi cause infections of various types, particularly in immunocompromised individuals. Based on the location of the infection, fungal diseases include superficial mycoses (located on the outer surface of hair, skin and nails, known as dermatophytosis), systemic mycoses (those which can invade the body tissues such as *Blastomyces* spp., *Histoplasma* spp., etc.) and opportunistic mycoses (fungi such as *Candida* that are normally harmless and reside in body, but can cause disease in immunocompromised hosts). Some fungal diseases can be zoonotic and remain as occupational hazards for humans (such as pet owners,

Textbook of Zoonoses, First Edition. Jasbir Singh Bedi, Deepthi Vijay, and Pankaj Dhaka.

veterinarians, herdsmen, agricultural workers, zoo keepers and horticulturists) who are exposed to and closely interact with infected animals. Contact with fungus-contaminated environments as well as objects used in animal rearing and restraint is considered important in natural dissemination of these diseases.

However, although the global burden of zoonotic fungal diseases is steadily increasing, many of these zoonotic fungal diseases are still 'neglected' and thus may be misdiagnosed because of lack of awareness and familiarity with them [3]. Public health policies and strategic plans for prioritising such infections are lacking in many resource-limited regions. Thus, there is a need for continuous research in zoonotic mycoses using a combination of classic and molecular surveillance and diagnostic tools. Further, level of awareness of these diseases need to be improved in order to better appreciate their public health burden across the globe.

References

1 Adebiyi, A.I. and Oluwayelu, D.O. (2018). Zoonotic fungal diseases and animal ownership in Nigeria. *Alexandria Journal of Medicine* 54 (4): 397–402.

2 Blanco, J.L. and Garcia, M.E. (2010). Animal as reservoir of fungal diseases (zoonoses?). In: *Combating Fungal Infections* (ed. I. Ahmad, M. Owais, M. Shahid and F. Aqil), 47–70. Berlin, Heidelberg: Springer.

3 Seyedmousavi, S., Guillot, J., Tolooe, A. et al. (2015). Neglected fungal zoonoses: hidden threats to man and animals. *Clinical Microbiology and Infection* 21 (5): 416–425.

43

Aspergillosis

Etiology

Aspergillus spp. are filamentous, environmental fungi that can cause a wide spectrum of infections in animals and humans. Among more than 250 species of *Aspergillus*, fewer than 40 are known to cause infections in humans, and of these, *Aspergillus fumigatus* is the most common cause of serious invasive infections in humans, primarily in immunocompromised individuals [1, 2].

Epidemiology and Transmission

Aspergillus fumigatus is a saprophytic and ubiquitous air-borne fungus, whose natural ecological niche is the soil. The presence of ambient temperature, moisture and organic matter promotes its development. Despite regular exposure to the fungi, infections in animals and humans are rare and mainly occur in immunocompromised individuals. *Aspergillus* spp. is associated with infections in various species of animals but transmission from animals to humans is rarely reported.

The invasive form of aspergillosis principally involves the sinopulmonary tract, reflecting that inhalation is the most common route of entry of *Aspergillus* spores, while other entry sites such as the gastrointestinal tract and skin occur on rare occasions. The major risk factors for invasive aspergillosis in humans include prolonged neutropenia (typically more than 7 days), long-term corticosteroid therapy, organ transplantation (especially bone marrow transplantation) and hereditary neutrophil dysfunction (e.g. chronic granulomatous disease).

Disease in Animals

In animals, aspergillosis is primarily a respiratory infection that can be generalised; however, tissue predilection is variable between species [3]. Aspergillosis may also occur in healthy animals under environmental stress and other immunocompromising conditions. Some important clinical manifestations in different species are listed below.

- **Dogs and cats:** Sinonasal, bronchopulmonary and disseminated infections are the major forms.
- **Ruminants:** *Aspergillus* spp., particularly *A. fumigatus*, are known to cause mycotic pneumonia, gastroenteritis, mastitis, placentitis and abortion in ruminants.

Textbook of Zoonoses, First Edition. Jasbir Singh Bedi, Deepthi Vijay, and Pankaj Dhaka.

- **Poultry:** All avian species are susceptible to *Aspergillus* species. *A. fumigatus* has been involved in significant deadly outbreaks of domestic and free-ranging wild birds causing huge economic losses.
- **Horses:** The fungi can cause guttural pouch infections, keratomycosis and pneumonia in horses.

Disease in Humans

Humans constantly inhale numerous conidia (spores) of this fungus, which are normally eliminated by mucociliary clearance and innate immune mechanisms of immunocompetent hosts. Depending on the immune status of the patient, *Aspergillus*-related diseases may present with acute invasive aspergillosis, chronic or allergic bronchopulmonary aspergillosis (ABPA) and/or with aspergilloma [4].

In immunocompetent patients, *Aspergillus* spp. can lead to allergic responses and chronic non-invasive forms of infection, ranging from the development of a fungus ball (aspergilloma) to chronic inflammatory and fibrotic processes classified as chronic pulmonary aspergillosis. The saprophytic colonisation of parenchymal lung cavity by *Aspergillus* spp. is referred to as aspergilloma, which consists of both dead and living mycelial elements, inflammatory cells, fibrin, mucus and components of degenerating blood and epithelia. The mycelial mass may lie free within the cavity or be attached to the cavity wall by inflammatory/granulomatous tissue.

A high risk of invasive aspergillosis occurs in patients with prolonged neutropenia, recipients of haematopoietic stem cell or solid organ transplants, and patients with advanced AIDS or chronic granulomatous disease. Symptoms such as fever, cough and dyspnoea are frequent, although non-specific findings of pulmonary aspergillosis, where the lung is the most common site of invasive aspergillosis may also occur. Vascular invasion of fungi may manifest as pleuritic chest pain from pulmonary infarction or as haemoptysis. Untreated infection may lead to extension to mediastinal and chest wall structures and haematogenous dissemination that can involve many organs. Involvement of the central nervous system (CNS) is associated with the devastating consequences of disseminated aspergillosis and may be manifested by seizures or neurological signs [5].

Diagnosis

The clinical diagnosis of aspergillosis remains difficult due to non-specific overlapping symptoms. Radiological findings can be suggestive but not confirmatory. Culture and microscopic examination remain the gold standard but lacks sensitivity.

Culture of the fungus from clinical samples has the advantage of isolating the specific aetiological agent and also allows antifungal susceptibility testing. However, a significant limitation is the fact that culture testing may take several days. Clinical specimens such as bronchoalveolar lavage (BAL), biopsies and sputum should preferably be cultured on Sabouraud-dextrose-agar (SDA), brain-heart-infusion-agar (BHI) or potato-dextrose-agar (PDA) at 30 °C and 37 °C for 72 hours. Supplementation of gentamicin plus chloramphenicol is also recommended for non-sterile specimens such as sputum [5].

The histological demonstration of invasive hyphae or a positive culture from a normally sterile environment (e.g. pleural fluid) indicates invasive fungal disease. Gomori's methenamine silver stain, periodic acid–Schiff or the application of fluorescent dyes such as Calcofluor white™, Uvitex 2B or Blancophor™ are some methods used for detection [5].

Newer antigen-based assays facilitate the diagnosis of invasive aspergillosis. Antigen assays such as cell wall component galactomannan in serum, BAL and urine, detection of the cell wall component 1,3-β-D-glucan (BDG) via factor G activation in serum, detection of *Aspergillus*-specific siderophores in BAL or urine, detection of *Aspergillus*-specific cell wall protein via a lateral flow device (LFD) test are in use for rapid detection of aspergillosis, yet these tests vary in sensitivity and specificity. Diagnosis via PCR assay for detection of *Aspergillus*-specific DNA in blood and BAL, although promising, is currently investigational.

Treatment

Prompt targeted systemic antifungal treatment remains the most important predictive factor for a successful outcome in immunocompromised individuals. Recent guidelines recommend voriconazole and/or isavuconazole for the primary treatment of invasive aspergillosis, with liposomal amphotericin B being the first alternative and posaconazole, as well as echinocandins, primarily recommended for salvage treatment [6].

Prevention and Control

It is difficult to avoid breathing in *Aspergillus* spores because the fungus is ubiquitous. Prevention of invasive aspergillosis relies on environmental infection control guidelines to reduce mould exposure and antifungal prophylaxis for at-risk groups. Immunocompromised persons can prevent exposure to spores by avoiding areas with a lot of dust, such as construction or excavation sites, and wearing N95 respirator while visiting risky sites. At-risk groups should avoid activities that involve close contact with soil or dust, such as yard work or gardening. To reduce the chances of developing a skin infection, clean any skin injuries well with soap and water, especially if they have been exposed to soil or dust. For the high-risk groups of invasive aspergillosis (e.g. in case of organ transplant or a stem cell transplant), antifungal prophylaxis may be recommended.

References

1. Geiser, D.M. (2009). Sexual structures in aspergillus: morphology, importance and genomics. *Medical Mycology 47* (suppl1): S21–S26.
2. Jenks, J. and Hoenigl, M. (2018). Treatment of aspergillosis. *Journal of Fungi 4* (3): 98.
3. Seyedmousavi, S., Bosco, S.D.M., De Hoog, S. et al. (2018). Fungal infections in animals: a patchwork of different situations. *Medical Mycology 56* (suppl 1): S165–S187.
4. Denning, D.W., Cadranel, J., Beigelman-Aubry, C. et al. (2016). Chronic pulmonary aspergillosis: rationale and clinical guidelines for diagnosis and management. *European Respiratory Journal 47* (1): 45–68.
5. Segal, B.H. (2009). Aspergillosis. *New England Journal of Medicine 360* (18): 1870–1884.
6. Latgé, J.P. and Chamilos, G. (2019). *Aspergillus fumigatus* and aspergillosis in 2019. *Clinical Microbiology Reviews 33* (1): e00140–e00118.

44

Blastomycosis

Etiology

Blastomycosis is caused by the thermally dimorphic fungus *Blastomyces dermatitidis*. It was previously known as Gilchrist disease, in honour of the scientist who first recognised it in Baltimore, USA, in 1894. Other synonyms of the disease are North American blastomycosis and Chicago disease [1].

Epidemiology

Outbreaks of blastomycosis are commonly reported from Mississippi, Missouri, the Ohio River valley and mid-Atlantic states of the USA, and from Canada in the focal areas of Ontario, Quebec and Manitoba. The disease has also been reported from other areas of North America and parts of Europe, Asia, Latin America and Africa.

Transmission

The fungus *B. dermatitidis* can exist in two forms: a yeast form and a mould form. The yeast form causes infections, but this form cannot be transmitted by direct contact or aerosols, whereas the mould form is highly infectious and is present at ambient temperatures in the environment. While routine contact with infected animals poses no risk, animal-to-human transmission of blastomycosis has been reported following dog bites. The incidence of blastomycosis in dogs is reported to be 8–10 times that of humans [2], therefore, dogs can be sentinels for human infections in endemic regions [3].

The inhalation of conidia into the alveoli remains the main route of disease transmission in humans, where the conidia undergo transition to yeasts, the forms that are seen in mammalian tissue and cultures at 37 °C. The spores are more likely to be air-borne when contaminated soil or organic matter containing microfoci of *B. dermatitidis* mycelia release infectious conidia, after disturbance by activities such as excavation, construction, digging or wood clearing. Other less common transmission routes include direct cutaneous inoculation via penetrating outdoor injury or bite from infected dogs. *B. dermatitidis* is not transmitted from animals to humans otherwise. The disease is not transmitted from person to person and therefore is not contagious [1].

Textbook of Zoonoses, First Edition. Jasbir Singh Bedi, Deepthi Vijay, and Pankaj Dhaka.

Disease in Humans

The clinical outcomes of infection with *B. dermatitidis* are protean, ranging from subclinical infection to the fatal disseminated form. Symptoms of the acute phase of the disease include fever, cough, myalgia, arthralgia and pleurisy. The extrapulmonary sites include cutaneous, osseous, genitourinary or central nervous system (CNS) sites [1].

Most human cases resolve spontaneously. However, without treatment, the prognosis is grave when the infection spreads beyond the lungs, especially among human immunodeficiency virus (HIV) patients, where it often disseminates to the CNS and is associated with high mortality rates.

Diagnosis

The clinical signs of *B. dermatitidis* infection need to be differentiated from those of other fungal pathogens, tuberculosis and malignant tumours. Isolation of the fungus from clinical samples (e.g. saliva, respiratory samples, lung biopsies, skin or other infected tissues) can be carried out in culture media, such as Sabouraud dextrose agar, potato dextrose agar, potato flake agar or inhibitory mould agar. For specimens that are likely to be contaminated with saprophytic fungi and/or bacteria, selective media containing cycloheximide to inhibit saprophytic fungi and antibacterial agents can be used. The inoculated plates need to be incubated at 25–30 °C for 4–6 weeks. Cytology smear (i.e. direct microscopic identification of broad-based budding yeast) and histopathology of surgical biopsies can be carried out. Urine antigen tests or serum antigen and antibodies tests are also available but have less reliability. Molecular PCR assays have been useful in the study of the molecular epidemiology of blastomycosis.

Treatment

Patients with chronic pulmonary or disseminated extrapulmonary blastomycosis and all immunocompromised patients with blastomycosis should receive antifungal therapy. The site(s) of disease, the severity of illness and the presence or absence of underlying immunosuppression influence the choice of antifungal drug and duration of treatment. A long course of amphotericin B is usually curative. Also, itraconazole is considered a highly effective and mainstay therapy for most patients with blastomycosis.

Prevention and Control

There is no vaccine available for blastomycosis, and it is not possible to completely avoid exposure to the fungus in endemic regions. Farmers, construction and forestry workers, veterinarians and other professionals working with infected dogs are considered at-risk groups for blastomycosis. People who have weakened immune systems should avoid activities that involve disrupting soil in contaminated areas. Additionally, dog bite avoidance and safe handling of sharps are other preventive measures.

References

1 Saccente, M. and Woods, G.L. (2010). Clinical and laboratory update on blastomycosis. *Clinical Microbiology Reviews* 23 (2): 367–381.

2 Herrmann, J.A., Kostiuk, S.L., Dworkin, M.S., and Johnson, Y.J. (2011). Temporal and spatial distribution of blastomycosis cases among humans and dogs in Illinois (2001–2007). *Journal of the American Veterinary Medical Association* 239 (3): 335–343.

3 George, A.S., Eckman, M.R., Davies, S.F., and Laskey, W.K. (1979). Canine blastomycosis as a harbinger of human disease. *Annals of Internal Medicine* 91 (5): 733–735.

45

Coccidioidomycosis

Coccidioidomycosis, also known as valley fever or desert rheumatism, is an infection caused by the soil-dwelling fungi of the genus *Coccidioides*. The disease is endemic to the semi-arid to arid life zones in the south western United States, northern Mexico and scattered areas of Latin America.

Etiology

The two species of genus *Coccidioides*, i.e. *Coccidioides immitis* and *C. posadasii*, are the aetiological agents for coccidioidomycosis. The fungus is dimorphic and can exist as mycelia or spherules (sac-like cells that give rise to endospores). These dimorphic fungi are considered true pathogens and change from their saprophytic mycelial form found in soil into the round, thick-walled spherule/endospore form inside animal hosts.

Epidemiology and Transmission

The fungi *Coccidioides immitis* is limited to the San Joaquin Valley in California and parts of Arizona, hence the infection is also named San Joaquin fever or California disease, whereas *C. posadasii* has a more widespread geographic distribution in the Americas. However, recent analysis using molecular tools has demonstrated that these species have distinct but overlapping geographic ranges and have recently hybridised and exchanged genes [1].

Coccidioidomycosis is the second most common fungal infection in the United States and around 350 000 new cases of coccidioidomycosis occur each year [2]. Endemic regions are usually dry arid areas, characterised by hot summers and relatively short winters with limited rainfall. The infection usually follows a cyclical pattern with a period of dormancy in winter and spring, followed by growth in summer and autumn. Therefore, primary coccidioidal infection occurs most frequently in summer and autumn, following the rainy seasons. Most fungal growth occurs during the rainy season in alkaline soil, rich in carbon and salt content and at low altitudes.

After promotion of hyphal growth by the wet environment, arthroconidia, the infectious particles of *Coccidiodes* species, become air-borne during wind storms or on disruption of soil by construction or farming activities or by burrowing animals. Large outbreaks of coccidioidomycosis have occurred after dust storms, earthquakes and other events that disturb and aerosolise the soil [3]. Archaeological excavations and digging of soil containing the organism have been reported

Textbook of Zoonoses, First Edition. Jasbir Singh Bedi, Deepthi Vijay, and Pankaj Dhaka.

to result in local outbreaks. In addition, transmission has been reported to occur by contaminated fomites, such as dusty clothing and farm products. Because of the ease by which arthroconidia become air-borne, the organism is dangerous to laboratory personnel and epidemics have resulted even from the inadvertent opening of culture plates.

After inhalation of the conidia, they transform into spherules filled with endospores (2–5 μm) in the lungs and tissues. This spherule can burst in the tissues. releasing endospores, which can disseminate infection within the body. However, other theories suggest that small, soil-dwelling animals might serve as the primary environmental reservoir for *Coccidioides*. The fungus is an endozoan which is able to live in the granulomata of infected mammals and, upon death of the host, the fungus can use local nutrients released in the surrounding soil for nourishment [4, 5].

Disease in Animals

Dogs are the most severely affected species, but other animals including cats, rodents, cattle and sheep can develop naturally acquired infections. Clinical outcomes in dogs are similar to those of humans, with subclinical infections, mild-to-severe primary pulmonary disease and disseminated disease. Osteomyelitis is the most common form of disseminated disease in dogs, while skin lesions predominate in cats [6]. In cattle, the disease resembles tuberculosis with nodular lesions in the bronchial and mediastinal lymph nodes. Disseminated infection and abortion have been reported from horses [7]. Animal-to-human transmission of the disease is rare.

Disease in Humans

Valley fever is usually a self-limited illness with cough, fever, chest pain or fatigue; however, some persons develop severe disease and in rare cases, death occurs [8]. Asymptomatic infections occur in about 60% of primary infections and 90% of non-disseminated infections are self-limited.

The disease typically presents as acute and chronic pulmonary disease, but infection may also disseminate widely, especially to cutaneous, osseous and central nervous system sites. Those at risk of severe disease include adults aged over 65 years, pregnant women, transplant recipients and people with underlying immunosuppressive conditions and certain ethnicity (i.e. African Americans and Filipinos) [8]. Disseminated disease occurs in an estimated 1% of cases and commonly affects the musculoskeletal system, soft tissues and meninges in high-risk patients. Disseminated coccidioidomycosis causes serious illness with a prolonged disease course, permanent tissue damage and a fatality rate exceeding 40% despite treatment [9].

Diagnosis

Coccidioidomycosis is diagnosed by culture, serological testing (antibody and antigen detection), polymerase chain reaction (PCR) on body fluids or tissue, and histopathological examination (a characteristic spherule is seen in tissue).

Coccidioides is classified as a bioterrorism agent and the mould form is highly infectious and must be handled using biosafety level 3 precautions. Definitive diagnosis involves culture of the fungus on standard media, where the organism grows as a white fluffy mould with small septate hyphae and barrel-shaped arthroconidia. The large spherules are readily identified using KOH or calcofluor white preparations on sputum or bronchoalveolar lavage fluid or smears from skin lesions. However, the two species of *Coccidioides* are phenotypically identical and can only be identified by molecular methods.

Serology is the common method for the diagnosis of coccidioidomycosis, where the detection of tube precipitin antibodies (IgM) in response to the polysaccharide antigen of the fungal cell is observed in 90% of patients in the first 3 weeks after exposure. Complement-fixing IgG antibodies in response to chitinase protein develop in the chronic stage of the infection [10]. Direct assays for *Coccidioides* are also available, and the measurement of β-1,3-d-glucan (BDG), a non-specific fungal assay, is widely available in clinical laboratories.

Treatment

There is no vaccine available and the treatment regime depends on the site and severity of the infection. The course of treatment is prolonged and relapses are common. Meningitis cases are almost invariably fatal, if untreated.

Common antifungal agents used include the azole group (e.g. fluconazole, itraconazole, posaconazole, voriconazole) or amphotericin B. Patients with disseminated disease and meningitis potentially require lifelong suppressive antifungal treatment because of high relapse rates. Titres can be followed to monitor response to therapy. Reactivation of primary infections may occur, especially in HIV-positive or immunocompromised hosts.

Prevention and Control

As there is no vaccine for *Coccidioides* and the fungus is an environmental pathogen, public awareness in endemic regions and among groups at risk for severe disease can be helpful in earlier disease recognition and management. People who live in endemic areas, particularly those who are at high risk, must try to avoid spending time in dusty places like construction or excavation sites. Avoid activities that involve close contact with dirt or dust such as gardening and digging. In endemic regions, N95 respirator can be used to avoid breathing in the fungal spores and dust storms need to be avoided by staying indoors [9]. To avoid any chance of wound infection with the spores, skin injuries must be cleaned well with soap and water. Preventive antifungal medication for at-risk groups can be recommended at the discretion of the physician.

References

1 Neafsey, D.E., Barker, B.M., Sharpton, T.J. et al. (2010). Population genomic sequencing of Coccidioides fungi reveals recent hybridization and transposon control. *Genome Research* 20 (7): 938–946.

2 Chiller, T. (2019). *Overview of Endemic Mycoses. Vaccine Strategies for Endemic Fungal Pathogens.* Rockville, MD: NIAID.

3 Schaechter, M. (2009). *Encyclopedia of Microbiology*. New York: Academic Press.

4 Taylor, J.W. and Barker, B.M. (2019). The endozoan, small-mammal reservoir hypothesis and the life cycle of Coccidioides species. *Medical Mycology* 57 (Suppl 1): S16–S20.

5 Ampel, N.M. (2020). Coccidioidomycosis: changing concepts and knowledge gaps. *Journal of Fungi* 6 (4): 354.

6 Shubitz, L.F. (2007). Comparative aspects of coccidioidomycosis in animals and humans. *Annals of the New York Academy of Sciences* 1111 (1): 395–403.

7 Langham, R.F., Beneke, E.S., and Whitenack, D.L. (1977). Abortion in a mare due to coccidioidomycosis. *Journal of the American Veterinary Medical Association* 170: 178–179.

8 Hurd-Kundeti, G., Cooksey, G.L.S., Jain, S., and Vugia, D.J. (2020). Valley fever (coccidioidomycosis) awareness – California, 2016–2017. *Morbidity and Mortality Weekly Report* 69 (42): 1512.

9 Odio, C.D., Marciano, B.E., Galgiani, J.N., and Holland, S.M. (2017). Risk factors for disseminated coccidioidomycosis, United States. *Emerging Infectious Diseases* 23 (2): 308.

10 Akram, S.M. and Koirala, J. (2017). *Coccidioidomycosis*. Treasure Island, FL: StatPearls Publishing.

46

Cryptococcosis

Cryptococcosis is an opportunistic fungal infection with worldwide distribution which is caused by pathogenic encapsulated yeasts of the genus *Cryptococcus*. *Cryptococcus* is an encapsulated, melanin-forming, basidiomycetous yeast that exists as a saprobe in nature. The fungal infection shows a wide array of clinical presentations and is considered as a leading cause of meningitis in HIV patients [1].

Aetiology

The heterogeneous genus *Cryptococcus* includes over 70 different species although few are human fungal pathogens. As per the recent classification, the genus *Cryptococcus* comprises two species: *C. neoformans* and *C. gattii*, which are commonly associated with human cryptococcosis. The species *C. gattii* was initially called *C. neoformans* var. *gattii* because of its characteristic similarity to *C. neoformans*. However, in 2002, the species was reclassified as a single species because of differences in phenotype, biology and genetic taxonomy from *C. neoformans* [2]. The genus comprises five serotypes (based on structural differences in the polysaccharide capsule): serotypes A, D and AD of *C. neoformans* and B and C of *C. gattii*. The genus is further classified into various molecular types and subtypes that can be identified by various molecular typing tools such as multilocus sequence typing (MLST), whole-genome sequencing (WGS) and quantitative trait loci (QTL) mapping [3]. Further, *C. neoformans* currently consists of two varieties: *C. neoformans* var. *grubii* (serotype A) and *C. neoformans* var. *neoformans* (serotype D).

Epidemiology

The serotypes A, D and AD of *C. neoformans* tend to be widely distributed throughout the environment. These are commonly associated with soil enriched with nitrogen-rich guano, particularly pigeon excreta. *C. gattii* is mainly found in decaying woods and other plant materials, particularly in and around various species of trees like river red gum tree (*Eucalyptus camaldulensis*), and recently, carob and olive trees have also been suggested as additional important environmental niches for *C. gattii* strains [4].

Cryptococcus neoformans var. *grubii* (serotype A), having a worldwide geographical distribution, is responsible for about 95% of cryptococcal infections. The infections caused by *C. neoformans* (serotype D) or *C. gattii* (serotypes B/C strains) account for the remaining 4–5% of cases [5].

Textbook of Zoonoses, First Edition. Jasbir Singh Bedi, Deepthi Vijay, and Pankaj Dhaka.

C neoformans var. *neoformans* (serotype D) is primarily observed in European countries and *C. gattii* has historically been geographically restricted to tropical and subtropical regions, such as southern California, Hawaii, Brazil, Australia, South-East Asia and central Africa. More recently, *C. gattii* has been identified in temperate climates such as Vancouver Island and the Pacific Northwest region of the United States and parts of Europe [6].

Cryptococcus neoformans was first identified as a human pathogen in the late nineteenth century, but *C. gattii* was only recognised as a human pathogen in the late 1970s by Gattii and Eeckels [7]. The species *C. neoformans* is more commonly associated with immunocompromised AIDS patients, although infections have also been reported from apparently immunocompetent hosts. Immunocompetent patients are at more risk of infections caused by *C. gattii* [5].

Cryptococcal meningitis is becoming a crucial public health issue, with up to 1 million new infections annually, and significant attributable morbidity and mortality as it is a major opportunistic infection in HIV patients, resulting in over 80% mortality [8, 9]. The incidence of cryptococcosis is decreasing in developed countries due to the availability of antiretroviral therapy. Although cryptococcosis cases in HIV-infected patients have been decreasing, an increase in the number of cases have been observed in non-HIV patients with haematological malignancies, organ transplant recipients and patients affected by autoimmune diseases [10].

Transmission

The cryptococcal infection is usually acquired by inhalation of the yeast into the lungs from an environmental source, such as soil contaminated with avian guano (for *C. neoformans* var. *neoformans* and var. *grubii*) or eucalyptus trees and decaying wood (for *C. gattii*). Viable *Cryptococcus* have been isolated from dried soil particles measuring less than 2 μm in diameter, and these small particles can easily become air-borne. The organism can colonise the respiratory tract without producing any symptoms and can be cleared or may enter a dormant stage. The yeast cells are also able to penetrate the pulmonary alveoli and disseminate through the bloodstream, causing soft tissue infections, pneumonia and most often meningoencephalitis [3]. In immunosuppressed individuals, fungi can reactivate and result in disseminated infections.

Disease in Animals

Naturally acquired infections occur in domestic animals, such as cats, dogs, cattle, pigs, rabbits, sheep and horses, wildlife species such as koalas and feral ungulates, and in many terrestrial and aquatic placental mammals, including marsupials, reptiles, amphibians and fishes. However, neither animal-to-human nor human-to-human infections have been reported. Cryptococcosis is usually a sporadic disease in individual animals and rarely in several animals at the same time in the same place. In animals, infection usually begins with involvement of the nasal cavity, paranasal tissues and lungs, and then disseminates into different organs, especially the skin, eyes and central nervous system.

Disease in Humans

In humans, the infection is mainly acquired through inhalation of desiccated yeast cells or basidiospores into the lungs. Cryptococcosis follows aspergillosis and candidiasis in frequency for invasive fungal infections and accounts for up to 7% of invasive fungal infections in solid organ transplant recipients [11].

Generally, *Cryptococcus* is recognised by its ability to cause meningoencephalitis, but the fungus can infect almost any organ in humans, with pulmonary infection being the second most common manifestation [12]. *C. neoformans* infections are usually characterised by dizziness, headache, nausea, changes in behaviour, impaired vision or hearing, coma or seizures. Most of the symptoms are due to meningoencephalitis with low immune response in HIV-infected patients. In *C. gatti* infection, brain and lung granulomas can be observed. Cryptococcal pneumonia is not clinically distinctive. Skin lesions such as ulcerated papules with exudates rich in cryptococci are found in disseminated infections in around 5% of patients, irrespective of HIV infection status. Bones and joints usually demonstrate osteolytic lesions and cold abscesses, and there is frequent lymph node involvement. Occasionally, keratitis, endocarditis, peritonitis and myositis have been reported.

Diagnosis

The presence of encapsulated yeasts under direct microscopic examination from clinical specimens such as CSF, urine, blood, sputum or brochoalveolar lavage, together with cryptococcal antigen testing in serum and CSF, are useful for diagnosis. The slow *in vitro* growth of the fungi in culture makes identification of cryptococcal infections difficult. The presence of virulence determinants such as polysaccharide capsule rich in glucuronoxylomannan, formation of melanin and urease activity distinguishes them from other pathogenic yeasts such as *Candida* [3]. The identification of *Cryptococcus* sp. can be confirmed by urease-positive yeast on Sabouraud dextrose agar, brain heart infusion agar and brown colonies on Niger seed agar.

Commonly used diagnostic tests such as India ink staining and antigen kit testing are relatively fast but cannot distinguish between the two species of *Cryptococcus*. Molecular tools such as polymerase chain reaction (PCR), matrix-assisted laser desorption/ionisation time-of-flight mass spectrometry (MALDI-TOF MS), gene chips and sequencing techniques are widely used for identification of *Cryptococcus* spp. from clinical specimens and can distinguish between *C. neoformans* and *C. gattii*. Novel methods such as use of positively charged silver nanoparticles as a substrate to distinguish between *C. neoformans* and *C. gattii* in clinical specimens directly via surface-enhanced Raman scattering (SERS) and spectral analysis have reported an accuracy of 100% after a 10-fold cross-over validation [7].

Treatment

Early diagnosis and treatment of cryptococcal meningitis is key to reduce mortality from cryptococcal disease. Assessment of disease severity, extent of dissemination such as CNS involvement or acute respiratory syndrome, and use of antigen titres decide the treatment course. Patients with asymptomatic infections or mild-to-moderate pulmonary infections can be treated with fluconazole. The severe disseminated form of cryptococcosis can be treated with amphotericin B and flucytosine.

Prevention and Control

Since the fungal spores are present in the environment in many regions of the world, regular targeted screening and pre-emptive antifungal therapy with fluconazole prophylaxis offer great promise in preventing cryptococcosis among at-risk populations in endemic areas. In addition, precautions to prevent the inhalation of fungal spores in endemic regions are important for susceptible populations. Avoidance of areas with dust that contain bird faeces may also help in preventing infections due to *C. neoformans*. Trees like eucalyptus and gum trees release propagules in higher concentration in endemic regions, which need to be avoided by at-risk groups.

References

1 Spadari, C.D.C., Wirth, F., Lopes, L.B., and Ishida, K. (2020). New approaches for cryptococcosis treatment. *Microorganisms 8* (4): 613.

2 Kwon-Chung, K.J., Boekhout, T., Fell, J.W., and Diaz, M. (2002). Proposal to conserve the name *Cryptococcus gattii* against *C. hondurianus* and *C. bacillisporus* (Basidiomycota, Hymenomycetes, Tremellomycetidae). *Taxon 51* (4): 804–806.

3 Kwon-Chung, K.J., Fraser, J.A., Doering, T.L. et al. (2014). *Cryptococcus neoformans* and *Cryptococcus gattii*, the etiologic agents of cryptococcosis. *Cold Spring Harbor Perspectives in Medicine 4* (7): a019760.

4 Danesi, P., Falcaro, C., Schmertmann, L.J. et al. (2021). *Cryptococcus* in wildlife and free-living mammals. *Journal of Fungi 7* (1): 29.

5 Maziarz, E.K. and Perfect, J.R. (2016). Cryptococcosis. *Infectious Disease Clinics 30* (1): 179–206.

6 Cogliati, M. (2013). Global molecular epidemiology of Cryptococcus neoformans and *Cryptococcus gattii*: an atlas of the molecular types. *Scientifica 2013*: 675213.

7 Hu, S., Gu, F., Chen, M. et al. (2020). A novel method for identifying and distinguishing *Cryptococcus neoformans* and *Cryptococcus gattii* by surface-enhanced Raman scattering using positively charged silver nanoparticles. *Scientific Reports 10* (1): 1–9.

8 Hagen, F., Khayhan, K., Theelen, B. et al. (2015). Recognition of seven species in the *Cryptococcus gattii/Cryptococcus neoformans* species complex. *Fungal Genetics and Biology 78*: 16–48.

9 Rajasingham, R., Smith, R.M., Park, B.J. et al. (2017). Global burden of disease of HIV-associated cryptococcal meningitis: an updated analysis. *Lancet Infectious Diseases 17* (8): 873–881.

10 Henao-Martínez, A.F. and Beckham, J.D. (2015). Cryptococcosis in solid organ transplant recipients. *Current Opinion in Infectious Diseases 28* (4): 300–307.

11 Pappas, P.G., Alexander, B.D., Andes, D.R. et al. (2010). Invasive fungal infections among organ transplant recipients: results of the Transplant-Associated Infection Surveillance Network (TRANSNET). *Clinical Infectious Diseases 50* (8): 1101–1111.

12 Zavala, S. and Baddley, J.W. (2020). Cryptococcosis. *Seminars in Respiratory and Critical Care Medicine 41* (01): 69–79.

47

Dermatophytosis

Dermatophytosis is caused by a group of highly specialised pathogenic fungi collectively referred to as 'dermatophytes' (literally meaning 'plants that live on skin'), which are the common agents of superficial mycoses in animals and humans. In 1841, David Gruby was the first person to demonstrate that an infection of the scalp called favus (Latin for 'honeycomb'), characterised by thick yellow honeycomb-like crust over hair follicles, was caused by a fungus.

Earlier, all pathogenic dermatophytes were classified into three genera: *Microsporum, Trichophyton* and *Epidermophyton*. However, with the advancement of diagnostic techniques, these dermatophytes were recently classified into six genera, with *Nannizzia, Lophophyton* and *Arthroderma* as the three new genera [1]. Dermatophytosis is also referred to as ringworm or tinea (Latin for 'worm') because of the classic ring-shaped patches that they cause, which are usually red and itchy, with worm-like borders. It causes infection of the stratum corneum of the epidermis and keratinised tissues such as skin, hair and nails of humans and animals. Some dermatophytes are adapted to humans (anthropophilic species) and are usually transmitted from person to person, e.g. *Trichophyton tonsurans*, *T. rubrum* complex, etc. Zoophilic species are adapted to animals. These zoophilic dermatophytes (e.g. *Microsporum canis*, *T. equinum*) may result in zoonoses when humans are exposed to these organisms [2]. A few geophilic species normally live in the environment, but occasionally act as parasites, e.g. *M. gypseum* and *M. nanum*.

Epidemiology and Transmission

Dermatophytosis is an important occupational mycozoonosis of dairymen, animal handlers, livestock farmers, pet owners, veterinarians, etc., where the disease is associated with huge socioeconomic losses. Unsanitary conditions as well as dietary deficiencies play a key role in the pathogenesis of dermatophytosis. The prevalence of superficial mycoses caused by zoophilic dermatophytes was found to be high especially in tropical countries with warm and humid climate, crowded living and poor sanitary conditions [3]. Generally, human infection results from direct contact with an infected animal, but may also be acquired indirectly through contact with contaminated environments, such as fungus-bearing hair and scales from infected animals.

The majority of zoonotic dermatophytes are caused by four species:

- *Microsporum canis* (usually derived from pet animals, particularly cats and dogs)
- *Trichophyton verrucosum* (usually derived from cattle)
- *Arthroderma vanbreuseghemii* (usually derived from cats and dogs)
- *Arthroderma benhamiae* (usually derived from guinea-pigs).

Textbook of Zoonoses, First Edition. Jasbir Singh Bedi, Deepthi Vijay, and Pankaj Dhaka.

People and animals become infected after contact with spores (conidia). Dermatophytes growing in a vertebrate host normally form only arthrospores (arthroconidia), the asexual spores that develop within the hyphae. In the environment and in laboratory culture, they can also produce microconidia and macroconidia, the asexual spores that develop outside the hyphae.

Clinical Signs

The pathogenicity of dermatophytes depends on their ability to produce enzymes, such as proteinases, collagenase and keratinases. Initially, the dermatophyte infects growing hair or the stratum corneum of the skin. These organisms do not usually invade resting hairs, since the essential nutrients they need for growth are absent or limited. Hyphae spread in the hairs and keratinised skin, eventually developing infectious arthrospores.

In Animals

Ringworm affects a wide variety of animals where the lesion appears as dry, grey, scaly patches. In dogs, *M. canis*, *M. gypseum* and *T. mentagrophytes* are mainly responsible for lesions like alopecia, broken hair, folliculitis and pustules. *M. canis* is responsible for the majority of cases in cats which results in focal alopecia, scaling and crusting [3]. In cattle and small ruminants, fungi like *T. verrucosum*, *T. mentagrophytes*, *M. gypseum*, etc. are associated with skin lesions. *T. equinum* is mainly associated with crust lesions in horses. In pigs, *M. nanum* produces rings of inflammation and brown discolouration.

In Humans

The incubation period varies from several days to weeks. The characteristic ring is typically observed in humans. Tinea infections in people are named after the area they infect. Some of the examples are provided below:

- Tinea barbae: ringworm of the beard (also known as barber's itch)
- Tinea capitis: ringworm of scalp
- Tinea corporis: ringworm of body
- Tinea cruris: ringworm of the groin (also known as jock itch)
- Tinea imbricata (or tokelau): characterised by the appearance of homogeneous sheets or concentric rings of scaling that may cover large areas of the body
- Tinea pedis: ringworm of feet (also known as athlete's foot)
- Tinea unguium: ringworm of the nail (also known as onychomycosis)

Diagnosis

Diagnosis is mainly based on the history, physical examination and microscopic examination of scrapings and hairs from the lesions. Other techniques such as Wood's lamp examination and histology of the tissues are also employed. A Wood's light emits 253.7 nm of ultraviolet light, which causes the tryptophan metabolites produced by some dermatophytes (e.g. *M. canis* and *Trichophyton quinckeanum*) to emit a bright apple green fluorescence.

Dermatophytes can often be detected by microscopic examination of infected hairs and skin or nail scrapings. Skin scrapings should be taken from the edge of the lesion, and hairs should be plucked (not cut) from this area. The best hairs to select are those that fluoresce under a Wood's lamp, or are broken or scaly. Nail scrapings are generally taken from the nail bed, or from deeper portions of the nail after removing the outer layers (except in cases where the infection is entirely superficial). Samples are usually cleaned with potassium hydroxide (KOH) or other agents to help visualise the organism. Various stains such as chlorazol black E, Parker blue-black ink, Swartz-Lamkin stain or Congo red stain may be added. Fluorescence microscopy, using calcofluor white or other stains, can also be used to visualise dermatophyte structures. Fungal cultures, which identify the species of dermatophyte, can be useful in understanding the source of infection and targeting preventive measures.

Culture may be necessary if the diagnosis is uncertain or the infection is resistant to standard treatment. Samples for culture include hair, skin and nails. Colonies appear in 5 days to 4 weeks, depending on the organism. Media commonly used include Sabouraud agar, but dermatophyte test medium or other fungal culture media can also be used for isolation. Bromocresol purple-milk solids glucose agar can be used for differentiation of *T. rubrum* and *T. mentagrophytes*.

Histology (biopsy) is occasionally helpful, especially in deep mycoses and some infections of the nails. The organisms are visualised best with periodic acid–Schiff (PAS) staining, although they may also be found in haematoxylin-eosin-stained preparations. Dermatophytes are closely related and morphologically similar, so are difficult to differentiate by histology. However, different species have unique macroconidia (large, multinuclear asexual spore), microconidia (small, single-celled asexual spore), and hyphae (filaments). For example:

- *Microsporum* spp. produce thick-walled, rough macroconidia and fewer microconidia
- *Trichophyton* spp. produce thin-walled, smooth macroconidia and numerous microconidia
- *Epidermophyton* spp. produce smooth, ovoid, clustered macroconidia and no microconidia.

Molecular diagnostic techniques like PCR assays for the diagnosis of dermatophytosis have evolved significantly over recent years, and are useful for rapid diagnosis of fungal strains.

Treatment

Various treatment options are available for dermatophytosis which can be used as monotherapy, combination therapy or sequential therapy. Dermatophytoses can be treated topically. Whitfield's ointment, which contains 3% salicylic acid and 3% benzoic acid, is a weak antifungal agent but is inexpensive and effective in treating all dermatophyte infections apart from scalp or nail disease, or kerion. Other treatment regimens involve primarily oral and/or topical formulations of azoles or allylamines, particularly itraconazole and terbinafine. Specific groups, such as pregnant women, children and the elderly, frequently require modified treatment algorithms due to their increased propensity for unacceptable adverse effects. Topical azoles are minimally or not absorbed systemically, and therefore can be prescribed at any stage of pregnancy. In extensive infections and infections that are refractory to topical therapy, oral treatment with agents such as terbinafine, itraconazole, fluconazole and griseofulvin is used. For tinea pedis, imidazole or tolnaftate powders may be used prophylactically [4].

Relapse of infection remains a problem, particularly with tinea pedis/unguium. Therefore, appropriate follow-up duration and education of patients on proper hygiene are important components in providing effective therapy [5].

Prevention and Control

Prevention and control measures for zoonotic dermatophytes include treatment of infected animals and disinfection of premises and fomites. Contact with infected animals should be limited, and gloves and protective clothing should be used if these animals are handled. Fungal colonisation is favoured by moisture, so keeping skin and hair clean and dry helps to minimise the infection. Better surveillance, improved living conditions and improved treatments can decrease the overall prevalence of anthropophilic dermatophytes, while hygiene and prevention of contact are helpful in individual cases.

References

1. de Hoog, G.S., Dukik, K., Monod, M. et al. (2017). Toward a novel multilocus phylogenetic taxonomy for the dermatophytes. *Mycopathologia* 182 (1–2): 5–31.
2. Moretti, A., Agnetti, F., Mancianti, F. et al. (2013). Dermatophytosis in animals: epidemiological, clinical and zoonotic aspects. *Giornale italiano di dermatologia e venereologia* 148 (6): 563–572.
3. Fehr, M. (2015). Zoonotic potential of dermatophytosis in small mammals. *Journal of Exotic Pet Medicine* 24 (3): 308–316.
4. Kaul, S., Yadav, S., and Dogra, S. (2017). Treatment of dermatophytosis in elderly, children, and pregnant women. *Indian Dermatology Online Journal* 8 (5): 310.
5. Begum, J., Mir, N.A., Lingaraju, M.C. et al. (2020). Recent advances in the diagnosis of dermatophytosis. *Journal of Basic Microbiology* 60 (4): 293–303.

48

Histoplasmosis

Histoplasmosis is a widely distributed non-contagious systemic fungal infection caused by *Histoplasma capsulatum*, a dimorphic fungus with two known varieties: *H. capsulatum* var. *capsulatum* and *H. capsulatum* var. *duboisii*. The disease was first described by Samuel Darling in the Canal Zone in Panama in 1906, where patients were described with clinical features suggestive of disseminated tuberculosis [1]. Darling named the organism *Histoplasma capsulatum* because the small yeasts within the cytoplasm of macrophages resembled encapsulated parasites.

Epidemiology

Cases of *H. capsulatum* var. *capsulatum* are sporadically distributed around the world. The disease is highly prevalent in areas along the Mississippi and Ohio valleys in the United States and in Central and South America. It is also endemic in India and South-East Asia. In the tropics, conditions that support the growth of *H. capsulatum* occur in bat roosting sites, including caves, where exposure in the confined space has resulted in epidemics. Infections are associated with outdoor activities and exposure to starling roost or soil upheaval.

H. capsulatum var. *duboisii* is mainly restricted to West and Central Africa and Madagascar, and the clinical condition caused by this fungus is often referred as African histoplasmosis, which is a misnomer because African patients can be infected with both variants of the fungus.

Transmission

Histoplasmosis is a disease originating from soil, i.e. infections often occur after human disruption of the soil that aerosolises the hyphae and conidia of the organism originating from the soil containing bat or bird guano (rich sources of nitrogen and phosphate compounds) [2]. *H. capsulatum* grows in its mycelial form at lower temperatures (25–30 °C). This phase is the saprobic state found in the environment which is characterised by hyphae with slender conidiophores and characteristic tuberculate macroconidia. When inhaled by mammalian hosts, the microconidia and short hyphal fragments of *Histoplasma* reach the alveoli, followed by rapid conversion to the yeast form that can persist in host tissues and may disseminate through the bloodstream and lymphatics to other organs, causing histoplasmosis. Occupational exposure to the fungus can occur during construction works, demolition drives, excavation and caving activities, as well as recreational ecotourism practices in endemic regions [3].

Textbook of Zoonoses, First Edition. Jasbir Singh Bedi, Deepthi Vijay, and Pankaj Dhaka.

Disease in Animals

Histoplasmosis have been reported in several species of small mammals, including wild rats and opossums [4]. The demonstration of histoplasmosis in animals helps to establish endemicity of the disease in a given area.

The disease is commonly reported among pet dogs and cats. In these companion animals, the infection may be clinically unapparent or develop into an acute or chronic disease, with local granulomatous response in the respiratory tract or fungal dissemination through lymphatic and haematogenous routes. Clinical signs in cats, such as weakness, lethargy, emaciation, ocular signs, skeletal involvement, fever, anorexia and respiratory signs, are often chronic and non-specific despite disseminated disease. Transmission of the fungus from companion animals to humans has never been reported. However, infected pets may act as sentinels for human exposure, and this is especially relevant if the animal resides with immunocompromised human beings.

Disease in Humans

Disease prognosis depends on host immune response, fungal inoculum size inhaled and fungal virulence. The primary attack site of fungal infection is the lung with affinity for the reticuloendothelial system.

The clinical forms of disease due to *H. capsulatum* var. *capsulatum* are also known with various synonyms including Darling' disease, American histoplasmosis, Ohio River valley fever, classic histoplasmosis and small form histoplasmosis [4]. *H. capsulatum* var. *capsulatum* generally causes subclinical infection in persons from endemic areas. However, after high exposure, acute primary pulmonary histoplasmosis (APPH) can develop even among immunocompetent hosts. The acute form is manifested by non-productive cough, dyspnoea, hoarseness, chest pain, cyanosis associated with fever, night sweats, muscle/joint pain, weight loss, malaise and fatigue. In patients with underlying chronic obstructive pulmonary disease, chronic cavitary pulmonary histoplasmosis may occur. Debilitated or immunocompromised persons can present with disseminated disease, where the clinical discourse varies from a fulminant, fatal disease marked by shock to a subacute disease with little systemic inflammation and localised organ-specific signs and symptoms [5]. Immunocompromised individuals, especially acquired immunodeficiency syndrome (AIDS) patients undergoing corticosteroid or other immunosuppressive therapy, can develop more severe forms of the disease due to fungal dissemination to several organs.

Infections caused by *H. capsulatum* var. *duboisii* (also known as African histoplasmosis and large form histoplasmosis) classically present with cutaneous and skeletal involvement. Skin lesions usually present as small papules that can develop an umbilicated centre, nodules, abscesses or ulcers. The underlying bone deposits are common in cases of large lesions.

Diagnosis

The demonstration of the yeast-like *H. capsulatum* cells on microscopic examination of fluids and tissue samples using specific staining techniques and the isolation of the fungus from culture of clinical specimens remain the gold standard method for the diagnosis of histoplasmosis. Staining of a paraffin-embedded clot section of bone marrow aspirate by periodic acid–Schiff (PAS), Gomori methenamine stain (GMS), Giemsa and Wright stains allows visualisation in granulomas.

However, these methodologies may require invasive medical procedures to obtain clinical specimens, and the culture test is time-consuming, requiring up to 8 weeks to reveal fungal growth and conversion to the yeast form.

As a result, alternative methods have been used as complementary diagnostic tools to detect anti-*Histoplasma* antibodies or *Histoplasma* antigens. These methods are less invasive and have greater sensitivity. Detection of galactomannan of *H. capsulatum* in serum, bronchoalveolar lavage and urine can be used in the diagnosis and therapeutic monitoring of disseminated histoplasmosis, particularly in HIV-infected patients. Complement fixation against the yeast phase is sensitive, and immunoprecipitating antibodies to the H antigen are specific for detection of the fungus.

Molecular methods using nucleic acid probes are currently under development for widespread application in clinical laboratories [6].

Treatment

Treatment of pulmonary histoplasmosis depends on the immune status of the host and extent of disease. Amphotericin B is the drug of choice for severe, refractory or relapsing infections; while the azoles (particularly itraconazole) have a prolonged treatment schedule.

Prevention and Control

In endemic regions, it can be difficult to avoid inhalation of *Histoplasma* spores through environmental exposure. However, susceptible individuals with weakened immune systems should avoid activities such as cleaning chicken coops, visiting bat-infested caves or other such sites, excavation, demolition and remodelling of old buildings, and cutting of dead trees which can lead to disruption of soil containing the organism and aerosolisation of microconidia.

References

1 Darling, S.T. (1908). Histoplasmosis: a fatal infectious disease resembling kala-azar found among natives of tropical America. *Archives of Internal Medicine 2* (2): 107–123.

2 Colombo, A.L., Tobon, A., Restrepo, A. et al. (2011). Epidemiology of endemic systemic fungal infections in Latin America. *Medical Mycology 49* (8): 785–798.

3 de Abreu Almeida, M., Almeida-Silva, F., Guimarães, A.J. et al. (2019). The occurrence of histoplasmosis in Brazil: a systematic review. *International Journal of Infectious Diseases 86*: 147–156.

4 Randhawa, H.S. and Gugnani, H.C. (2018). Occurrence of histoplasmosis in the Indian subcontinent: an overview and update. *Journal of Medical Research and Practice 7* (3): 71–83.

5 Deepe, G.S. and Buesing, W.R. (2012). Deciphering the pathways of death of histoplasma capsulatum-infected macrophages: implications for the immunopathogenesis of early infection. *Journal of Immunology 188* (1): 334–344.

6 Azar, M.M. and Hage, C.A. (2017). Laboratory diagnostics for histoplasmosis. *Journal of Clinical Microbiology 55* (6): 1612–1620.

49

Mucormycoses

Aetiology

The term 'mucormycoses' is used to describe a spectrum of infections caused by fungi of the order Mucorales of the class Zygomycetes. Mucormycosis (also known as zygomycosis and deadly black fungus infection) can be a serious life-threatening infection which is mainly associated with haematological malignancies, haematopoietic stem cell transplantation, solid organ transplantation, etc. [1]. The common agents causing mucormycosis are *Rhizopus* spp., *Mucor* spp., *Rhizomucor* spp. and *Leichtheimia* spp. The disease is characterised by extensive necrotising vasculitis, resulting in thrombosis and subsequent tissue infarction.

Transmission

Mucormycosis is a rare fungal infection caused by exposure to mucor mould commonly found in soil, manure, plants, decaying fruits and vegetables, air and even in the mucus of healthy people. The main modes of infection of mucormycosis is inhalation of spores, consumption of contaminated food and inoculation of the fungi into abrasions or cuts on the skin [2]. In addition, nosocomial outbreaks have been linked to contamination of medical devices, ventilation systems and hospital disposables [3]. Some notable risk factors for infection include diabetes, neutropenia, organ or stem cell transplantation, trauma and burns, haematological disorders, steroid use, metabolic acidosis, intravenous drug usage, renal insufficiency, increase in iron in the system, malnutrition, usage of broad-spectrum antibiotics, voriconazole, etc. However, the fungus does not spread from contact with infected humans or animals.

Disease in Humans

The primary site and discourse of infection vary according to the different genera included in the order *Mucorales* as well as with the underlying immune status of the patient [4]. The infection can affect the sinus, brain and lungs and can be life-threatening in diabetic or severely immunocompromised individuals. In immunocompromised patients, Mucorales have a tropism for angioinvasion, resulting in dissemination, tissue infarction and necrosis. In contrast, the cutaneous disease rarely disseminates and is associated with less severe outcomes. Based on the location of their occurrence, mucormycosis can be classified into six forms: rhino-orbital cerebral mucormycosis (ROCM), pulmonary, cutaneous,

Textbook of Zoonoses, First Edition. Jasbir Singh Bedi, Deepthi Vijay, and Pankaj Dhaka.

gastrointestinal, disseminated and uncommon sites [3]. Although mucormycosis represents a rare disease, its consequences can be devastating in terms of high mortality rates, ranging from 20% to 50% in localised infections and up to 70–90% with disseminated disease [5]

An upsurge in cases of mucormycosis (black fungus infection) was observed in India and nearby South Asian countries during the COVID-19 pandemic. Studies indicated that patients hospitalised for COVID-19 and particularly those who require oxygen therapy and corticosteroid treatment are at much higher risk of mucormycosis [6]. Earlier symptoms include greyish-black pigmentation in the nose or oral cavity and blockage of the nasal cavity. Lodgement of fungal spores near the eyes leads to ocular swelling, and a few patients may get lesions over the cheeks. At a later stage, this fungus can make its way to the brain, resulting in fatality rates of up to 50%.

Diagnosis

Early diagnosis and prompt treatment and surgical debridement (as needed) are crucial for improving outcomes of patients with mucormycosis. Common diagnostic methods include biopsy and fungal staining (KOH mount). Culture of clinical specimens (e.g. tissue, bronchoalveolar lavage fluid (BAL)) on standard medium is considered the gold standard test. Imaging tests such as CT scan of lungs, sinuses or other parts of body, depending on the location of the suspected infection, may also be used to support the diagnosis. Recently, non-invasive PCR-based procedures have been used to detect Mucorales DNA in samples such as plasma or serum or even urine. Mucorales may now be reliably identified using matrix-assisted laser desorption ionisation–time of flight mass spectrometry (MALDI-TOF MS) techniques.

Treatment

Mucormycosis is difficult to treat. It may sometimes require both intravenous antifungal therapy and surgical excision, thus necessitating a multidisciplinary team approach in a facility setting. Liposomal amphotericin B is the drug of choice and needs to be initiated early. Other antifungals like posaconazole or isavuconazole have also been described for treatment [7].

Prevention and Control

It is difficult to avoid breathing in fungal spores because the fungi that cause mucormycosis are common in the environment. There is no vaccine to prevent mucormycosis. People who have weakened immune systems may adopt preventive measures including the following.

- Try to avoid areas with lots of dust such as construction or excavation sites. If such visits are unavoidable, use an N95 respirator.
- Avoid activities that involve close contact with soil or dust, such as gardening. If this is not possible, then wear protective shoes, gloves, long trousers and long-sleeved shirts during outdoor activities.
- To reduce the chances of developing a skin infection, clean skin injuries with disinfectant soap and water, especially if they have been exposed to soil or dust.

Prevention of COVID-associated mucormycosis needs to focus on addressing the underlying risk factors [7], such as better glycaemic control among diabetic patients, appropriate use of systemic corticosteroids and prevention of unnecessary use of antibiotics, antifungals and other immunomodulators. Other infection prevention and control (IPC) measures at the hospital facility level are essential to prevent the environmental spread of this pathogen. These methods include [7]:

- proper sterilisation and disinfection of equipment used by multiple patients (tracheal tubes, ventilators) and ventilation systems (poor ventilation in the hospital can contribute to dampness and dust)
- proper wound management (bandage, tape, adhesives, ostomy devices must be sterilised and changed regularly)
- proper line management in health facilities.

References

1 Jeong, W., Keighley, C., Wolfe, R. et al. (2019). The epidemiology and clinical manifestations of mucormycosis: a systematic review and meta-analysis of case reports. *Clinical Microbiology and Infection 25* (1): 26–34.

2 Mahalaxmi, I., Jayaramayya, K., Venkatesan, D. et al. (2021). Mucormycosis: an opportunistic pathogen during COVID-19. *Environmental Research 201*: 111643.

3 Simbli, M., Hakim, F., Koudieh, M., and Tleyjeh, I.M. (2008). Nosocomial post-traumatic cutaneous mucormycosis: a systematic review. *Scandinavian Journal of Infectious Diseases 40* (6-7): 577–582.

4 Serris, A., Danion, F., and Lanternier, F. (2019). Disease entities in mucormycosis. *Journal of Fungi 5* (1): 23.

5 Sipsas, N.V., Gamaletsou, M.N., Anastasopoulou, A., and Kontoyiannis, D.P. (2018). Therapy of mucormycosis. *Journal of Fungi 4* (3): 90.

6 Singh, A.K., Singh, R., Joshi, S.R., and Misra, A. (2021). Mucormycosis in COVID-19: a systematic review of cases reported worldwide and in India. *Diabetes & Metabolic Syndrome: Clinical Research & Reviews 15* (4): 102146.

7 World Health Organization (2021). Mucormycosis fact sheet. www.who.int/india/emergencies/coronavirus-disease-(covid-19)/mucormycosis (accessed 17 February 2021)

50 Sporotrichosis

Aetiology

Sporotrichosis (also known as rose gardener's disease) is caused by several species of *Sporothrix*, such as *Sporothrix schenckii*, *S. braziliensis* and *S. globosa*, which are widely distributed as soil saprophytes. The classic species *S. schenckii* have worldwide distribution, especially in tropical and subtropical zones, with endemicity in Japan, India, Mexico, Brazil, Uruguay and Peru [1]. The recently described species *S. brasiliensis* and *S. globosa* are prevalent in South America and East Asia, respectively.

Transmission

Sporothrix schenckii resides naturally as a saprophyte on decaying vegetation, animal excreta and soil. Infection generally occurs through traumatic inoculation of soil, plants and/or organic matter contaminated with the fungus. Occupational and leisure activities such as horticulture, gardening, fishing, hunting, farming, mining and others that facilitate exposure to the fungus are mainly associated with transmission of sporotrichosis. Zoonotic transmission to humans is not considered as the predominant mode of transmission [2]. However, from the early 2000s, cases of sporotrichosis have also been associated with animal scratches and bites, mainly felines [3]. The presence of infected felines in densely populated urban areas precedes human infection, and is also associated with increased numbers of cases. As cat transmission to humans is the most common form of zoonotic sporotrichosis, veterinarians, and cat owners are considered as populations at risk of infection.

Disease in Animals

In dogs and cats, three distinct presentations are recognised: the localized or fixed cutaneous form, the cutaneous-lymphatic form and the disseminated form. The cutaneous form is the most commonly reported, in which multiple firm nodules, ulcerated plaques with raised borders or annular crusted and alopecic areas are present, especially on the head, pinnae and trunk. The cutaneous-lymphatic form involves the skin, subcutaneous tissues and lymphatics. The disseminated form usually occurs as a rare sequel to the cutaneous-lymphatic form. In these

Textbook of Zoonoses, First Edition. Jasbir Singh Bedi, Deepthi Vijay, and Pankaj Dhaka.

cases, liver and lungs are the primary sites of dissemination. The spleen, kidneys, eyes, central nervous system, gastrointestinal tract and mammary gland have also been reported as sites of dissemination [4].

Disease in Humans

Sporotrichosis is a chronic fungal infection principally affecting the skin, lymphatics and subcutaneous tissues. The pulmonary and disseminated forms, with the involvement of the lungs, osteoarticular and musculoskeletal tissues, viscera, mucous membranes and central nervous system (CNS), are rare.

The most common form is lymphocutaneous, in which a small, firm, movable subcutaneous nodule develops at the site of inoculation. The nodule later becomes soft and breaks down to form a persistent friable ulcer or chancre. Mostly the lesions remain localised, but disseminated cutaneous lesions have been reported in immunocompromised patients with AIDS.

Diagnosis

Classic cutaneous lymphatic sporotrichosis is distinctive but the variability of other forms can make diagnosis difficult.

Direct mycological examination using potassium hydroxide (KOH) or differential staining has low sensitivity for the diagnosis of human sporotrichosis due to the scarcity of fungal elements in the lesions, particularly in lymphocutaneous and fixed cutaneous forms. However, Gram, Giemsa, periodic acid–Schiff (PAS) and Grocott-Gomori (silver) staining can be successfully used in disseminated manifestations. On the other hand, in feline sporotrichosis, there is a high fungal load in the lesions favouring direct examination for rapid diagnosis of the disease.

The gold standard for diagnosing *Sporothrix* is conventional culture of clinical specimens obtained from active lesions, pus, secretions or biopsy. Samples are cultured on Sabouraud agar which may be followed by antifungal susceptibility testing and additional phenotypic characterisation on a case-by-case basis. Phenotypic identification often requires 7–14 days for culture and 10–21 additional days for physiological assays. Moreover, morphological characteristics are insufficiently diagnostic for clinically relevant species. Molecular tools are required for the recognition of cryptic entities.

Molecular assays based on species-specific DNA amplification can easily detect *Sporothrix* sp. from clinical samples or small amounts of cells in culture, thereby improving sensitivity and considerably shortening the time required for identification to a few hours.

Treatment

Most cases of sporotrichosis are not life-threatening and only involve the skin or tissues underneath the skin. However, these lesions must be treated with appropriate antifungal medicines such as itraconazole. Supersaturated potassium iodide is also a treatment option for skin sporotrichosis. In cases of severe disseminated infection, intravenous amphotericin B medicine is recommended followed by azole antifungal treatment. Individuals with pulmonary sporotrichosis may also need surgery to cut away the infected tissue.

Prevention and Control

There are no available vaccines to prevent sporotrichosis. Susceptible individuals can reduce the risk of sporotrichosis by wearing protective clothing such as gloves and long sleeves when handling wires, rose bushes, bales of hay, pine seedlings or other materials that may cause minor cuts or punctures in the skin. It is also advisable to screen pets for sporotrichosis and avoid skin contact with suspected infectious pets in endemic areas.

References

1 Barros, M.B.D.L., de Almeida Paes, R., and Schubach, A.O. (2011). *Sporothrix schenckii* and Sporotrichosis. *Clinical Microbiology Reviews 24* (4): 633–654.

2 Barros, M.B.D.L., Schubach, A.D.O., do Valle, A.C.F. et al. (2004). Cat-transmitted sporotrichosis epidemic in Rio de Janeiro, Brazil: description of a series of cases. *Clinical Infectious Diseases 38* (4): 529–535.

3 Conceição-Silva, F. and Morgado, F.N. (2018). Immunopathogenesis of human sporotrichosis: what we already know. *Journal of Fungi 4* (3): 89.

4 Mascarenhas, M.B., Lopes, N.L., Pinto, T.G. et al. (2018). Canine sporotrichosis: report of 15 advanced cases. *Pesquisa Veterinária Brasileira 38*: 477–481.

51

Other Important Fungal Infections

Disease	Aetiology	Distribution	Route(s) of human transmission	Animal hosts	Clinical signs in human
Adiaspiromycosis	*Emmonsia crescens* and *Emmonsia parva*	Case reports from Asia, Australia, Europe and North America	Inhalation of *Emmonsia* conidia	Wild rodents, fossorial mammals and their predators	A rare human infection. As in other mammals, infection in humans usually involves the lungs, with only a few cases of infection at other sites
Basidiobolomycosis	*Basidiobolus ranarum*	Environment saprophyte found worldwide. Prevalence is highest in tropical and subtropical zones in Africa, Asia and Latin America	Traumatic implantation or inhalation of the fungus present in debris. Ingestion of food contaminated with soil or animal faeces is also a route of infection	It is occasionally present in the gastrointestinal tracts of amphibians, reptiles, fish and mammals (e.g. horses, dogs, insectivorous bats and humans)	Produces a hard and enlarged lump under the skin, often in the legs and arms. Infection is more common in children and adolescents than in adults. If not treated, the fungus may spread to the deeper tissues, and sometimes affects vital organs like the brain which can result in death

Textbook of Zoonoses, First Edition. Jasbir Singh Bedi, Deepthi Vijay, and Pankaj Dhaka.

Disease	Aetiology	Distribution	Route(s) of human transmission	Animal hosts	Clinical signs in human
Candidiasis	*Candida albicans*	Candidiasis occurs throughout the world	*C. albicans* is a common saprophyte on mucosal surfaces, particularly in the mouth, gastrointestinal tract and vagina	Distributed worldwide in a variety of animals. *C. albicans* is a normal inhabitant of the nasopharynx, gastrointestinal tract and external genitalia of many species of animals and is opportunistic in causing disease	*Oral candidiasis (thrush)*: This is common in the elderly, infants and denture wearers. It can follow immunosuppression or antibiotic therapy and can be an important marker of AIDS. *Vaginal candidiasis*: Vaginal infection with *Candida* is common, and although it can be associated with diabetes and the third trimester of pregnancy, most of those affected do not have an underlying abnormality. The symptoms are irritation and discomfort associated with a creamy discharge. *Paronychia and Candida onychomycosis*: Infection of the nail folds by *Candida* species is a cause of paronychia. The periungual skin is usually raised and painful, and a prominent gap develops between the fold and the nail plate. Rarely, invasion of the nail plate with onycholysis occurs. *Candida intertrigo*: The name given to a painful or irritative inflammatory dermatosis confined to body folds. Secondary bacterial infections can contribute to the process. Infection is most common in overweight or diabetic subjects

(Continued)

Disease	Aetiology	Distribution	Route(s) of human transmission	Animal hosts	Clinical signs in human
Chromoblastomycosis (chromomycosis)	Caused by several species of related fungi. The most common are *Fonsecaea pedrosoi*, *F. compactum*, *Phialophora verrucosa* and *Cladophialophora carrionni*	The disease has a worldwide distribution with a high prevalence in Costa Rica and Madagascar	Mainly through traumatic inoculation by implantation from an environmental source, leading to an initial cutaneous lesion at the inoculation site	It is mainly a human disease. Scarce reports occur in other animals, such as amphibians and mammals	The initial lesion is a warty papule on an exposed site, e.g. leg or arm, that enlarges slowly to form a verrucous plaque. In some instances, the primary lesion is a pustule, a flat plaque or ulcer. As infection progresses, ulceration and serous exudation occur. Non-painful, large, hyperkeratotic plaques up to 3 cm thick with central scar formation occur. Superinfection may be responsible for lymphostasis and resultant elephantiasis
Lobomycosis	*Lacazia loboi*	South and Central America, Canada, Europe, South Africa	Trauma is considered the pivotal event to start an infection	Can cause primary skin infection in dolphins	The disease affects primarily the subcutaneous tissue manifested by a chronic granulomatous reaction. Keloid-like lesions are the most common clinical presentation
Malassezia infection (pityriasis)	*Malassezia* spp.	Worldwide distribution	*Malassezia* yeasts are commensals of human skin (part of the normal microbiota)	Domestic animals such as dogs, cats, cows, sheep, pigs, horses, and wild animals can be affected	Chronic superficial disease of the skin (pityriasis versicolor), folliculitis, seborrhoeic dermatitis, dandruff and fungaemia
Mycetoma (maduromycosis, Madura foot)	Mycetoma is a chronic, localised, slowly progressive, subcutaneous infection caused by species of actinomycetes or fungi	Most commonly reported in Africa, Central and South America, India	Infection is initiated by traumatic implantation, often by the piercing of skin or mucosal surfaces with thorns or wood splinters	Mycetoma is primarily a human infection, though natural infection in some animals has been reported	It is characterised by destructive granuloma, suppuration and draining sinus tracts that can communicate with each other and with the skin surface. In affected tissues, filaments of the causal agents form compact grains or granules

Disease	Aetiology	Distribution	Route(s) of human transmission	Animal hosts	Clinical signs in human
Paracoccidioidomycosis	*Paracoccidioides brasiliensis*, *P. lutzii*	Mainly prevalent in South America	Inhalation of the fungus, injuries of the skin and mucosal membranes	Dogs, domesticated and wild animals (armadillos and monkeys)	Mucocutaneous, pulmonary or disseminated forms of infection are observed
Talaromycosis (formerly known as penicilliosis)	*Talaromyces* (formerly *Penicillium*) *marneffei*	South-East Asia, southern China and north-eastern India	The fungus is transmitted to humans through inhalation of spores from soil	Bamboo rats, domestic animals such as dogs, cats	Bumps on the skin are a common symptom. These bumps are usually small and painless. Other symptoms include fever, swollen lymph nodes, dyspnoea, abdominal pain, etc.
Pneumocystosis (*Pneumocystis* pneumonia)	*Pneumocystis carinii* (mammals), *P. jirovecii* (human)	Worldwide	Inhalation of air-borne conidia	Rodents, dogs, cats, cattle	*Pneumocystis jirovecii* causes an acute or subacute, potentially life-threatening pneumonia in immunocompromised individuals, typically those with AIDS. The symptoms are dyspnoea, non-productive cough, fever and fatigue that gradually progress over several days to weeks
Rhinosporidiosis	The causative organism has been identified as a member of the aquatic Protista rather than a fungus	Most reported cases are from India and Sri Lanka	Transmission is thought to occur through water or dust from which the endospore penetrates the nasal cavity mucosa and matures into sporangia	The infection is reported in dogs, cats, cattle and horses; other mammalian and avian species may also be affected	Rhinosporidiosis is a chronic, localised granulomatous condition that presents with polyp-like or wart-like lesions on the nasal and ocular mucous membranes

Section 5

Rickettsial Zoonoses

Introduction

Rickettsial diseases are zoonoses caused by Gram-negative obligate intracellular bacteria which are grouped in the order Rickettsiales. The name of the genus *Rickettsia* was introduced by Henrique da Rocha Lima in honour of Howard Taylor Ricketts, who first described these pathogens in connection with studies on the Rocky Mountain spotted fever in 1909 [1]. Unfortunately, in 1910 this young scientist was infected with epidemic typhus and died at the age of 39 [2]. In the past, bacteria in the order Rickettsiales were described as short, Gram-negative rods that retained basic fuchsin when stained by the Gimenez staining method; however, with the advent of 16S rDNA sequencing methods, the taxonomy has undergone reorganisation [2] and several bacteria of the order Rickettsiales have been reclassified as described below [3, 4].

- *Coxiella burnetii* and *Rickettsiella grylli* have been moved to the Legionellaceae.
- *Eperythrozoon* sp. and *Haemobartonella* sp. have been moved to the Mycoplasmataceae.
- *Wolbachia persica* has shifted to the γ-subdivision of Proteobacteria, close to *Francisella* sp.
- *Wolbachia melophagito*, *Bartonella* sp., *Rochalimaea* sp. and *Grahamella* sp. have been moved to the Bartonellaceae.

As per the recent classification, the order Rickettsiales comprises two families [5].

- Family Rickettsiaceae (includes *Rickettsia* and *Orientia*)
- Family Anaplasmataceae (includes *Anaplasma*, *Ehrlichia*, *Neorickettsia* and *Wolbachia*)

Family Rickettsiaceae

Based on the lipopolysaccharide (LPS) profile, the genus *Rickettsia* are classically divided into two antigenic and genetic groups [2].

1) Typhus group (include *Rickettsia prowazekii* and *R. typhi*)
2) Spotted fever group (includes various species which have been associated with human illnesses, e.g. *Rickettsia rickettsii*, *R. honei*, *R. conorii*, *R. africae*, *R. parkeri*, *R. akari* and *R. felis*).

Differences between typhus group and spotted fever group of Rickettsiae

Textbook of Zoonoses, First Edition. Jasbir Singh Bedi, Deepthi Vijay, and Pankaj Dhaka.

Characteristics	Typhus group	Spotted fever group
Optimal growth temperature	35 °C	32–34 °C
G-C content	29%	32–33%
Polymerisation of actin in the host cell	These are not able to polymerise actin, thus cannot enter the nuclei, and are found in the cytoplasm of host cells	They can polymerise actin and thus move into the nuclei of host cells
Cultivation in cell monolayers	They produce plaque smaller than 1 mm in 8–10 days	They produce plaque with a diameter of 2–3 mm in 5–8 days
Vectors or reservoirs	Associated with human body lice (*R. prowazekii*) and fleas (*R. typhi*)	Mostly are associated with ticks (two exceptions: *R. akari* is transmitted by mites and *R. felis* is transmitted by fleas)
Transmission	The flea- and louse-borne rickettsiae do not have transovarial transmission, thus have mammals as reservoirs	The transstadial and transovarial transmission of the pathogen occurs in ticks. Therefore, ticks serve as a reservoir of the organism

Generally, rickettsiae are not stable outside the host body (except for the stable forms of *R. prowazekii* which can survive for several weeks in louse faeces) and are rapidly inactivated at 56 °C. Most rickettsial organisms are transmitted by the bites or infectious fluids (such as faeces) inoculated into the skin from ectoparasites such as fleas, lice, mites and ticks. Rickettsiae divide by binary fission and can be cultivated in living tissues. Although rare, the transmission of some rickettsial pathogens (e.g. *R. rickettsii*) can occur from transfusion of infected blood products or by organ transplantation [6]. The major antigens of rickettsiae are lipopolysaccharides, lipoproteins, heat shock proteins and outer membrane proteins of the surface cell antigen (SCA) family [7].

Family Anaplasmataceae

Anaplamataceae comprise a group of intracellular α-proteobacteria. The organisms are pathogenic to certain mammals, including humans, where they grow within cytoplasmic vacuoles containing one to many individual organisms, resembling a mulberry structure, hence the name 'morulae'. The bacteria within the family Anaplasmataceae have long been considered to be only of veterinary importance; however, in recent years some species of the family have been implicated in human diseases, as described below.

Human granulocytic anaplasmosis (HGA)

HGA was first described in the USA in 1994. Currently, *Anaplasma phagocytophilum* is considered as the causative agent for HGA [5]. The pathogen is transmitted by *Ixodes persulcatus* complex ticks which have worldwide distribution. Important animal reservoirs include small mammals, such as mice, voles and cervids (for example, the white-tailed deer, *Odocoileus virginianus*, is a major reservoir in the USA) [8]. The disease is characterised by fever, headache, myalgia, anaemia and thrombocytopenia in humans. In horses, it causes granulocytic ehrlichiosis and in ruminants, it causes 'tick-borne fever' or 'pasture fever'.

Human monocytic ehrlichiosis (HME)

HME was first described in 1987 in the USA and later in 1991, *Ehrlichia chaffeensis* was described as the causative agent of HME. The pathogen is mainly transmitted by *Amblyomma americanum* (the lone star tick), which is mainly prevalent in USA. The lone star tick can feed on different hosts, including humans. The white-tailed deer (*O. virginianus*) is the major reservoir of the pathogen on which all three life stages of *A. americanum* can feed. The clinical manifestation of HME ranges from mild febrile illness to serious multisystem organ failure.

Canine granulocytic ehrlichiosis (CGE)

Ehrlichia ewingii was found to be the causative agent of CGE in humans in 1999. Cases have been reported from many regions of USA, where the epidemiological and ecological conditions are nearly identical to those for *E. chaffeensis* due to the shared tick vector, *A. americanum*.

References

1 Ricketts, H.T. (1991). Some aspects of Rocky Mountain spotted fever as shown by recent investigations (1909). *Reviews of Infectious Diseases* 13: 1227–1240.
2 Parola, P., Paddock, C.D., and Raoult, D. (2005). Tick-borne rickettsioses around the world: emerging diseases challenging old concepts. *Clinical Microbiology Reviews* 18 (4): 719–756.
3 Diop, A., El Karkouri, K., Raoult, D., and Fournier, P.E. (2020). Genome sequence-based criteria for demarcation and definition of species in the genus rickettsia. *International Journal of Systematic and Evolutionary Microbiology* 70 (3): 1738–1750.
4 Raoult, D., Fournier, P.E., Eremeeva, M. et al. (2005). Naming of Rickettsiae and rickettsial diseases. *Annals of the New York Academy of Sciences* 1063 (1): 1–12.
5 Dumler, J.S., Barbet, A.F., Bekker, C.P. et al. (2001). Reorganization of genera in the families Rickettsiaceae and Anaplasmataceae in the order Rickettsiales: unification of some species of Ehrlichia with Anaplasma, Cowdria with Ehrlichia and Ehrlichia with Neorickettsia, descriptions of six new species combinations and designation of Ehrlichia equi and 'HGE agent' as subjective synonyms of Ehrlichia phagocytophila. *International Journal of Systematic and Evolutionary Microbiology* 51 (6): 2145–2165.
6 Wells, G.M., Woodward, T.E., Fiset, P., and Hornick, R.B. (1978). Rocky Mountain spotted fever caused by blood transfusion. *JAMA* 239 (26): 2763–2765.
7 Blanc, G., Ngwamidiba, M., Ogata, H. et al. (2005). Molecular evolution of rickettsia surface antigens: evidence of positive selection. *Molecular Biology and Evolution* 22 (10): 2073–2083.
8 Bakken, J.S. and Dumler, S. (2008). Human granulocytic anaplasmosis. *Infectious Disease Clinics of North America* 22 (3): 433–448.

Part A

Typhus Group

52

Epidemic Typhus

Synonyms

Louse-borne typhus, red louse disease, historical typhus, classic typhus, sylvatic typhus, jail fever.

Aetiology

Historically, epidemic typhus is considered one of the deadliest arthropod-borne diseases, caused by *Rickettsia prowazekii*. The organism is named in honour of Ricketts and von Prowazek, who both died of typhus while carrying out their research studies on the pathogen. The Centers for Disease Control and Prevention (CDC) classified *R. prowazekii* as a category B bioterrorism agent due to its ability to transmit through the aerosol route in addition to efficient arthropod transmission. The pathogen can survive for a long duration in dried louse faeces and the severe clinical outcome is associated with untreated cases of epidemic typhus.

Vectors and Reservoirs

In 1909, Charles Nicolle, the Nobel Prize recipient, demonstrated the role of the body louse (*Pediculus humanus corporis*) in the transmission of *R. prowazekii*. The body louse is a strictly haematophagous ectoparasite which feeds around five times per day and has a lifespan of about 4–12 weeks [1]. Body lice live in clothing, and their prevalence is favoured by cold and humid climates, poverty and lack of personal hygiene. It is important to note that the lice deposit their infected faeces near the bite lesion and during blood sucking, the proteins in the lice saliva provoke an allergic reaction which can lead to pruritus, and scratching of the affected area facilitates faecal transmission of the pathogen. Therefore, transmission of the pathogen does not occur directly by bites but via contamination of bite sites, conjunctivae and mucous membranes with the faeces or crushed bodies of infected lice.

The lice are host specific and lack mobility, so close contacts between human hosts are needed for their efficient transmission. Other important characteristics of body lice for disease transmission include the following.

- The physiology of the louse is dependent on temperature; therefore, the lice tend to leave febrile hosts and seek new healthy individuals.
- The faeces of lice contain large amounts of ammonium, which can act as an attractant for other lice to the host.

Textbook of Zoonoses, First Edition. Jasbir Singh Bedi, Deepthi Vijay, and Pankaj Dhaka.

- *R. prowazekii* can remain viable for 100 days in the faeces of the lice [2]. Infection through faecal dust aerosols have been reported as an important risk factor for transmission of epidemic typhus in close contact groups.
- The lice also suffer from *R. prowazekii* infection, where the pathogen multiplies in the louse gut epithelium and is released on rupture of infected epithelial cells. As a result of loss of the epithelial lining, the blood enters the louse body cavity and the louse becomes red. This is why typhus is also called 'red louse' disease. The infected red lice die within 1 week [3].

As the louse does not survive the infection and is unable to transmit the infection to its progeny (no transovarial transmission), *R. prowazekii* requires vertebrate hosts to maintain its life cycle.

To add complexity to the epidemiology of epidemic typhus, those who survive epidemic typhus can remain infected with *R. prowazekii* for their entire life, and under stressful conditions or with a waning immune system, the person may experience a recrudescence of the disease known as 'Brill–Zinsser disease'. Brill–Zinsser disease is generally milder but associated with bacteraemia. Thereby, if conditions facilitate louse infestation of the patient, it can be the source of a new outbreak. Thus, humans with latent *R. prowazekii* infection are considered as the main reservoir hosts enabling bacterial survival and maintenance in nature [1].

In the USA, flying squirrels (*Glaucomys volans*) and their ectoparasites have been identified as reservoirs for *R. prowazekii*. However, the lice of flying squirrels are highly host specific and do not bite humans; therefore, the infection may only spread to humans through aerosolised ectoparasite faeces. The role of other animal reservoirs in the global burden of typhus is currently not well defined [1]. An overview of the transmission cycle of epidemic typhus is presented in Figure 52.1.

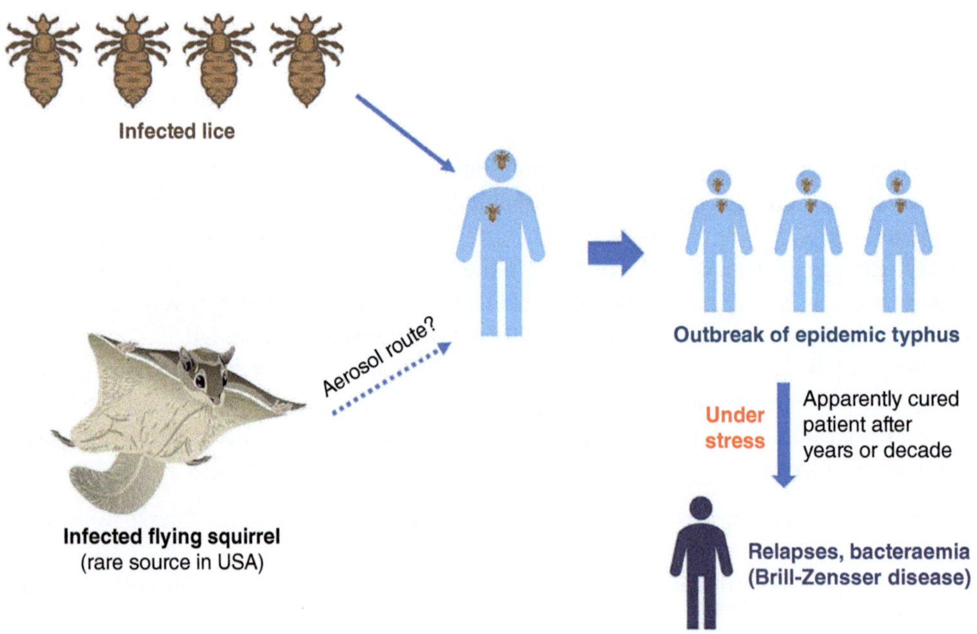

Figure 52.1 Transmission cycle of epidemic typhus.

Epidemiology and Risk Factors

Epidemic typhus is one of the oldest pestilential diseases of humankind, especially in regions where crowded and poor sanitary conditions were conducive to the proliferation of lice in the wake of wars, famines, mass migrations and social upheaval [1]. Historically, the disease cost many lives during wars, and high mortality rates were reported during the Napoleonic wars, World War I and World War II. There were more than 30 million cases of epidemic typhus during and immediately after World War I, resulting in an estimated 3 million deaths [4]. Since then, a rapid decline in cases of epidemic typhus have been observed due to the advocacy of sanitary practices and wide use of the potent insecticide dichlorodiphenyltrichloroethane (DDT) in the early 1950s to kill the lice. However, the disease has been observed in war-disrupted areas and refugee populations of many resource-limited regions/countries [5].

Clinical Signs

The name typhus is derived from the Greek word *tuphos* (meaning 'smoke'), referring to the delirium commonly seen in affected individuals. The incubation period of epidemic typhus is usually 10–14 days [6]. After entering the body, *R. prowazekii* spreads through the blood and lymph and thereby infects endothelial cells of the small capillaries, which leads to endothelial damage and associated vasculitis. The vasculitis can also be associated with thrombi in small vessels and surrounding inflammatory infiltrates. The vasculitis of *R. prowazekii* infection is generalised and thus any organ may be involved. The vasculitis may also occur focally throughout the central nervous system (CNS), known as 'typhus nodules'. Therefore, neurological features are commonly associated with epidemic typhus infection.

In general, epidemic typhus manifests as an acute febrile illness with non-specific symptoms such as headache and myalgia. In the absence of treatment, during a later stage, neurological manifestations, rash, vasculitis and gangrene of extremities can occur. The rashes initially appear as non-confluent erythematous and blanching areas but non-blanching macules, petechiae and even purpura appear in more than one-third of patients. The skin lesions are distributed mostly on the trunk, starting in the axilla, and may spread centrifugally to involve the extremities; however, eschars are generally absent. In up to 80% of untreated cases, CNS manifestations, such as delirium that interrupts stupor, coma, seizures and hearing loss, can occur. The mortality rate is variable and was estimated up to 60% in the preantibiotic era, but is now approximately 4% if the correct antibiotics are given [1].

Treatment

Epidemic typhus is infamously known for its high mortality rate throughout human history, particularly before the advent of modern sanitary practices and the availability of antimicrobial drugs. Vaccines against epidemic typhus have existed since 1920 and the attenuated strain *R. prowazekii* Madrid E has been used as a vaccine. However, the limited market for vaccines and the availability of effective antibiotics and other control strategies have restricted vaccine development efforts and their usage. There is currently no commercial vaccine available for epidemic typhus.

Clinical cases of epidemic typhus can be treated with doxycycline. The appropriate antibiotic therapy is highly effective when given soon after symptoms begin.

Prevention and Control

The elimination of lice remains the central theme in the prevention and control of epidemic typhus outbreaks. Body lice are generally prevalent in overcrowded areas with substandard personal hygiene. Therefore, proper personal hygiene is the key to prevention of lice infestation. In endemic regions, proper delousing of clothes and bedding by destroying them or washing in boiling water or dusting the appropriate pediculicides (e.g. 10% DDT, 1% malathion, 1% permethrin) is important. During the washing of lice-infested clothes and bedding, the temperature of the water is critical, as soap and detergent alone will not kill the lice; therefore, washing at 50 °C is considered sufficient to kill body lice [4]. Clothing and items that are not washable can be dry-cleaned or sealed in a plastic bag and need to be stored for 2 weeks. In areas where flying squirrels can be the reservoir of the pathogen, people should avoid contact with flying squirrels and their nests.

References

1 Bechah, Y., Capo, C., Mege, J.L., and Raoult, D. (2008). Epidemic typhus. *Lancet Infectious Diseases 8* (7): 417–426.

2 Silverman, D.J., Boese, J.L., and Wisseman, C.L. (1974). Ultrastructural studies of *Rickettsia prowazekii* from louse midgut cells to feces: search for "dormant" forms. *Infection and Immunity 10* (1): 257–263.

3 Houhamdi, L., Fournier, P.E., Fang, R. et al. (2002). An experimental model of human body louse infection with *Rickettsia prowazekii*. *Journal of Infectious Diseases 186* (11): 1639–1646.

4 Raoult, D. and Roux, V. (1999). The body louse as a vector of reemerging human diseases. *Clinical Infectious Diseases 29* (4): 888–911.

5 Raoult, D. and Roux, V. (1997). Rickettsioses as paradigms of new or emerging infectious diseases. *Clinical Microbiology Reviews 10* (4): 694–719.

6 Raoult, D., Woodward, T., and Dumler, J.S. (2004). The history of epidemic typhus. *Infectious Disease Clinics 18* (1): 127–140.

53

Endemic Typhus

Synonyms

Murine typhus and flea-borne typhus.

Aetiology

Endemic typhus is a febrile zoonosis caused by *Rickettsia typhi* (previously known as *R. mooseri*). *R. typhi* is transmitted by the oriental rat flea (*Xenopsylla cheopis*) and cat flea (*Ctenocephalides felis*), and also been reported from the mouse flea (*Leptosyllia segnis*) [1].

Epidemiology and Transmission

Murine typhus occurs worldwide in tropical and subtropical climates, mainly South-East Asia, North America, the Mediterranean and African regions. In humans, the disease is predominantly transmitted by fleas through rodent reservoirs. The cat flea is prevalent worldwide and commonly parasitises cats, dogs, opossums and many animals of similar size, but it can readily switch to different hosts, including humans. The organism resides in the epithelial cells of the midgut of the flea and is thereby shed through flea faeces and deposited during feeding. In addition, the organism can infect the flea's reproductive tract which leads to transovarian infection.

Globally, the rat–flea–rat cycle remains the major route of infection. The rat flea does not routinely bite humans but will do so in the absence of their normal hosts. Humans acquire the infection when infected flea faeces (also known as flea dirt) come into contact with damaged skin due to a scratch or other injury. The rodent reservoir not only serves as a host for the flea vector but also makes rickettsiae available in the blood for fleas, which transmit rickettsiae back to a rat host during subsequent feeding [2]. In urban areas, cats and opossums also harbour infected fleas, and are effective in the maintenance and transmission of murine typhus [3]. An overview of the transmission cycle of endemic typhus is presented in Figure 53.1.

Clinical Signs

Murine typhus is usually considered as a mild illness with a low fatality rate in treated patients. The incubation period of the disease is around 6–14 days, with the primary outcome as a classic triad of fever, headache and rash. The disease can be serious in untreated cases and cause

Textbook of Zoonoses, First Edition. Jasbir Singh Bedi, Deepthi Vijay, and Pankaj Dhaka.

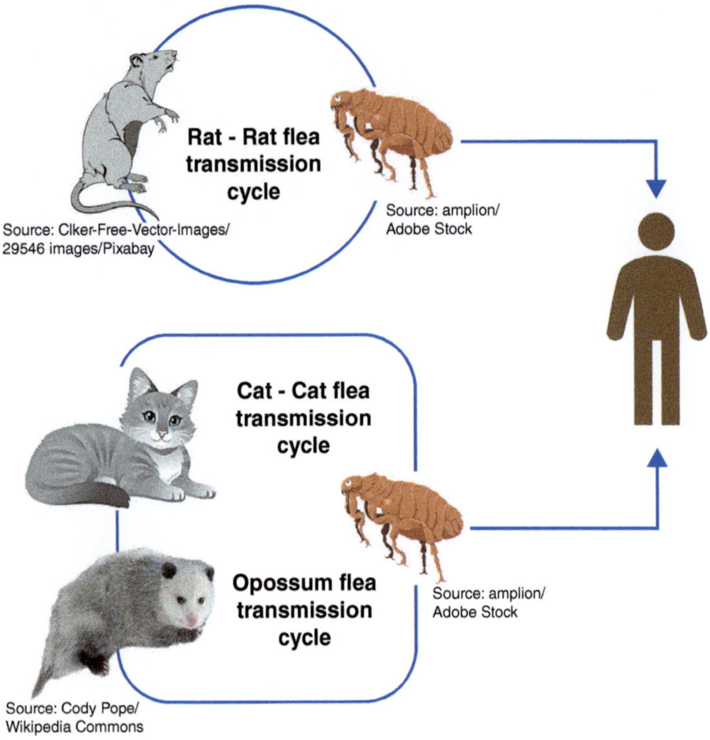

Figure 53.1 Transmission cycle of endemic typhus.

systemic vasculitis with severe complications, including pulmonary, central nervous system and renal system involvement [4].

Treatment

Murine typhus can be treated well with the antibiotic doxycycline. The timely treatment of cases is important to prevent adverse health outcomes.

Prevention and Control

There is no effective vaccine to prevent murine typhus [5]. The risk of infection can be avoided through flea control measures on rats and pets, especially domesticated cats. Pet owners should use flea control products for cats and dogs, such as flea collars or oral medication. Food sources, such as open rubbish bins, fallen food and pet food that could encourage stray animals or wild animals to take up residence around the home, should be avoided. Rodent control methods like rat trapping and the use of rodenticides should be in place in endemic regions [5].

References

1 Azad, A.F. (1990). Epidemiology of murine typhus. *Annual Review of Entomology 35* (1): 553–570.

2 Parola, P., Davoust, B., and Raoult, D. (2005). Tick-and flea-borne rickettsial emerging zoonoses. *Veterinary Research 36* (3): 469–492.

3 Civen, R. and Ngo, V. (2008). Murine typhus: an unrecognized suburban vectorborne disease. *Clinical Infectious Diseases 46* (6): 913–918.

4 Howard, A. and Fergie, J. (2018). Murine typhus in South Texas children: an 18-year review. *Pediatric Infectious Disease Journal 37* (11): 1071–1076.

5 Centers for Disease Control and Prevention. (2019). Flea-borne (murine) typhus. www.cdc.gov/typhus/murine/index.html (accessed 17 February 2022).

Part B

Spotted Fever Group

54

Tick-Borne Spotted Fever

Rocky Mountain Spotted Fever

Rocky Mountain spotted fever (RMSF) is a life-threatening tick-borne zoonosis caused by an obligately intracellular bacterium, *Rickettsia rickettsii*. The disease is considered the prototype and most severe of all the known spotted fever rickettsioses [1]. The pathogen can cause systemic illness that can involve endothelial cells of capillaries and small to medium-sized vessels of all tissues and organs.

Epidemiology and Transmission

The geographical distribution of RMSF is restricted to countries of the Western hemisphere (e.g. USA, western Canada, western and central Mexico, Panama, Costa Rica, north-western Argentina, Brazil, Colombia). The disease is the most common tick-borne rickettsial disease in the USA [2].

Rickettsia rickettsii is transmitted by the bite of an infected tick, which acts as both a reservoir and vector of the pathogen. The hard ticks (family Ixodidae) of various genera and species are the natural reservoirs of *R. rickettsii*. The predominant tick species acting as a vector can vary geographically (e.g. in the USA, it is the American dog tick [*Dermacentor variabilis*]; in Canada and the Rocky Mountain region, it is the Rocky Mountain wood tick [*D. andersoni*]; in Mexico, it is the brown dog tick [*Rhipicephalus sanguineus*]). In ticks, the pathogen is maintained through transstadial (between developmental life stages) and transovarial (from an infected female tick to her progeny) routes.

During the attachment and feeding of ticks on humans, a reactivation phenomenon is observed where the dormant form (avirulent stage) of *R. rickettsii* transforms to the pathogenic form. This reactivation process requires an attachment period, commonly ranging from 4 to 6 hours, although it may be as long as 24 hours [3].

The pathogen has been found in domestic and wild mammals but the role of these animals as reservoirs is not well documented [4]. Other possible routes of transmission, although rare, include blood transfusion and accidental inoculation of the pathogen through mucous membranes following contact with contaminated hands.

Clinical Signs

Rocky Mountain spotted fever is among the most virulent infections identified in human beings, and its diagnosis often presents a dilemma for physicians. During the late nineteenth century, the first clinical description of RMSF (so-called spotted fever of Idaho) was provided by Edward E. Maxey as: 'a febrile disease, characterized clinically by continuous moderately high fever, and profuse or

Textbook of Zoonoses, First Edition. Jasbir Singh Bedi, Deepthi Vijay, and Pankaj Dhaka.

purpuric eruption in the skin, appearing first on ankles, wrists, and forehead, but rapidly spreading to all parts of the body' [5]. In contrast to other intracellular bacteria causing disease in human beings, *R. rickettsii* is not surrounded by a host cell membrane and the pathogen can be found in the nucleus or cytoplasm of the host cell [6]. Patients with RMSF display a diverse range of systemic, cutaneous, cardiac, pulmonary, gastrointestinal, renal, neurological, ocular and skeletal muscle manifestations.

The mean incubation period of RMSF is 7 days (range: 2–14 days) [7]. The initial clinical signs and symptoms are similar to those observed in other tick-borne rickettsial diseases so clinical diagnosis is difficult in the early phase when treatment would be most effective. Initially, the disease is characterised by sudden onset of fever, malaise and severe headache, usually accompanied by myalgia, anorexia, nausea, vomiting, abdominal pain and photophobia. Two weeks after the tick bite, the classic clinical triad (fever, headache, rash) can be seen in 60–70% of patients [2].

The typical rash appears 2–5 days after the onset of fever. Initially, the rash appears as small (1–5 mm diameter), blanching erythematous macules on the wrists and ankles, with subsequent centrifugal progression to the palms and soles. Later, the rash spreads centripetally from the wrists and ankles to the arms, legs and trunk. By the end of the first week, the eruption becomes maculopapular with central petechiae. In severe cases, the continuous skin and tissue damage caused by *R. rickettsii* may result in skin necrosis and gangrene, which may require amputation [8]. Some patients who recover from severe RMSF can develop long-term or permanent disabilities such as cognitive deficits, ataxia, hemiparesis, blindness, deafness or amputation following gangrene [9].

Treatment

The high fatality due to RMSF is often associated with delayed or incorrect diagnosis and treatment. Tetracyclines and chloramphenicol are effective drugs for the treatment of RMSF. However, the use of tetracyclines in the treatment of tick-borne rickettsial diseases in children is controversial because of the risk of permanent tooth discolouration [10].

Prevention and Control

In the absence of an effective vaccine, the prevention of tick bites remains the central preventive measure. Some other preventive strategies include the following [11].

- Avoid tick habitats in endemic regions, such as grassy fields, highly wooded areas, grassy edges of forests, stream banks and trails.
- Adopt personal protective measures to prevent possible tick exposure. People in endemic regions are advised to wear light-coloured, long-sleeved clothing, trousers and footwear.
- As the transmission of *R. rickettsii* requires a minimum period of attachment, early tick removal is crucial to diminish the possibility of infection. For example, the 'grace period' (i.e. the interval during which the attached tick(s) can be removed before transmission of the pathogen to a vertebrate host) for *D. andersoni* ranges from 2 to 20 hours (average 10 hours) [12]. Therefore, frequent examination for any attached ticks and proper removal by grasping the tick carefully with fine forceps, as close to the point of attachment as possible, and pulling with steady constant pressure, is important. Always disinfect the bite wound after the tick removal.
- Chemoprophylaxis in the form of tick repellent (DEET: N, N-diethylmetatoluamide) on exposed skin should be carried out in high-risk areas. The application of permethrin on clothes as an acaricide may also be useful. Removal and decontamination of clothes immediately after leaving tick-infested areas is also advised.

Other Important Tick-Borne Spotted Fever Rickettsioses

Sl. No.	Disease	Causative agent	Tick vector	Epidemiological and clinical characteristics
1.	Mediterranean spotted fever (MSF)	*Rickettsia conorii*	Brown dog tick (*Rhipicephalus sanguineus*)	The disease is endemic in the Mediterranean area, including northern Africa and southern Europe. It is also known as 'boutonneuse fever' because of the papular rather than macular rashes. The main vector of MSF, the brown dog tick, lives in a peridomestic environment with dogs but has relatively low affinity for humans. The clinical form includes classic single eschar (rarely multiple) and maculopapular generalised rashes. In recent years, more fatal cases of MSF ('malignant MSF') have been reported. The severe forms may include neurological manifestations and multiorgan involvement
2.	Indian tick typhus	*R. conorii indica*	*Rh. sanguineus*	The disease is prevalent in India. The rashes are frequently purpuric and the eschar at the tick bite site is rarely identified. No fatal forms have been observed
3.	African tick-bite fever	*Rickettsia africae*	*Amblyomma variegatum*, *Amblyomma hebraeum*	The disease is prevalent in sub-Saharan Africa and West Indies. It is an acute febrile illness frequently accompanied by headache, prominent neck muscle myalgia, inoculation eschars and regional lymphadenitis
4.	Astrakhan fever	*R. conorii caspia*	*Rh. sanguineus*, *Rh. pumilio*	The disease is mainly identified in patients living in rural areas of Astrakhan (region of Russia located by the Caspian Sea). The symptoms include eschar, maculopapular rash and conjunctivitis. No fatal cases have been reported
5.	Israeli spotted fever	*R. conorii israelensis*	*Rh. sanguineus*	Prevalent in rural areas of Israel. Eschars are less frequent and resemble a small pinkish papule. The clinical discourse ranges from mild to severe illness
6.	Siberian tick typhus	*R. sibirica*	*Dermacentor nuttalli*, *D. marginatus*, *D. silvarum*, *Haemaphysalis concinna*	The disease is well documented in rural settings of the former USSR and western China. Siberian tick typhus is an acute infectious disease characterised by fever, eschar, typical maculopapular rash and lymphadenopathy
7.	Far-Eastern tick-borne rickettsiosis	*Rickettsia heilongjiangensis*	*D. silvarum*	Mainly occurs in far-eastern territories of Russia and northern China. Clinical signs include rash, eschar and lymphadenopathy. No fatal cases have been reported

(Continued)

Sl. No.	Disease	Causative agent	Tick vector	Epidemiological and clinical characteristics
8.	Queensland tick typhus	*R. australis*	*Ixodes holocyclus, I. tasmani*	Queensland tick typhus is prevalent on the eastern coast of Australia and east of the Great Dividing Range. The disease is characterised by sudden fever, headache and myalgia. Within 10 days of infection, vesicular rashes appear along with eschar and lymphadenopathy
9.	Japanese or Oriental spotted fever	*R. japonica*	*Haemaphysalis flava, H. longicornis, Dermacentor taiwanensis, Ixodes ovatus*	The disease is endemic in Japan, predominantly in rural settings associated with agricultural activities. Important clinical outcomes include abrupt onset of fever, headache and chills. The macular rash and eschar are commonly associated with disease outcomes
10.	Flinders Island spotted fever	*Rickettsia honei*	*Aponomma hydrasauri, Amblyomma cajennense, Ixodes granulatus*	The disease mainly occurs in rural areas of Flinders Island. Symptoms include maculopapular eruption, eschar and lymphadenopathy
11.	Lymphangitis-associated rickettsiosis	*R. sibirica mongolitimonae*	*Haemaphysalis asiaticum, H. truncatum, Hyalomma anatolicum excavatum, Rhipicephalus pusillus*	The disease has been reported from Algeria, China, France, Niger and South Africa. It is characterised by fever, headache, rash, multiple eschars and lymphangitis
12.	Tick-borne lymphadenopathy (TIBOLA) and *Dermacentor*-borne-necrosis-erythema lymphadenopathy (DEBONEL)	*Rickettsia slovaca*	*Dermacentor reticulatus, D. marginatus*	Cases have been reported from France, Spain, Hungary, Slovakia, Bulgaria, Italy and Germany. Important clinical signs include typical scalp eschar with cervical lymphadenopathy often accompanied by alopecia and chronic fatigue. The TIBOLA cases with eschar on the scalp are designated as scalp eschar and neck lymphadenopathy (SENLAT)

Other agents causing tick-borne spotted fever include:

- *R. parkeri* (tick vectors: *Amblyomma maculatum, A. tigrinum, A. triste*)
- *R. aeschlimannii* (tick vectors: *Hyalomma marginatum marginatum, Hy. marginatum rufipes, Rh. sanguineus appendiculatus*)
- *R. massiliae* (tick vectors: *Rh. sanguineus, Rh. turanicus, Rh. muhsamae, Rh. lunulatus, Rh. sulcatus*)
- *R. helvetica* (tick vectors: *Ixodes ricinus, I. ovatus, I. persulcatus, I. monospinus*).

References

1 Childs, J.E. and Paddock, C.D. (2007). Rocky Mountain spotted fever. *Infectious Disease and Therapy Series 43*: 97.

2 Dantas-Torres, F. (2007). Rocky Mountain spotted fever. *Lancet Infectious Diseases 7* (11): 724–732.

3 Thorner, A.R., Walker, D.H., and Petri, W.A. Jr. (1998). Rocky Mountain spotted fever. *Clinical Infectious Diseases 27*: 1353–1359.

4 Azad, A.F. and Beard, C.B. (1998). Rickettsial pathogens and their arthropod vectors. *Emerging Infectious Diseases 4* (2): 179–186.

5 Maxey, E.E. (1899). Some observations on the so-called spotted fever of Idaho. *Medical Sentinel 7*: 433–438.

6 Walker, D.H. (1989). Rocky Mountain spotted fever: a disease in need of microbiological concern. *Clinical Microbiology Reviews 2* (3): 227–240.

7 Lacz, N.L., Schwartz, R.A., and Kapila, R. (2006). Rocky Mountain spotted fever. *Journal of the European Academy of Dermatology and Venereology 20* (4): 411–417.

8 Kirkland, K.B., Marcom, P.K., Sexton, D.J. et al. (1993). Rocky Mountain spotted fever complicated by gangrene: report of six cases and review. *Clinical Infectious Diseases 16* (5): 629–634.

9 Regan, J.J., Traeger, M.S., Humpherys, D. et al. (2015). Risk factors for fatal outcome from Rocky Mountain spotted fever in a highly endemic area – Arizona, 2002–2011. *Clinical Infectious Diseases 60* (11): 1659–1666.

10 Grossman, E.R., Walchek, A., Freedman, H., and Flanagan, C. (1971). Tetracyclines and permanent teeth: the relation between dose and tooth color. *Pediatrics 47* (3): 567–570.

11 Gottlieb, M., Long, B., and Koyfman, A. (2018). The evaluation and management of Rocky Mountain spotted fever in the emergency department: a review of the literature. *Journal of Emergency Medicine 55* (1): 42–50.

12 Spencer, R.R. and Parker, R.R. (1923). Rocky Mountain spotted fever: infectivity of fasting and recently fed ticks. *Public Health Reports 38*: 333–339.

55

Flea-Borne Spotted Fever

Flea-borne spotted fever (also known as 'cat flea typhus') is considered as an emerging rickettsial disease. It is the only one of the spotted fever group (SFG) that is transmitted by fleas. The causative organism of flea-borne spotted fever, *Rickettsia felis*, was first described in 1990 when cat fleas (*Ctenocephalides felis*) were examined for *Rickettsia typhi* [1]. It was originally named as ELB agent after the laboratory in which it was first isolated, i.e. El Labs (ELB) in the United States. Since then, the pathogen has been associated with fleas throughout the world with wide geographic distribution.

The primary reservoir and vector of *R. felis* is *C. felis*, where it is vertically transmitted to progeny (for up to 12 generations) with little adverse effect on the vector's fitness [2]. The infection by *R. felis* has been attributed to contact with contaminated flea saliva rather than faeces, like *Rickettsia typhi* [3].

The expansion of *R. felis* hosts and potential vectors to include mites, lice and ticks (both ixodid and argasid) further highlights the emerging potential of this pathogen [4]. Generally, *R. felis* infection causes mild-to-moderate clinical outcomes characterised by fever, fatigue, headache, cutaneous rash (sometimes with an inoculation eschar), and neurological and digestive symptoms. Treatment of the patient in the early stages with doxycycline remains effective.

As there is no effective vaccine available, preventive measures include control of the main reservoirs such as cat fleas and rodents.

References

1 Adams, J.R., Schmidtmann, E.T., and Azad, A.F. (1990). Infection of colonized cat fleas, *Ctenocephalides felis* (bouche), with a rickettsia-like microorganism. *American Journal of Tropical Medicine and Hygiene 43* (4): 400–409.

2 Wedincamp, J. Jr. and Foil, L.D. (2002). Vertical transmission of *Rickettsia felis* in the cat flea (*Ctenocephalides felis* Bouché). *Journal of Vector Ecology 27* (1): 96–101.

3 Azad, A.F. (1990). Epidemiology of murine typhus. *Annual Review of Entomology 35* (1): 553–570.

4 Yazid Abdad, M., Stenos, J., and Graves, S. (2011). *Rickettsia felis*, an emerging flea-transmitted human pathogen. *Emerging Health Threats Journal 4* (1): 7168.

Textbook of Zoonoses, First Edition. Jasbir Singh Bedi, Deepthi Vijay, and Pankaj Dhaka.

56

Mite-Borne Spotted Fever (Rickettsial Pox)

Rickettsial pox is a mite-borne zoonosis caused by *Rickettsia akari*. The disease cycles among house mice (*Mus musculus*) and house mouse mites (*Liponyssoides sanguineus*) [1]. Cases of rickettsial pox have been reported from the United States, Ukraine, Croatia, Turkey, South Korea, Mexico and the Netherlands [2]. The disease probably occurs throughout many other regions of the world where *M. musculus* and *L. sanguineus* co-exist. The transovarial and transstadial transmission of the organism occurs in *L. sanguineus* to implicate the mite as the most likely reservoir host of *R. akari*. Humans become infected with *R. akari* only when a mite infected with the pathogen cannot locate its natural host and is forced to obtain a blood meal from humans. Because of its small size, this mite is rarely seen by patients and goes unnoticed [1].

The incubation period ranges from 6 to 15 days after the bite of an infected mite [1, 3]. The disease is characterised by an inoculation eschar at the site of the bite, followed by fever, malaise, headache, myalgia and maculopapular or vesiculopapular rashes. Tetracyclines, particularly doxycycline, remain the drug of choice for treatment. There is no vaccine available against rickettsial pox. Preventive measures usually involve rodent control measures and the use of acaricides [2].

References

1 Paddock, C.D., Zaki, S.R., Koss, T. et al. (2003). Rickettsialpox in New York City: a persistent urban zoonosis. *Annals of the New York Academy of Sciences 990* (1): 36–44.

2 Paddock, C.D. and Eremeeva, M.E. (2007). Rickettsialpox. In: *Rickettsial Diseases* (ed. D. Raoult), 75–98. CRC Press.

3 Rose, H.M. (1949). The clinical manifestations and laboratory diagnosis of rickettsialpox. *Annals of Internal Medicine 31* (5): 871–883.

Textbook of Zoonoses, First Edition. Jasbir Singh Bedi, Deepthi Vijay, and Pankaj Dhaka.

Part C

Scrub Typhus

57

Scrub Typhus

Scrub typhus is a clinically important, but neglected, worldwide rickettsial infection. It is a mite-borne infectious disease caused by a Gram-negative obligate intracellular bacterium called *Orientia* (formerly *Rickettsia*) *tsutsugamushi* (the Japanese word *tsutsuga* means 'dangerous' and *mushi* means 'bug') [1]. *O. tsutsugamushi* is transmitted to humans by the bite of the larva of trombiculid mites (chiggers) which are almost microscopic, so difficult to notice during biting. The word 'scrub' in the disease name denotes the predominant type of vegetation that maintains the chigger–mammal relationship even though other ecological regions can also support the rodents and mites.

Epidemiology and Transmission

Scrub typhus affects almost a million people every year and mainly occurs in rural populations that encounter scrub vegetation as part of their occupation. The infection is endemic in Asia, northern Australia and islands in the Indian and Pacific Oceans (this region is also known as the 'tsutsugamushi triangle'). In addition, there is growing evidence of the disease being present in Africa, France and South America [2]. There are estimated to be more than a billion people at risk of contracting the disease in these regions [3]. In addition, many cases have been reported among tourists returning from these endemic regions.

The pathogen can be transmitted by the bite of larval trombiculid mites inhabiting scrub vegetation. The infected chiggers are mainly found in scrub vegetation during the egg-laying rainy season, so the disease is also known as 'river fever' or 'flood fever' [1]. Transovarial and transstadial transmission are the main mechanisms for maintaining *O. tsutsugamushi* in the mite. Rodents play an important role in maintaining the population density of chiggers via the chigger–rodent cycle, especially in the rice fields of endemic regions. The transmission cycle of scrub typhus is presented in Figure 57.1.

Clinical Signs

Most cases of scrub typhus go undiagnosed because of the non-specific symptoms and unavailability of specific diagnostics in rural tropical regions. The chigger bite is painless and hence often goes unnoticed during the bite. An eschar, approximately 5–20 mm in diameter, is formed at the site bitten by trombiculid mites, where the initial multiplication occurs before widespread dissemination of the pathogen. The eschar, which begins as a small papule, subsequently increases in size and

Textbook of Zoonoses, First Edition. Jasbir Singh Bedi, Deepthi Vijay, and Pankaj Dhaka.

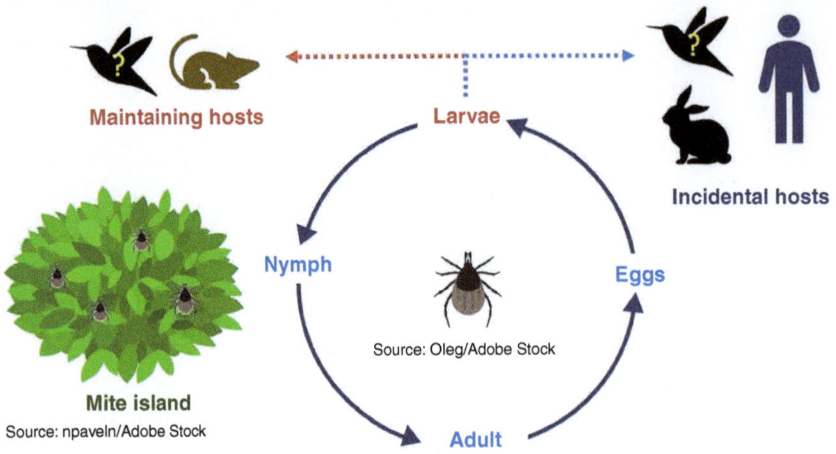

Figure 57.1 Transmission cycle of scrub typhus.

undergoes central necrosis and acquires a black crust resembling a cigarette burn. Therefore, a thorough examination should be carried out for the presence of an eschar during diagnosis. Another clinical sign is conjunctival suffusion, which is helpful in diagnosis but not specific [4].

After an incubation period of 6–21 days, the disease usually presents as an acute febrile illness with headache, myalgia, cough and gastrointestinal symptoms. However, in severe cases, it can cause disseminated vasculitis and perivascular inflammatory lesions which may result in significant vascular leakage and organ injuries. Severe complications include acute respiratory distress syndrome (ARDS), hepatitis, renal failure, meningoencephalitis and myocarditis with shock in a varying proportion of patients [5].

Treatment

The timely diagnosis of scrub typhus is crucial in preventing mortality and morbidity, as in untreated cases the case fatality rate can be as high as 70% [6]. Cases of scrub typhus should be treated with the antibiotic doxycycline which remains the drug of choice.

Prevention and Control

There is no vaccine available to prevent scrub typhus. Therefore, avoiding contact with infected chiggers remains the most important strategy to reduce infection, especially among occupational risk groups and tourists. Always wear appropriate clothing during outdoor activities, including long-sleeved shirts, long trousers, boots and hats to reduce exposure. In endemic regions, people should apply insect repellent containing dibutyl phthalate, benzyl benzoate, diethyltoluamide or other chemicals to their skin, and permethrin to their clothing, to prevent chigger bites. Farmers and field workers can employ various measures like sanitation, clearing of vegetation, rodent control, use of insecticides, etc. These steps can impede the propagation of chiggers and block the transmission cycle [4].

References

1 Hornick, R.B. (2000). Rickettsial diseases. In: *Goldman: Cecil Textbook of Medicine*, 21e (ed. J.C. Bennett and F. Plum), 1911–1192. Philadelphia, PA: WB Saunders.

2 Jiang, J. and Richards, A.L. (2018). Scrub typhus: no longer restricted to the tsutsugamushi triangle. *Tropical Medicine and Infectious Disease 3* (1): 11.

3 John, R. and Varghese, G.M. (2020). Scrub typhus: a reemerging infection. *Current Opinion in Infectious Diseases 33* (5): 365–371.

4 Xu, G., Walker, D.H., Jupiter, D. et al. (2017). A review of the global epidemiology of scrub typhus. *PLoS Neglected Tropical Diseases 11* (11): e0006062.

5 Watt, G. and Parola, P. (2003). Scrub typhus and tropical rickettsioses. *Current Opinion in Infectious Diseases 16* (5): 429–436.

6 Taylor, A.J., Paris, D.H., and Newton, P.N. (2015). A systematic review of mortality from untreated scrub typhus (*Orientia tsutsugamushi*). *PLoS Neglected Tropical Diseases 9* (8): e0003971.

58

Diagnosis of Rickettsioses

Most of the human rickettsioses are diagnosed by careful clinical examination and epidemiological investigation of patients. To reduce morbidity and mortality, early diagnosis is important in order to facilitate early antibiotic treatment. The clinical manifestations of rickettsial diseases range from mild, self-limiting to severe or fatal illness. Clinically, the existence of specific rashes and eschar (mainly for the spotted fever group [SFG]) remains crucial for the diagnosis of rickettsioses. However, it may be clinically difficult to differentiate rickettsial diseases from other acute febrile illnesses. Moreover, these diseases are largely endemic in low-resource countries that lack diagnostic capacity.

Some of the important diagnostic methodologies for rickettsial diseases are described below (Based on Luce-Fedrow et al. [1]).

Staining and Culture Techniques

Staining methods remain historically important in clinical settings; however, the use of stains in diagnostic capacity and research laboratories is not so common. Some of the common stains used for the detection of *Rickettsiae* are Giemsa, Gimenez, Macchiavello, Castaneda, Stamp and/or acridine orange stains.

The obligate, intracellular nature of rickettsial organisms restricts their culture to cell lines, embryonated chicken eggs and laboratory animals. However, most of the time, the isolation approach is not clinically practical and requires biosafety level 3 laboratory facilities, but culture remains imperative to the identification and characterisation of new species and strains. The important clinical samples for detection and isolation of rickettsial organisms include whole blood, buffy coats, plasma, necropsy tissues, skin biopsies and/or arthropods as samples. The important cell lines for the culture of the organism are Vero (African Green monkey kidney epithelial cells), L929 (mouse fibroblast cells), HEL (human embryonic lung cells), XTC-2 (*Xenopus laevis* cells) and MRC5 (human fetal lung fibroblast cells).

Serological Tests

Globally, serological assays for the diagnosis of rickettsial diseases are widely used. Some of the important serological techniques are described below.

Textbook of Zoonoses, First Edition. Jasbir Singh Bedi, Deepthi Vijay, and Pankaj Dhaka.

Detection of Antigens

Group-specific detection of rickettsiae can be carried out using direct immunofluorescence assays (DFA) and/or indirect immunofluorescence assays (IFA).

Antibody Detection

The detection of antibodies as indicators of current and/or past exposure to the pathogen is a commonly used method for diagnosing rickettsial diseases and conducting epidemiological surveillance. The paired serum samples should be tested when diagnosing rickettsial diseases in order to eliminate background antibody levels from previous infection(s) and to prevent misdiagnosis because of lack of seroconversion in a single sample.

The commonly used tests for antibody detection include the following.

- **Weil–Felix test:** This agglutination test was first described by Edmund Weil and Arthur Felix in 1916. Due to its low sensitivity and specificity, the test is no longer recommended in routine practice [2]; however, it still has great importance in resource-limited regions where advanced methods are not available. The diagnosis is based on the principle that certain serotypes of *Proteus* bacteria display antigenic cross-reactivity with *Rickettsia* species. The important serotypes of *Proteus* bacteria and the respective cross-reactivity for *Rickettsial* groups are described below.
  - *P. vulgaris* OX19 antigen reacts with antibodies to typhus group rickettsiae (i.e. *Rickettsia prowazekii*, *R. typhi*).
  - *P. mirabilis* OXK antigen reacts with antibodies to the scrub typhus group (i.e. *Orientia tsutsugamushi*).
  - *P. vulgaris* OX2 and OX19 antigens react with antibodies to the SFG (e.g. *R. rickettsiae*, *R. conorii*).
- **Complement fixation test**: Based on the interaction of serum antibodies with known antigens, of which their binding is proportional to the amount of complement that is 'fixed' in the reaction.
- **Indirect immunofluorescence assays (IFA):** Considered the 'gold standard' in testing for rickettsial diseases. The IFA can detect group-specific IgM and/or IgG in patient samples.
- **Indirect immunoperoxidase** (IIP) **assay:** Similar to the IFA, but utilises peroxidase instead of a fluorescently labelled antibody. This allows for the assay to be interpreted using a light microscope instead of a fluorescent microscope.
- **Enzyme-linked immunosorbent assay** (ELISA)**:** This is another commonly used serological assay that can detect rickettsial group-specific IgM, IgG or both.
- **Others:** The recent dipstick, immunochromatographical rapid diagnostic tests (RDT) and immunodot assays produce rapid results and are relatively inexpensive. They are useful in rural areas where sophisticated diagnostics like IFA may not be available.

Limitations

The cross-reactivity that might occur between the antigens of organisms within the same genus and in different genera remains the major limitation for serodiagnosis. Therefore, serological results must be supported by proper epidemiological investigations, particularly if no rickettsiae have ever been isolated or detected in the tested region. When the cross-reaction is suspected, other methods such as a difference in dilution as well as cross-absorption of sera and Western blotting can be adopted to differentiate rickettsial antigens.

Molecular Methods

Molecular detection of rickettsial organisms is becoming highly useful in clinical settings, as these methods are rapid, sensitive and specific. Molecular detection can be performed on various human samples (e.g. blood, skin biopsy, etc.). Ticks, fleas, lice and other vectors may also be used as epidemiological tools to detect the presence of pathogen activity in targeted regions. The commonly used molecular assays include conventional polymerase chain reaction (PCR), nested PCR, real-time PCR and loop-mediated isothermal amplification (LAMP) assays. In addition, methods for further molecular characterisation include modified PCR assays, restriction enzyme fragment length polymorphism (RFLP) analysis, multilocus sequence typing/multilocus sequence analysis (MLST/MLSA), multispacer typing (MST) and whole-genome sequencing.

References

1. Luce-Fedrow, A., Mullins, K., Kostik, A.P. et al. (2015). Strategies for detecting rickettsiae and diagnosing rickettsial diseases. *Future Microbiology* 10 (4): 537–564.
2. Kularatne, S.A.M. and Gawarammana, I.B. (2009). Validity of the Weil–Felix test in the diagnosis of acute rickettsial infections in Sri Lanka. *Transactions of the Royal Society of Tropical Medicine and Hygiene* 103 (4): 423–424.

Section 6

Prion Diseases

59

Prion Diseases

Prions are proteinaceous infectious particles that can induce abnormal folding of the host-encoded cellular non-pathogenic prion proteins, which are found abundantly in the neurons of both humans and animals [1]. Prions are defined as 'small proteinaceous infectious particles that are resistant to inactivation by most procedures that modify nucleic acids' [2]. When the pathogenic isoform (denoted as PrP^{Sc}) with a β-sheet enriched three-dimensional structure comes in contact with the normal α-helical protein (denoted as PrP^{C}) encoded on the gene locus *PRNP* in the genome of hosts, an autocatalytic conversion process converts PrP^{C} into thermodynamically stable PrP^{Sc} by inducing abnormal folding and aggregation of proteins [3]. This process repeats over time whenever contact between both the isoforms occurs, and thereby PrP^{Sc} accumulates in the body, resulting in the induction of transmissible spongiform encephalopathies (TSEs) [4]. Though the functions of normal prion proteins are still not completely understood, the abnormal folding of the prion proteins leads to brain damage and associated characteristic signs and symptoms of the disease.

Epidemiology and Transmission

In the early 1980s, Stanley B. Prusiner coined the term 'prion' for proteinaceous infectious particles and proposed the 'prion hypothesis' pointing to protein only mechanism of agent replication, suggesting protein agent replication without nucleic acid, unlike viruses and viroid [2]. In 1997, Dr Prusiner was awarded the Nobel Prize in Physiology or Medicine, for his discovery of prions.

The prion diseases are invariably fatal TSEs which are a family of rare neurodegenerative disorders. These diseases have occurred in a wide range of mammalian species, including humans. There are considerable differences between individual TSEs in their host range, routes of transmission and factors influencing host susceptibility (such as genotype). However, all the prion diseases are often characterised by a long incubation period and neuropathological signs with motor, sensory and cognitive deficits due to spongiform vacuolation, astrogliosis and deposition of PrP^{Sc} amyloid plaques in the central nervous system (CNS). In addition, prion diseases do not elicit a typical immune response by the host, and the mechanism of brain damage is poorly understood. The prions are highly resistant to many physicochemical treatments, such as heat, and exposure to ionising or ultraviolet radiation [5].

The human prion diseases may occur in *sporadic* (Creutzfeldt–Jakob disease [CJD]), *genetic* (genetic CJD, Gerstmann–Sträussler–Scheinker syndrome and fatal familial insomnia) and

Textbook of Zoonoses, First Edition. Jasbir Singh Bedi, Deepthi Vijay, and Pankaj Dhaka.

acquired (kuru, variant CJD and iatrogenic CJD) forms. CJD, a rare form of adult dementia, is the most common human prion disease. In about 85% of patients, CJD occurs as a sporadic disease with no recognisable pattern of transmission. A smaller proportion of patients (5–15%) develop CJD because of inherited mutations of the prion protein gene (PRNP) on the short arm of chromosome 20. These inherited forms also include Gerstmann–Sträussler–Scheinker syndrome and fatal familial insomnia, all of which are autosomal dominant diseases. Iatrogenic CJDs have been reported to spread via the use of prion-infected donor tissues, including human growth hormone, corneal transplants and dura mater grafts, as well as through the use of contaminated neurosurgical instruments. Variant CJD (vCJD) is caused by the same strain of agent that causes BSE; although the transmission route of vCJD is yet to be fully proven, it is widely accepted that it is transmitted through exposure to food contaminated by the bovine BSE agent. Kuru, a rare form of human TSE, was associated with ritual cannibalism in some tribes of Papua New Guinea, with prevalence as high as 2% [6].

The animal prion diseases mainly include scrapie in sheep, chronic wasting disease (CWD) in cervids, bovine spongiform encephalopathy (BSE) in cattle, transmissible mink encephalopathy (TME) in mink, feline spongiform encephalopathy (FSE) in felines, exotic ungulate spongiform encephalopathy (EUE) in ungulates and spongiform encephalopathy of primates. Most cases of animal prion diseases are usually acquired through the transmission of an infectious agent (prion), except for some cases of sporadic atypical scrapie and BSE.

Throughout the eighteenth and nineteenth centuries, scrapie, the most ancient animal TSE was reported in many breeds of sheep in Europe. No risk to humans from sheep scrapie has yet been demonstrated even after centuries of human and sheep co-habitation [6]. In 1985 in the UK, the emergence of a new TSE called BSE was reported. The massive epidemic of BSE throughout the country affected more than 4 million cattle between 1986 and October 2004, pathologically characterised by brainstem grey matter vacuolation, resulting in progressive neurological disorder, changes in sensation, posture and movement [7]. The outbreak was thought to be initiated by scrapie infection of cattle, but the epidemic propagated within the cattle population via the use of recycled infected cattle as feed. Apart from classic BSE, rare and atypical forms of BSE (L-type and H-type) are also reported in older cattle [8].

Transmissible mink encephalopathy, a rare TSE of farmed mink, was first recognised in Wisconsin and Minnesota in 1947. The agents of TME and L-BSE were found to be similar via epidemiological and experimental evidence [9]. CWD is a TSE of wild cervids, first identified in Colorado in the US in 1967, and has now been reported from around 26 states of the USA, three Canadian provinces, South Korea, and also from free-ranging reindeer and moose in Norway, Finland and Sweden [10]. CWD is now the only prion disease of wild free-ranging animals and continues to affect several Cervidae species across the world. FSE and EUE have been attributed to the feeding of BSE-contaminated food to animals. FSE, reported for the first time in 1990, is the TSE of domestic and captive feline species. In addition, TSEs have also been reported in non-human primates [11] and dromedary camels in Algeria [12].

Although cross-species transmission of prion diseases seems to be limited by an apparent 'species barrier', the occurrence of BSE and its transmission to humans in the form of a novel human TSE (vCJD) in the late 1990s indicated that animal prion diseases can pose a significant public health risk [13]. Secondary person-to-person spread of vCJD via blood products further illustrates the potential public health impacts of BSE.

Except for BSE, there is insufficient epidemiological evidence that other animal TSEs are associated with human prion disease. However, experimental studies in non-human primates and human PrP transgenic mice suggest some prion diseases including classic scrapie, L-type atypical BSE (L-BSE) and CWD have zoonotic potential [14]. Risk factors such as game hunting and venison consumption may expose humans to diseases like CWD by the oral route.

Disease in Animals

Disease and species affected	Mode of transmission	Incubation period	Clinical signs
Scrapie Sheep and goats	Oral infection with prions of unknown origin and horizontal transmission with secretions and excretions of affected animals and tissues like placenta are the major source of infection. It can also transmit maternally from ewe to lamb, before or at the time of parturition	The incubation period is 2–5 years and death occurs within 2 weeks to 6 months after clinical onset	**Typical scrapie:** Behavioural changes, blindness, ataxia, inco-ordination, hyperexcitability and tremors. Intense pruritus is the most common symptom leading to wool loss by rubbing and scraping **Atypical scrapie:** Pruritus is uncommon. The major clinical symptoms are ataxia and inco-ordination
Transmissible mink encephalopathy Mink and racoons	Considered as a food-borne disease with exposure to a scrapie-like agent in feed. Cases have also been reported through cannibalism or biting of each other among caged minks	The incubation period may range from 6 to 12 months, and death usually occurs within 2–8 weeks after the onset of clinical symptoms	The clinical signs include hyperirritability, ataxia, compulsive biting, arching their tails over their backs and ultimately losing locomotor co-ordination, somnolence, coma and death
Chronic wasting disease Mule deer, white-tailed deer, black-tailed deer, Rocky Mountain elk, moose, etc.	Horizontally transmitted between animals by direct contact (e.g. through saliva) and indirectly through pasture or water body contamination with saliva, urine or faeces	Incubation periods lie in the range of 16 months to 5 years. Death usually occurs within 1 year after the onset of clinical signs	Clinical signs include progressive weight loss, pronounced behavioural changes, excessive salivation and ataxia with head tremors
Bovine spongiform encephalopathy or 'mad cow disease' Cattle (typical BSE and atypical BSE, H-& L-types)	Mainly food-borne through contaminated meat and bone meal (MBM) contaminated with infectious mammalian pathogenic prions	The incubation period is 2–8 years and most BSE cases occur in 4-5 years old dairy cattle	Clinical signs include tremors, gait abnormalities particularly of the hindlimb (ataxia), aggressive behaviour, apprehension and hyper-reactivity to stimuli
Exotic ungulate spongiform encephalopathy (EUE) Exotic ruminants of the family Bovidae	Transmission through food-borne route by contaminated meat and bone meal (MBM) derived from ruminants	The clinical course of EUE varies between species. All EUE cases are fatal	Clinical symptoms vary according to species and are distinct from those of BSE and scrapie
Feline spongiform encephalopathy Domestic cats and wild members of the family Felidae	Oral transmission by infection with BSE prions through the use of infected bovine spleen and CNS tissue as pet feed	The incubation period is in the range of 4.5–8 years in cheetahs	Clinical signs include behavioural changes like fear, uncharacteristic aggressiveness or unusual timidity and hiding, hyperaesthesia to touch or noise, depression, restlessness, abnormal or hypermetric gait, and ataxia, mainly of the hindlimbs, etc.

Disease in Humans

Disease form	Mode of transmission	Incubation period	Clinical signs
Sporadic Creutzfeldt–Jakob disease (CJD)	The cases are sporadic	The mean age of onset is 60 years, and the length of survival is 4 months	Rapidly developing dementia, difficulty in walking, changes in gait, hallucinations, muscle stiffness. Confusion, fatigue and difficulty in speaking are common clinical symptoms
Familial/ genetic CJD	Inherited autosomal dominant mutations in *PRNP* gene locus	Earlier age of onset and longer clinical course than sporadic CJD	
Iatrogenic CJD	Through contaminated surgical instruments/ hormones/ grafts	Occurs in 16 months to 18 years after exposure	
Variant CJD	Consumption of BSE-contaminated meat	The mean age of onset is 29 years, and the length of survival is 14 months	The prominence of psychiatric and sensory symptoms, and long course of infection
Gerstmann–Sträussler–Scheinker syndrome	Inherited mutation	Onset at 20–40 years of age, and the clinical course may last to 5–11 years	Characterised by progressive cerebellar ataxia and spastic paraparesis
Fatal familial insomnia	Inherited mutation	The incubation period may be as long as 30 years; death generally occurs within 1 year of the onset of symptoms	The symptoms include progressive insomnia, autonomic dysfunction and dementia
Kuru	Cases are found to be associated with ritual cannibalism	The mean incubation period is between 10.3 and 13.2 years	Progressive cerebellar ataxia within a few months; the cognitive changes develop only in advanced stages of the disease

Diagnosis

The reliable diagnosis of prion diseases is possible only through autopsy. In live animals/humans, the level of prions in the peripheral nervous system is too low to detect by any of the available diagnostic tests.

Animal Prion Diseases

Most of the laboratory diagnostic tests detect the infectious agent in dead animals in the tissues of the central nervous system, including the brain and spinal cord. However, the antemortem screening of sheep for scrapie by immunohistochemistry of tonsils or third eyelid lymphoid tissues is suitable for preclinical diagnosis in live animals [15]. The abnormal prion protein can be detected using some of the approved screening tests such as:

- **Enzyme-linked immunosorbent assay (ELISA):** PrP^{Sc} antigen detection in fresh brain tissue
- **Western blot:** PrP^{Sc} antigen detection in fresh brain tissue

- **Immunohistochemistry** (IHC): In CNS and/or lymphoid tissues (i.e. third eyelid or rectoanal lymphoid tissue, tonsil or lymph node, cerebellum or other brain tissue)
- **Microscopic evaluation:** Detection of spongiform changes, neuronal vacuolation and degeneration by hematoxylin and eosin-stained sections of formalin-fixed tissues of the CNS through electron microscopy.

Human Prion Diseases

Although the prion diseases have relatively characteristic symptoms, their clinical profiles are not unique, with the initial symptoms being similar in many neurological or neuropsychological complications. Moreover, none of the diagnostic tests is 100% sensitive or specific. Some of the routinely used diagnostic tests are listed below.

- **EEG/MRI:** Characteristic patterns on MRI and the synchronised biphasic or triphasic sharp-wave complexes on the electroencephalogram support the diagnosis of CJD.
- **Cerebrospinal fluid** (CSF) **protein tests**: Although the test requires a lumbar puncture, the sensitivity of a CSF 14-3-3 test for sporadic CJD is as high as around 90% [16]
- **Tonsil biopsy:** Tonsil biopsy is a useful test for vCJD because of the deposition of PrP^{Sc} in lymphoreticular tissues in vCJD.
- **PMCA (protein misfolding cyclic amplification):** An amplification method that uses brain tissue extract as the substrate and the output is detected by Western blot.
- **RT-QuIC (real-time quaking-induced conversion) test:** CSF RT-QuIC is a highly sensitive and specific test for sporadic CJD. Skin biopsy and olfactory epithelium (obtained by nasal brushing or swabbing) using RT-QuIC to detect PrP are now used in routine clinical practice.
- **Transgenic mouse bioassays:** The transmission of prions to humans can be modelled by the inoculation of humanised transgenic mice 129-M lines [17].

Treatment

Prion diseases cannot be cured by any form of treatment, so supportive therapy is recommended.

Prevention and Control

The control of animal prion diseases can be initiated by withdrawal of the source of contamination from animal diets, such as contamination of specified risk material (SRM) like bovine CNS tissue in animal feed. Other methods include movement restrictions on affected herds and culling of test-positive animals. The selective breeding of sheep for genetic resistance to prions has been successful for classic scrapie in sheep. However, scrapie and CWD are self-sustaining epidemics and their control necessitates the development of therapeutics that can block the cellular propagation of prions. Moreover, prions are very stable and can remain in the environment for prolonged periods. This poses serious practical questions about the decontamination of infected premises.

The proper sterilisation of medical equipment can prevent the spread of the iatrogenic form of the disease in humans. The instruments need to be sterilised by immersing in 1 N NaOH or sodium hypochlorite (20 000 ppm available chlorine) for 1 hour, followed by autoclaving and routine sterilisation [18]. Organ donation or grafts from CJD patients need to be avoided. To reduce any risk of acquiring vCJD from food, travellers to areas with indigenous cases of BSE may consider either avoiding beef and beef products altogether or selecting beef or beef products, such as solid pieces of muscle meat (rather than brains or beef products like burgers and sausages), that might have a reduced opportunity for contamination with tissues that may harbor the BSE agent. Milk and milk products from cows are not believed to pose any risk of transmitting the BSE agent [19].

References

1 Colby, D.W. and Prusiner, S.B. (2011). Prions. *Cold Spring Harbor Perspectives in Biology* 3 (1): a006833.

2 Prusiner, S.B. (1982). Novel proteinaceous infectious particles cause scrapie. *Science* 216 (4542): 136–144.

3 Haik, S. and Brandel, J.P. (2014). Infectious prion diseases in humans: cannibalism, iatrogenicity and zoonoses. *Infection, Genetics and Evolution* 26: 303–312.

4 Igel-Egalon, A., Moudjou, M., Martin, D. et al. (2017). Reversible unfolding of infectious prion assemblies reveals the existence of an oligomeric elementary brick. *PLoS Pathogens* 13 (9): e1006557.

5 Aguzzi, A. and Calella, A.M. (2009). Prions: protein aggregation and infectious diseases. *Physiological Reviews* 89 (4): 1105–1152.

6 World Health Organization (2021). Prion Diseases. www.who.int/zoonoses/diseases/prion_diseases (accessed 17 February 2022).

7 Smith, P.G. and Bradley, R. (2003). Bovine spongiform encephalopathy (BSE) and its epidemiology. *British Medical Bulletin* 66 (1): 185–198.

8 Greenlee, J.J. and Greenlee, M.H.W. (2015). The transmissible spongiform encephalopathies of livestock. *ILAR Journal* 56 (1): 7–25.

9 Cassmann, E.D., Moore, S.J., Smith, J.D., and Greenlee, J.J. (2019). Sheep are susceptible to the bovine adapted transmissible mink encephalopathy agent by intracranial inoculation and have evidence of infectivity in lymphoid tissues. *Frontiers in Veterinary Science* 6: 430.

10 Rivera, N.A., Brandt, A.L., Novakofski, J.E., and Mateus-Pinilla, N.E. (2019). Chronic wasting disease in cervids: prevalence, impact and management strategies. *Veterinary Medicine: Research and Reports* 10: 123.

11 Bons, N., Mestre-Frances, N., Belli, P. et al. (1999). Natural and experimental oral infection of nonhuman primates by bovine spongiform encephalopathy agents. *Proceedings of the National Academy of Sciences* 96 (7): 4046–4051.

12 Babelhadj, B., Di Bari, M.A., Pirisinu, L. et al. (2018). Prion disease in dromedary camels, Algeria. *Emerging Infectious Diseases* 24 (6): 1029.

13 Belay, E.D. and Schonberger, L.B. (2005). The public health impact of prion diseases. *Annual Review of Public Health* 26: 191–212.

14 Houston, F. and Andréoletti, O. (2018). The zoonotic potential of animal prion diseases. In: *Handbook of Clinical Neurology*, vol. 153 (ed. M. Pocchiari and J. Manson), 447–462. St Louis, MO: Elsevier.

15 O'Rourke, K.I., Baszler, T.V., Besser, T.E. et al. (2000). Preclinical diagnosis of scrapie by immunohistochemistry of third eyelid lymphoid tissue. *Journal of Clinical Microbiology* 38 (9): 3254–3259.

16 Collins, S.J., Sanchez-Juan, P., Masters, C.L. et al. (2006). Determinants of diagnostic investigation sensitivities across the clinical spectrum of sporadic Creutzfeldt–Jakob disease. *Brain* 129 (9): 2278–2287.

17 Safar, J.G., Scott, M., Monaghan, J. et al. (2002). Measuring prions causing bovine spongiform encephalopathy or chronic wasting disease by immunoassays and transgenic mice. *Nature Biotechnology* 20 (11): 1147–1150.

18 World Health Organization (2000). WHO infection control guidelines for transmissible spongiform encephalopathies: report of a WHO consultation, Geneva, Switzerland, 23–26 March 1999. www.who.int/csr/resources/publications/bse/whocdscsraph2003.pdf (accessed 17 February 2022)

19 Centers for Disease Control and Prevention (2021). Preventing vCJD. www.cdc.gov/prions/vcjd/preventing.html (accessed 17 February 2022).

Appendix 1

Important Global Health Days

Sl. No.	Name of the event	Date/week
1)	World Cancer Day	4 February
2)	World Water Day	22 March
3)	World Tuberculosis Day	24 March
4)	World Health Day	7 April
5)	World Earth Day	22 April
6)	World Malaria Day	25 April
7)	World Immunisation Week	24–30 April
8)	World Hand Hygiene Day	5 May
9)	World No Tobacco Day	31 May
10)	World Milk Day	1 June
11)	World Environment Day	5 June
12)	World Food Safety Day	7 June
13)	World Zoonoses Day	6 July
14)	World Hepatitis Day	28 July
15)	World Ozone Day	16 September
16)	World Rabies Day	28 September
17)	World Obesity Day	11 October
18)	World Food Day	16 October
19)	World Polio Day	24 October
20)	International One Health Day	3 November
21)	World Diabetes Day	14 November
22)	World Antimicrobial Awareness Week	18–24 November
23)	World AIDS Day	1 December

Textbook of Zoonoses, First Edition. Jasbir Singh Bedi, Deepthi Vijay, and Pankaj Dhaka.

Appendix 2

List of Important Zoonoses Related to Farm Animals and Pets

Zoonotic Diseases Associated with Cattle

1) Anthrax: *Bacillus anthracis*
2) Bovine spongiform encephalopathy (BSE): Prion
3) Bovine tuberculosis: *Mycobacterium bovis*
4) Brucellosis: *Brucella abortus*
5) Campylobacteriosis: *Campylobacter jejuni*, *Campylobacter coli*, *Campylobacter fetus*
6) Chlamydiosis: *Chlamydia abortus*
7) Colibacillosis: *Escherichia coli* (mainly enterohaemorrhagic *E. coli*)
8) Cryptosporidiosis: *Cryptosporidium* spp.
9) Cysticercosis/taeniasis: *Taenia saginata*
10) Dermatophilosis: *Dermatophilus congolensis*
11) Dermatophytosis: *Microsporum* spp., *Trichophyton* spp. (specifically *Trichophyton verrucosum*)
12) Echinococcosis: *Echinococcus granulosus* sensu lato complex (cystic echinococcosis), *E. multilocularis* (alveolar echinococcosis)
13) Leptospirosis: *Leptospira* spp. (mainly Hardjo and Pomona serovars)
14) Listeriosis: *Listeria monocytogenes*
15) Mange/acariasis: *Sarcoptes scabiei* var. *bovis*
16) Pseudocowpox: Parapoxvirus
17) Q fever: *Coxiella burnetii*
18) Rabies: Lyssavirus
19) Salmonellosis: *Salmonella* spp. (specifically serovar Dublin)
20) Staphylococcosis including methicillin-resistant *Staphylococcus aureus* (MRSA)
21) Streptococcosis: *Streptococcus zooepidemicus*, *Streptococcus pyogenes*

Zoonotic Diseases Associated with Sheep and Goats

1) Anthrax: *B. anthracis*
2) Brucellosis: *Brucella melitensis*
3) Campylobacteriosis: *C. jejuni*, *C. coli*, *C. fetus*
4) Chlamydiosis: *Chlamydia abortus*
5) Colibacillosis: *E. coli* (Shiga toxin-producing *E. coli*; mainly enterohaemorrhagic *E. coli*)
6) Cryptosporidiosis: *Cryptosporidium* spp.
7) Cysticercosis/taeniasis: *Taenia* spp.
8) Dermatophilosis: *D. congolensis*

Textbook of Zoonoses, First Edition. Jasbir Singh Bedi, Deepthi Vijay, and Pankaj Dhaka.

9) Echinococcosis: *Echinococcus granulosus* sensu lato complex (cystic echinococcosis), *E. multilocularis* (alveolar echinococcosis)
10) Leptospirosis: *Leptospira* spp.
11) Listeriosis: *L. monocytogenes*
12) Mange/acariasis: *Sarcoptes scabiei* var. *ovis* (sheep)
13) Q fever: *Coxiella burnetii*
14) Rabies: Lyssavirus
15) Ringworm/dermatophytosis: *Microsporum* spp., *Trichophyton* spp.
16) Salmonellosis: *Salmonella* Typhimurium and *Salmonella* Enteritidis
17) Staphylococcosis including methicillin-resistant *S. aureus* (MRSA)
18) Toxoplasmosis: *Toxoplasma gondii*
19) Tularaemia: *Francisella tularensis*

Zoonotic Diseases Associated with Pigs

1) Ascariais: *Ascaris suum*
2) Brucellosis: *Brucella suis*
3) Campylobacteriosis: *C. jejuni*, *C. coli*
4) Colibacillosis: *E. coli*
5) Cryptosporidiosis: *Cryptosporidium* spp.
6) Cysticercosis/taeniasis: *Taenia* spp.
7) Erysipelas: *Erysipelothrix rhusiopathiae*
8) Giardiasis: *Giardia duodenalis* or *Gasterophilus intestinalis*
9) Hepatitis E
10) Japanese encephalitis: Flavivirus
11) Leptospirosis: *Leptospira* spp.
12) Mange/acariasis: *Sarcoptes scabiei* var. *suis*
13) Nipah virus infection
14) Salmonellosis: *Salmonella* spp.
15) Staphylococcosis including methicillin-resistant *S. aureus* (MRSA)
16) Streptococcosis: *Streptococcus suis*
17) Swine influenza: Influenzavirus A (most common: H1N1, H3N2 variant H1N2)
18) Toxoplasmosis: *Toxoplasma gondii*
19) Trichinellosis: *Trichinella* spp.
20) Trichuriasis: *Trichuris suis*
21) Vesicular stomatitis: Vesiculovirus
22) Yersiniosis: *Yersinia enterocolitica*

Zoonotic Diseases Associated with Horses

1) Anthrax: *B. anthracis*
2) Brucellosis: *B. abortus*, *B. suis*
3) Campylobacteriosis
4) Colibacillosis: *E. coli*
5) Dermatophilosis (rain rot): *D. congolensis*
6) Dermatophytosis (ringworm): *Microsporum* spp., *Trichophyton* spp.
7) Eastern, Western and Venezuelan equine encephalitis: Alphavirus
8) Glanders: *Burkholderia mallei*

9) Hendra virus: Henipavirus
10) Influenza A
11) Japanese encephalitis: Flavivirus
12) Leptospirosis: *Leptospira* spp.
13) Rabies: Lyssavirus
14) Salmonellosis: *Salmonella* spp.
15) Staphylococcosis including methicillin-resistant *S. aureus* (MRSA)
16) Streptococcosis: *Streptococcus equi* subsp. *zooepidemicus*
17) West Nile fever: Flavivirus

Zoonotic Diseases Associated with Poultry

1) Avian chlamydiosis/ornithosis: *Chlamydia psittaci*
2) Avian influenza: Influenzavirus A
3) Avian tuberculosis: *Mycobacterium avium*
4) Campylobacteriosis: *C. jejuni*
5) Colibacillosis: *E. coli*
6) Cryptococcosis: *Cryptococcus neoformans*
7) Erysipelas: *E. rhusiopathiae*
8) Favus/avian ringworm: *Microsporum gallinae*
9) Newcastle disease: Avian paramyxovirus
10) Salmonellosis: *Salmonella* spp.

Zoonotic Diseases Associated with Dogs

1) Brucellosis: *Brucella* spp. (mainly *B. canis*)
2) Campylobacteriosis: *Campylobacter* spp.
3) *Capnocytophaga* infection: *Capnocytophaga canimorsus*
4) Dermatophytosis (ringworm): *Microsporum* spp. (mainly *M. canis*), *Trichophyton* spp.
5) Larva Migrans: Hookworms
6) Leptospirosis: *Leptospira* spp.
7) Q fever: *Coxiella burnetii*
8) Rabies: Lyssavirus
9) Salmonellosis: *Salmonella* spp.

Zoonotic Diseases Associated with Cats

1) Campylobacteriosis: *Campylobacter* spp.
2) Cat scratch disease: *Bartonella henselae*
3) Cryptococcosis: *Cryptococcus neoformans*, *Cryptococcus gattii* species complex
4) Dermatophytosis (ringworm): *Microsporum* spp. (mainly *M. canis*), *Trichophyton* spp.
5) Larva Migrans: Hookworms
6) Plague: *Yersinia pestis*
7) Q fever: *Coxiella burnetii*
8) Rabies: Lyssavirus
9) Salmonellosis: *Salmonella* spp.
10) Sporotrichosis: *Sporothrix schenckii*
11) Toxoplasmosis: *Toxoplasma gondii*

Appendix 3

Bioterrorism Agents

Category A

High-priority agents include organisms that pose a risk to national security because they:

- can be easily disseminated or transmitted from person to person
- result in high mortality rates and have the potential for major public health impact
- might cause public panic and social disruption
- require special action for public health preparedness.

Diseases/Agents

1) Anthrax (*Bacillus anthracis*)
2) Botulism (*Clostridium botulinum* toxin)
3) Plague (*Yersinia pestis*)
4) Smallpox (Variola major)
5) Tularemia (*Francisella tularensis*)
6) Viral haemorrhagic fevers, including filoviruses (Ebola, Marburg) and arenaviruses (Lassa, Machupo)

Category B

Second highest priority agents include those that:

- are moderately easy to disseminate
- result in moderate morbidity rates and low mortality rates
- require specific enhancements of CDC's diagnostic capacity and enhanced disease surveillance.

Diseases/Agents

1) Brucellosis (*Brucella* species)
2) Epsilon toxin of *Clostridium perfringens*
3) Food safety threats (*Salmonella* species, *Escherichia coli* O157:H7, *Shigella*)
4) Glanders (*Burkholderia mallei*)
5) Melioidosis (*Burkholderia pseudomallei*)
6) Psittacosis (*Chlamydia psittaci*)

Textbook of Zoonoses, First Edition. Jasbir Singh Bedi, Deepthi Vijay, and Pankaj Dhaka.

7) Q fever (*Coxiella burnetii*)
8) Ricin toxin from *Ricinus communis* (castor beans)
9) Staphylococcal enterotoxin B
10) Typhus fever (*Rickettsia prowazekii*)
11) Viral encephalitis (alphaviruses, such as eastern equine encephalitis, Venezuelan equine encephalitis and western equine encephalitis)
12) Water safety threats (*Vibrio cholerae, Cryptosporidium parvum*)

Category C

Third highest priority agents include emerging pathogens that could be engineered for mass dissemination in the future because of:

- availability
- ease of production and dissemination
- potential for high morbidity and mortality rates and major health impact.

Diseases/Agents
Emerging infectious diseases such as Nipah virus and hantavirus.

Source: CDC/Bioterrorism Agents/Diseases/Public Domain

Index

Page numbers in **bold** indicate tables; page numbers in *italic* refer to figures.

Textbook of Zoonoses, First Edition. Jasbir Singh Bedi, Deepthi Vijay, and Pankaj Dhaka.

e

i

n

S